Qualitative Methods

A *Field Guide for*

APPLIED RESEARCH

IN SEXUAL AND

REPRODUCTIVE HEALTH

PRISCILLA R. ULIN • ELIZABETH T. ROBINSON

ELIZABETH E. TOLLEY • ERIN T. McNEILL

FAMILY HEALTH INTERNATIONAL

Library of Congress Cataloging-in-Publication Data

Qualitative methods : a field guide for applied research in sexual and
reproductive health / Priscilla R. Ulin ... [et al.].
        p. cm.
Includes bibliographical references and index.
ISBN 0-939704-74-9
1. Reproductive health—Research—Methodology. 2.
Sexology—Research—Methodology. 3. Qualitative research. I. Ulin,
Priscilla R.
RA788 .Q354 2002
612.6'07'2—dc21

                                                    2001008311

Family Health International (FHI) is a nonprofit organization working
to improve lives worldwide through research, education, and services in
family health.

ISBN: 0-939704-74-9
Library of Congress: 2001008311

 Funding for this manual is provided by the U.S. Agency for
International Development (USAID). The contents do not
necessarily reflect FHI or USAID policy.

Qualitative Methods:
A Field Guide for Applied Research in Sexual and Reproductive Health

CONTENTS

List of Appendixes

List of Boxes, Figures, and Tables

List of Field Perspectives

Preface

When the central objectives of an inquiry are to explore and explain behavior rather than to describe it, when the subject matter is unfamiliar and insufficiently researched, or when a suitable vocabulary with which to communicate with respondents is not available, researchers are well advised to address their research questions through the use of qualitative methods. Investigation into most aspects of sexual and reproductive health falls into one or the other of these categories, and hence frequently calls for qualitative designs. The potential contributions of this approach to research are many. Qualitative design can lead us to underlying behaviors, attitudes, and perceptions that determine reproductive health; it can help us explain social and programmatic impediments to informed choice or the use of services; it can be used to shed light on the success of our interventions; and it can facilitate better understanding of the policy, social, and legal contexts in which reproductive choices are made. Furthermore, qualitative design is flexible, encouraging discovery and further investigation of the unexpected. The value of combining qualitative and structured survey methods in a single design and allowing each to inform and reinforce the other cannot be sufficiently stressed.

Qualitative Methods: A Field Guide for Applied Research in Sexual and Reproductive Health fills an enormous need. Despite the merits of qualitative research, the field has thus far lacked a clear and systematic set of guidelines for planning and conducting qualitative research in sexual and reproductive health and behavior, the contexts in which each occurs, their antecedents and consequences, and their insights for program development. This volume does so commendably. It presents practical strategies and methods for using qualitative research, along with the basic logic and rationale for qualitative research decisions. With its user-friendly but rigorous approach, this guide makes researchers aware of the complexities, advantages, and limitations of qualitative methods. Its eight chapters cover a wide range of topics and guide readers through every phase of research — from defining the language and logic of qualitative research, to study design, data collection, analysis, interpretation, and even dissemination. It emphasizes the importance of addressing gender issues in research on sexual and reproductive health and describes in practical ways how a strong gender focus can be incorporated in research. The guide provides useful examples where necessary, and contains insightful views by a range of experts who share their experiences and perspectives on qualitative research themes. It is systematically organized and attractively presented, enabling readers to access material that responds to their particular interests and research needs.

explain behavior

Although written largely in nonacademic language, the guide conveys the complexities of solid qualitative research and dispels any hopes that qualitative research is simple, quick, or easy to conduct. It is clear that this guide is not intended to be an introductory research text. Rather, it is intended for those with formal training in the social sciences or those who are experienced in the practice of research and are interested in expanding their repertoire to include qualitative methods. It complements *Social Science Methods for Research on Reproductive Health*, a guide published in 1999 by the World Health Organization's Special Programme of Research, Development and Research Training in Human Reproduction (Campbell et al. 1999).

The volume will undoubtedly make a mark. It appears at a time when the field is asking new and difficult questions on factors underlying risk behaviors that require qualitative explanations. It provides researchers with the tools to make realistic decisions on complex research questions, highlights the value of emphasizing qualitative research capacity-building within research teams, and describes ways in which to promote dissemination and timely utilization of study findings.

The four authors bring together a range of strengths and experiences and have synthesized these into a cogent and instructive, yet elegantly and clearly written guide. *Qualitative Methods: A Field Guide for Applied Research in Sexual and Reproductive Health* is essential reading for researchers interested in explaining sexual and reproductive behaviors and understanding program effectiveness. I am confident that the volume will contribute to the generation of new and sound information on, and explanations of, reproductive choice, sexual risk and protection, gender relations, and other critical areas related to population, health, and disease. It should be disseminated widely.

Shireen J. Jejeebhoy

Acknowledgments

It takes a village to raise a child, and as we have experienced with this field guide, it takes a community of colleagues, friends, and scholars to capture new and old wisdom in a useful text. We thank each contributor for participation, large or small, in the process that has taken this effort from the initial spark to a printed book. Antonio Machado wrote, "Se hace el camino al andar" (paths are made by walking),* and we have appreciated your presence, your questions, the challenges your ideas have posed as this field guide has evolved to completion.

We would like to thank the many people at the U.S. Agency for International Development (USAID), CARE International, the Horizons Project, the MEASURE Project, and Mothercare who shaped the content and form of this guide through their responses to the needs assessment FHI conducted in preparation. USAID colleagues who provided advice include Dr. Felice Apter, Dr. Paul Delay, Dr. Duff Gillespie, Dr. Sarah Harbison, Dr. Laurie Krieger, Mr. Jeffrey Spieler, and Dr. Patricia Stephenson. USAID's Office of Population provided funding for the development and publication of this guide; we hope their confidence in our approach and the material support expressed in their decision is justified by the results. In particular, Dr. Harbison's commitment to develop a tool to help researchers apply qualitative methods to the study of reproductive health was pivotal in the development of this field guide. We also thank Dr. Katherine Bond for helpful comments on network analysis.

The expert reviewers who provided detailed critiques of the guide improved the conceptual and technical mettle of the work, and challenged us to address the practical constraints and information needs of researchers new to qualitative methods. We thank Dr. Sarah Harbison (USAID), Drs. Valerie J. and Terence H. Hull (Australia National University, Canberra), Dr. Shireen J. Jejeebhoy (World Health Organization, Geneva), Dr. John Knodel (University of Michigan, Ann Arbor), Dr. Kate MacQueen (formerly of the U.S. Centers for Disease Control, now at Family Health International, Research Triangle Park); Dr. Susan Paulson (Miami University, Oxford, Ohio), Dr. Lawrence J. Severy (University of Florida, Gainesville), and Dr. Cynthia Woodsong (formerly of the Research Triangle Institute, now at Family Health International, Research Triangle Park). Their insights, thoughtfulness, and candor are deeply appreciated. Our respect for their knowledge and experience is immeasurable.

---

* *Proverbios y cantares*, verse XXIX.

Scientists at FHI who read and commented on early drafts deserve our particular thanks. They include Ms. JoAnn Lewis, a true believer in the notion that better research builds a better world and that understanding the perspectives of individuals is key to improving public health; Ms. Karen Katz, whose advice reflected her unflagging commitment to meeting developing country needs; Dr. Jason B. Smith, who offered insights into reconciling theory and practice; Dr. Lorie Broomhall, who advised on ethnographic methods; Dr. Emilita L. Wong, who provided advice on quantitative methods; and Dr. Patricia Bailey, Dr. David Sokal, Dr. Nancy Williamson, and Dr. Cindy Waszak.

Authors of the Field Perspectives who shared the benefit of their experience include Dr. Sri Moertiningsih Adioetomo, Mr. Edmond Bagdé Dingamhoudou, Dr. Patricia Bailey, Dr. Deborah E. Bender (with Dr. Dina C. Castro), Ms. Marge Berer, Dr. Sarah Castle, Dr. Boachang Gu, Dr. Theresa Hatzell, Dr. Barbara Janowitz, Ms. Naveeda Khawaja, Dr. Kate MacQueen, Dr. Susana L. Rance, Dr. Suzanne Smith Saulniers, Dr. Iqbal Shah, Dr. Michele G. Shedlin, Dr. Nancy Stark, and Dr. Cynthia Woodsong. Their written contributions, and patience with editorial revisions as we wove their Field Perspectives with the main text of the guide, are much appreciated. They helped us ground our work in the reality of field conditions and reminded us again of the importance of resourcefulness and flexibility in high-quality qualitative research.

Sine qua non colleagues, those FHI staff without whose help we could not have compiled this guide, include Mr. William Barrows, for systematically identifying scientific journals that publish qualitative studies on reproductive health, and for writing a section on how to include standardized cataloguing information in qualitative research reports; Ms. Catherine Bocher, for researching book publishers that produce collections on qualitative research on health topics, assembling the text, correcting our errors, making sure reviewers received the most current drafts, and being consistently gracious and helpful as we finalized the material; Ms. Leda Hardesty, Ms. Sonia McCoy, and Ms. Kathy Tomasik, for their cheerful and expert assistance typing and formatting rogue pages; Ms. Laura Johnson for her early help getting materials organized into electronic files; Ms. Carol Manion, who used her reference library skills to serve as our poetry consultant; Ms. Nell Mincey, for creating an initial reference list; Ms. Catherine Mapp, for driving to Chapel Hill to locate obscure books in the University of North Carolina libraries; and Ms. Margaret Shiels, for being the Sherlock Holmes of the online world, identifying sources for submission of qualitative data sets and reports that make study findings accessible to researchers around the world.

We wish to acknowledge Ms. Karen Dickerson for copyediting the book, managing graphic production with grace and aplomb, identifying publishers' contact information, establishing bibliographic order in the references, and providing expert photo research. She has our sincere thanks. We appreciate Mr. Nash Herndon's keen advice on editorial organization of complex material and his frank suggestions on what to leave out. We also appreciate Mr. William R. Finger's assistance in editing several Field Perspectives.

We are grateful to Ms. Erica King, who developed the graphic design and helped typeset the text. Her artistic talent and calm professionalism made her a joy to work with. Ms. Patsy Norman steered us through the intricacies of contracting with printers and other vendors.

Finally, we thank our families for supporting our work on this book — Alan, Noah, and Zoë Dehmer; Carn, Zoë, and Ninian Gibson; Mark, Elise, and Kyle Healy; and Richard, Donald, and Marjorie Ulin and the Ulin grandchildren. They hold a special place in our hearts for listening to our stories, making do with our absences, and sharing in our excitement as we put it all into words.

Priscilla R. Ulin
Elizabeth T. Robinson
Elizabeth E. Tolley
Erin T. McNeill

text n. 1. original words of author [especially as opposed to para-phrase of or commentary on them ... from Latin textus, tissue, literary style (in medieval Latin = Gospel); from Latin textere text — weave]

textile a & n 1. a. of weaving ... woven, suitable for weaving, (textile fabrics, materials). 2. n. textile material; any cloth ...

textual a. of or in the text ...

texture a. & v. t. 1. arrangement of threads, etc. in textile fabric, characteristic feel due to this; arrangement of small constituent parts, perceived structure (of skin, rock, soil, organic tissue, liter-ary work, etc.); representation of structure and detail of objects in art ... 2.v.t. make by weaving; provide with texture [from Latin textura weaving] ...

Adapted from Sykes JB, editor. *The Concise Oxford Dictionary of Current English.* Seventh Edition. Oxford: Clarendon Press; 1982. [emphasis added]

Text, textile and texture all share the same root, and their definitions have in common the notion of things interwoven — threads, ideas, or themes. The core material of qualitative research is the fabric of social life, and what emerges from qualitative research is very often text of one kind or another. Qualitative methods elicit narratives and discourse expressed as text, essentially stories. *To tell a good story is to spin a fine yarn.* The regular weaving and textual metaphors are not an accident in qualitative methods work. Social history can be interpreted as cloth with a warp and a weft made up of different threads, interlocking to produce a structure that is stronger and more permanent than its constituents. The pattern is often unique yet nevertheless recognizable. Counting the number and color of threads, or detailing the composition of the yarn alone, does not enable the observer to see the whole image produced by the final fabric in context.

The work of the qualitative researcher is to interpret the pattern or texture of that text — to discern the inherent pattern in the expressed ideas or images and actions. The art of qualitative research involves both weaving together the ideas and words of study participants and seeing or revealing to others the structure of the social fabric and its characteristics or "feel." Qualitative research is a means of looking at and better understanding life's rich tapestry to reach insights into the human heart and mind.

Invitation to Explore

1

The field of reproductive health is full of puzzling questions, complicated relationships, and slowly evolving events — phenomena leaving gaps in understanding that invite qualitative methods to fill.

(Rubin and Rubin 1995, 51)

Why do some sexual and reproductive health programs succeed and others fail? Why do many women want to space pregnancies but continue to bear children at intervals too close? Why do countless couples know how to protect themselves from sexually transmitted infection — but do not? Questions like these may be all too familiar to readers of this field guide — reproductive health practitioners, researchers, and program planners, many of whom have worked for years to protect health and prevent disease in highly vulnerable populations.

Invitation to Explore

Advances in the biomedical and population sciences have brought the means to better sexual and reproductive health within reach of people around the world. Yet evidence of unmet need for family planning and escalating rates of sexually transmitted infection (STI) in many countries tell us that there is still much we do not know. How do women and men understand and actually use the technical information they receive to make critical decisions that affect their lives and the lives of their children? By opening windows on cultural understandings of reproductive health and disease, methods of qualitative research can help us comprehend some of these old problems in new ways.

Our Purpose

The purpose of this field guide is to make the methods of qualitative science more accessible to researchers and health practitioners who study sexual and reproductive health problems and related gender issues. Our intention is to offer our combined experiences with qualitative methods, hoping that readers will find this approach useful for reformulating and answering critical questions that arise in their work. We write especially for social scientists, epidemiologists, health providers, public health professionals, and others whose training and experience may be predominantly in quantitative methods. Our readers will be researchers from many fields who are looking for ways to probe more deeply the "whys" and "hows" of questions they have partially answered in terms of "how much" and "how many." They will want to know what qualitative methods can offer to improve their practice. They may also be training others to ask these questions, to listen, and to observe.

Many disciplines have contributed in different ways to the field of sexual and reproductive health. Demography, sociology, anthropology, psychology, women's studies, education, nursing, and various fields of public health have brought their unique perspectives and methods to a multidisciplinary understanding of reproductive health problems. Parallel advances in these disciplines have resulted in different ways of conceptualizing and addressing such issues as family planning, sexual risk, method acceptability, couple decision-making, and gender relations. Similar advances in service delivery research and evaluation have given us a broader understanding of providers' knowledge and values, client-provider communication, and issues related to the accessibility and quality of reproductive health care for populations at risk.

Much of this work has focused on objective questions, such as numbers of births, patterns of contraceptive use, trends in disease prevalence, and factors that can predict certain behavioral outcomes. Research designs traditionally have been quantitative, describing measurable phenomena, projecting trends, and sometimes discovering causal relationships. Psychological research in sexuality and fertility behavior has developed primarily from a quantitative perspective, contributing useful rating scales and behavioral indicators, along with case study methods and tools for observation. Anthropologists and qualitative sociologists have approached some of the same problems from different perspectives, focusing on cultural norms and relationships that influence how people interact and act on everyday experiences (Bernard 1995; Knodel 1997). Their methods rely primarily on techniques of observation, participation, guided discussion, in-depth interviewing, life histories, and secondary analysis of documentary data.

Box 1.1
If You Want to Know, Ask Them

A country plagued with high rates of STI and low condom use invited a team of experts to introduce a new contraceptive option: the female condom. This new barrier device, they argued, was an effective alternative to the male condom and would at last give women the control they needed to protect themselves or their partners against infection.

Working with local counterparts, the team initiated a program to strengthen STI prevention and treatment services, inform people about the female condom, train providers in its use, stock the shelves of clinics and dispensaries, and recruit lay outreach workers to carry the message to women in the communities. Six months later, encouraging results showed that rates of infection had dropped; women and men were indeed seeking treatment for STI symptoms. Twelve months later, treatment rates were still up, but rates of new infection were not declining as expected.

The team was forced to conclude that introduction of the female condom was not a cost-effective strategy because it had little sustained impact on the incidence of STI. The team leader, however, began to suspect that there might be more to the story. She invited a social scientist with qualitative research skills to investigate further the failure of the female condom to lower STI rates. This researcher designed a follow-up study that used in-depth interviews, focus groups, and clinic observation to explore the meaning of the new device to different community groups. He and his trained interviewers soon learned that clinicians were not distributing the female condom because they feared being accused of lacing the condoms with HIV virus — a rumor that was circulating in the community. Data from providers about the popular belief that the female condom could carry HIV were reinforced by comments from women. Talking with women revealed that most women knew about the method but did not ask for it, believing that providers (who rarely suggested it) either did not have it or thought it was ineffective, or even dangerous.

In both men's and women's focus groups, participants discussed what the female condom meant to them. Men were candid in their criticism of giving women control over pregnancy and therefore license to engage in extramarital affairs. They surprised the researchers with their anger at a program that "encouraged promiscuity" while claiming to promote reproductive health. They also questioned the motives of women "who would want to collect a man's semen" in a condom. Against a backdrop of cultural beliefs in the power of witchcraft to bring harm to one's enemies, men's anxiety concerning illicit use of the female condom was a serious and understandable obstacle to the program.

Women felt caught between program messages urging them to try the female condom and partner resistance. While most were attracted to the idea of independent protection, they also understood that control carried its own risks. By accepting the female condom, they possibly would trade the risk of infection for the risk of abandonment by partners who could accuse them of infidelity.

Listening to people tell how they made their decisions gave program developers the information they needed to understand and address specific social and cultural issues in female condom promotion. But even more important was the realization that the forces motivating sexual and reproductive decisions are complex and often more powerful than competing health promotion messages. We may not know why some programs succeed and others fail, but the simple lesson from this situation is that if you want to understand how and why people make the decisions they do, ask them.

Yet there is much overlap among different disciplinary approaches. Quantitative researchers at times use qualitative methods to guide a sampling design or to develop a sensitive data collection tool. Anthropologists and qualitative sociologists turn to quantitative methods when they want to describe a population or measure some tendency they may have observed qualitatively. Quantitative research with representative samples can produce hard, factual, reliable outcome data that usually are generalizable to wider populations (Steckler et al. 1992). But most quantitative studies lack contextual detail and reflect a limited range of responses (Carey 1993). On the other hand, qualitative methods elicit rich, contextual data, but their small samples and flexible design usually are not appropriate if the study objective is to describe larger populations with statistical accuracy (Patton 1990). As a result, researchers increasingly are exploring creative new ways to combine techniques, letting the strengths of one method compensate for the limitations of another to yield a more powerful methodology (Wolff et al. 1991).

We have written this guide not to promote one methodology over another, but because many quantitatively trained health professionals, policymakers, and researchers are looking for ways to expand their methodological options with new tools for answering difficult questions.

In searching the literature on qualitative research, we found it divided between manuals that summarize specific techniques for designing and conducting health-related studies (Yoddumnern-Attig et al. 1993; Hudelson 1996; Campbell et al. 1999) and more comprehensive texts for general academic audiences (Denzin and Lincoln 1994; Patton 1990; Rossman and Rallis 1998). Missing from most manuals was a theoretical basis for qualitative decisions, and few texts included strategies to address practical reproductive health research issues and problems that arise in the field. Nor did we find clear guidelines for dealing with the large volume of transcripts that qualitative data collection on

qualitative data not generalizable

sensitive topics often generates. Another gap in the literature was the lack of direction for writing and disseminating qualitative results. Our intent, therefore, is to show first how qualitative methods can shed new light on perplexing questions in sexual and reproductive health and second, to provide basic skills to design, conduct, and disseminate the research.

What Is Qualitative Research?

A challenge to the author of any book on qualitative research is to answer the commonsense question: What is it? Although there is no short, comprehensive definition, the unique organizing framework is a theoretical and methodological focus on complex relations between: (1) personal and social meanings; (2) individual and cultural practices; and (3) the material environment, or context. Similarly, there is no universal blueprint for doing qualitative research, but the availability of rigorous methods for qualitative inquiry can take us down many rewarding paths to understanding life in ways that consider the perspectives and experiences of people who live it. Note that while qualitative analysis can answer questions about how people make sense of the world, it also can address many objective dimensions of human action and interaction, relating these findings to the contexts in which they occur.

Qualitative researchers seek answers to their questions in the real world. They gather what they see, hear, and read from people and places and from events and activities … their purpose is to learn about some aspect of the social world and to generate new understandings that can be used by that social world.

(Rossman and Rallis 1998, 5)

The problems most central to the study of sexual and reproductive health are deeply embedded in their cultural contexts. Each individual confronts decisions and challenges that are conditioned by membership in multiple social groups — whether or not to use contraception, where to get family planning information and services, how to protect oneself from STIs, how to get through pregnancy and childbirth safely, and how to give young people the skills and confidence they will need for healthy adulthood. Running through the fabric of sexual and reproductive lives is the pervasive influence of gender, a theme that resonates in the voices of the women and men in our research.

The fact that people differ in the ways they interpret — and consequently act on — ordinary situations has profound implications for sexual and reproductive health research. If it is true that what people define as real is real in its consequences (Thomas 1929), then applied research in reproductive health must have the capacity to uncover multiple perspectives and to understand their implications for sexual decision-making. Qualitative researchers have taken seriously this charge, with the result that we now have at our disposal powerful techniques for "hearing data" (Rubin and Rubin 1995), listening to what people are saying about their own lives in their own words.

Qualitative researchers know that there are always at least two key players: the participant who contributes the information and the researcher who, as learner and co-interpreter, guides the process toward the knowledge they seek. Together they form a partnership for exploring different social understandings of reality. Creating a qualitative research partnership requires a high level of skill. It also carries with it profound ethical obligations, because it is a relationship based on trust and mutual understanding of a common goal.

Application of Research to Action

We have chosen to focus on applied research because it informs action and enhances decision-making on practical issues, unlike basic research, which is conducted to generate theory and produces knowledge for its own end. While applied research can add immeasurably to our understanding

Table 1.1

Characteristics of Qualitative Research

- Asks why, how, and under what circumstance things occur
- Seeks depth of understanding
- Views social phenomena holistically
- Explores and discovers
- Provides insight into the meanings of decisions and actions
- Uses interpretive and other open-ended methods
- Is iterative rather than fixed
- Is emergent rather than prestructured
- Involves respondents as active participants, rather than subjects
- Defines the investigator as an instrument in the research process

of human behavior, its outcomes are "judged by their effectiveness in helping policymakers, practitioners, and the participants themselves make decisions and act to improve the human condition" (Rossman and Rallis 1998, 6). Most well-designed qualitative studies have elements of both the basic and the applied, since rigorous applied research has a theoretical base, and scholars ground their theory in concrete findings. Unfortunately, however, too many examples of hastily constructed qualitative research attempt to apply faulty findings to policy or program issues. Such studies often have an inadequate theoretical base or they use data collection techniques that are inappropriate to the purpose of the research. These misguided efforts do not constitute science and seldom contribute significantly to solutions to problems.

At least three important developments are fueling the demand for qualitative expertise in the reproductive health arena:

- advances in knowledge of reproductive health and behavior
- global health crises
- increased awareness of issues in human rights

These are discussed below.

Advances in reproductive health research

Sophisticated quantitative methods have produced an extensive base of knowledge for understanding such phenomena as population growth, disease patterns, and many aspects of human behavior that are determinants of health and sickness. But each new finding leads to more questions and new research problems that often require a different approach to data collection and analysis. For example, knowing the contraceptive prevalence rate in a population leads us to ask why fertility is still high in some sectors. Or, with the availability of effective barrier methods, why are people who are at risk of STI not using them? Qualitative methods are adding a new dimension to the ongoing search for answers to these and other complex questions.

Designs for quantitative surveys increasingly are incorporating qualitative techniques in an effort to improve the validity of interview tools through better understanding of the language and perspectives of study populations. Hearing customary language for sexual issues helps the survey researcher compose standardized items in familiar words or prestructure response categories from actual experience. Program planners, too, are finding that participation of local people in qualitative data collection and in analysis of local problems leads to more relevant programs and a greater sense of community ownership. In Zambia, for example, CARE International used a participatory approach to design a peer outreach program to reduce sexual and reproductive health morbidity and mortality among peri-urban adolescents.* The active participation of young people and others in in-depth interviewing was instrumental in the design of the project and its successful implementation (Shah 1999).

Responding to global health crises

Demographic and health statistics speak to the urgent need for solutions to public health problems in disadvantaged regions. The world population has gone beyond the six billion mark, including an estimated 1.7 billion youth, with promise of further escalation in years to come. Sexual activity in the teen years is becoming more common, yet large numbers of young people use no protection against pregnancy or STIs. Complications of pregnancy, childbirth, and unsafe abortion claim the lives of approximately 600,000 women annually, 99 percent of them in developing countries (World Health Organization 1996).

Meanwhile, in some of the poorest nations, the AIDS pandemic is worsening. In 16 sub-Saharan African countries, more than 10 percent of 15- to 49-year-olds are infected with HIV, and in the hardest-hit countries, the toll exceeds one-third of the population (UNAIDS 2000b). Moreover, reproductive health experts are only just beginning to acknowledge the full impact of many social problems like gender-based violence, the feminization of poverty, economic crises, persistent regional conflict — all played out in a climate of increasing globalization and overburdened resources. Qualitative research is not a solution, but rather a route to better understanding of the human condition, with the hope of contributing to more rational decision-making for improved health program effectiveness and impact. Given the magnitude of problems we face, we must use all the tools at our disposal, and use them well.

---

* The Partnership for Adolescent and Sexual Reproductive Health (PALS) Project.

Supporting human rights and social justice

Researchers in the reproductive health field, along with women's advocates, program planners, and others, are responding to commitments made at international conferences. The 1994 International Conference on Population and Development (ICPD) in Cairo was the impetus for a new global consensus on population and development, human rights, and gender. In its wake came growing recognition that if we hope to address pressing needs for improved health and social development, we urgently need to understand better the complexities of human reproductive behavior. The resulting *Programme of Action for the International Conference on Population and Development* (United Nations 1994), followed a year later by the Fourth World Conference on Women in Beijing (United Nations 1995), put forth sweeping goals for program implementation in sexual and reproductive health and rights and in gender equity, equality, and empowerment. The reports from these conferences challenge the international reproductive health community to find new ways to address old, intractable questions. The United Nations' subsequent review of progress toward ICPD goals calls for action to improve the status of women. Meanwhile, government and nongovernment representatives alike continue to search for better understanding of key developmental processes such as gender socialization and role awareness, raising new questions that invite a more qualitative approach to research.

Concern for the status of women is a critical element in development policy, but human rights and the ethics of inclusion add another dimension. We are seeing a gradual shift of priorities toward new goals for community participation, human rights advocacy, and gender equity, broadly defined. This trend has strengthened research outcomes by influencing how research is conceptualized and conducted. Our research questions are more likely now to include attention to gender relations in reproductive health decision-making, and to status and power as significant factors in the study of health

service delivery. Qualitative methods enable researchers to explore more fully the nature and consequences of gender identities and relations in reproductive health. As they become more aware of the powerful role of status in everyday life, researchers themselves are adopting participatory approaches to research that are consistent with qualitative work. This shift is creating new collaborative relationships with study participants and heightened awareness of the researcher's ethical responsibility in the data collection partnership.

Getting Started

This volume takes you step-by-step through the qualitative research process, from its theoretical base to its application in problems of sexual and reproductive health and finally to dissemination of findings for program and policy change. Key elements in the process will be interaction and interpretation. By interaction, we mean broadly the art and science of asking, observing, listening, reflecting, probing — always with the purpose of engaging people in meaningful dialogue. We advocate qualitative techniques, independent of, or in association with, quantitative methodology, as a way of discovering how people act and interact in the familiar contexts of their lives. Our purpose is to share what we have learned with other researchers in applied sexual and reproductive health who are similarly committed to systematic policy and program development for healthier and more empowered populations.

The chapters that follow build the qualitative process — understanding, designing, implementing, and using methods to answer questions and solve problems that challenge workers in reproductive health. Chapter 2, "The Language and Logic of Qualitative Research," begins with a brief overview of the theoretical basis for qualitative research, emphasizing the practical application of theory to research design and analysis. To help the reader locate qualitative research in the theoretical universe, we review three important paradigms, or theoretical frameworks, that have guided methodological decisions in sexual and reproductive health. We emphasize the complementarity of these frameworks and the added value of linking them in well-coordinated designs to solve complex problems. Chapter 2 also reviews key qualitative concepts, explaining what they mean and how they are inter-related. We conclude Chapter 2 with a discussion of standards for judging the scientific rigor of qualitative research. We maintain that different assumptions and purposes make the criteria for evaluating quality in quantitative and qualitative studies analogous but not interchangeable.

Chapter 3, "Designing the Study," reviews the basic steps in research design, from defining the area of inquiry and the purpose and problem of the research to analyzing, writing, and disseminating the findings. We also discuss conceptual and initial frameworks that link concepts and relationships to qualitative data collection strategies. We then review aspects of informed consent that are particularly relevant to qualitative studies, including the ethical responsibility of the researcher in an open-ended interview or discussion. To underscore the point that combining qualitative and quantitative methods can increase the power of the design and result in a more comprehensive understanding of the topic of study, we present a practical strategy for mixed-method design.

Chapter 4, "Collecting Qualitative Data: The Science and the Art," describes the principal methods of data collection. We identify three fundamental methods — observation, in-depth interviewing, and focus group discussion. Observation is further divided into nonreactive (including documentary research) and participant observation. Techniques of in-depth interviewing and focus group discussion are presented in detail, along with participatory research methods and other selected structured qualitative approaches: freelisting and pile sorts,

photo narrative, storytelling, network analysis, and body mapping. We recommend a semi-structured approach to data collection and discuss the construction and use of topic guides.

In **Chapter 5,** "Logistics in the Field," we focus on implementation. This chapter contains practical recommendations for introducing a study, building a research team, working with stakeholders and policy-makers, selecting and training data collectors, developing field materials, and recording, transcribing, and translating data.

Chapter 6, "Qualitative Data Analysis," is a comprehensive overview in which the reader learns how to process and interpret text using manual methods as well as a coding technique appropriate for conducting computer searches and synthesizing findings. Included in this discussion are some guidelines for analysis of data in mixed-method studies. We then detail the concept of rigor in qualitative studies, showing how qualitative concepts analogous to validity and reliability can be used to judge the trustworthiness of the findings.

Chapter 7, "Putting It All into Words: Reporting Qualitative Research Results," discusses the steps in writing up qualitative study findings. These steps incorporate ethical norms that govern how we present results, integrate thematic ideas into a meaningful narrative, determine one's audiences, and select a presentation format that is both appropriate to the study methods and relevant to potential readers. The chapter offers practical advice on how to organize qualitative findings in written reports, how to report combined qualitative and quantitative results, and how to enhance the credibility and communicability of qualitative writing.

Chapter 8, "Disseminating Qualitative Research," outlines ways to effectively disseminate and promote the use of results. We suggest some possible outcome indicators for dissemination and utilization of study findings and challenge researchers to reconsider their roles in dissemination planning and implementation.

Finally, one of our objectives in writing this field guide is simply to share with readers the rewards and frustrations of doing qualitative research. Therefore, we offer numerous examples from our own research and from the practical experiences of others who have already embarked on this journey. Throughout the book you will find short Field Perspectives written by some of these colleagues. They speak to you from lessons they have learned in their own experiences with qualitative methods, offering stories, ideas, reflections, and advice to help you on your way.

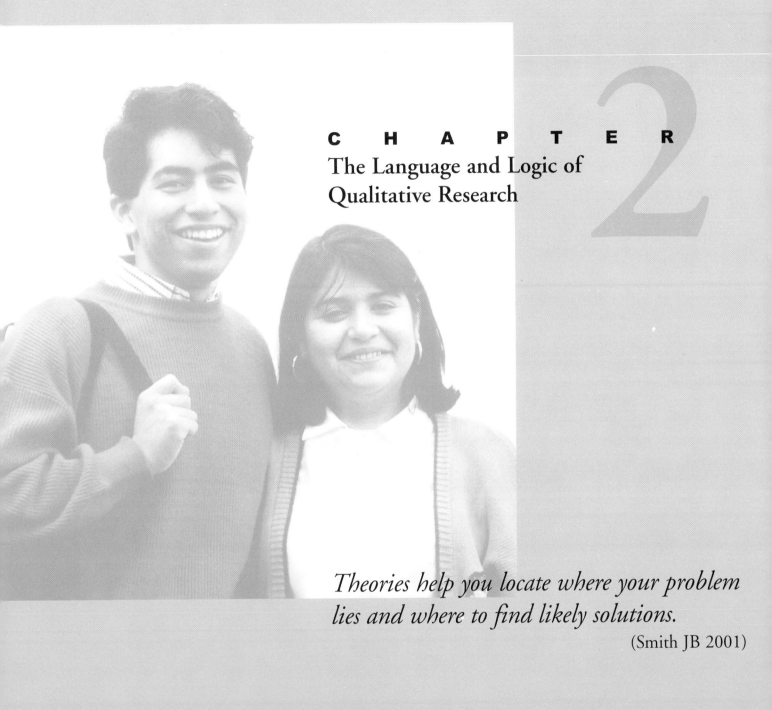

The Language and Logic of
Qualitative Research

*Theories help you locate where your problem
lies and where to find likely solutions.*

(Smith JB 2001)

R eproductive health researchers and practitioners daily confront a myriad of challenging questions. How do people make fertility decisions? How are health promotion messages understood by individuals at risk? How can an HIV-negative woman have a safe relationship with an infected partner? It is useful to have an idea of how a new contraceptive product will be received, how people will react to public health messages, how a woman will negotiate the use of condoms during sex with an infected partner, or how couples decide how many children to have.

The Language and Logic of Qualitative Research

We cannot know for certain how any individual will respond to any of these issues, but if we turn to the lessons learned from countless observations and studies of related human behavior, we begin to have some idea of a range of responses. Thus we have the beginning of our research questions, and from the set of more general statements from many lessons learned, we develop conceptual and theoretical frameworks. These frameworks provide the logic and the language that guide our research. Through a common understanding of how the world works (or doesn't work), theory provides researchers and practitioners with reference points for understanding human behavior in a more general context.

The purpose of theory in the social sciences is to make sense of the world and to understand and anticipate how people will react to each other and to events. For most applied researchers in sexual and reproductive health, <u>the test of a good theory is how well it helps us define our research problems, design our studies, and produce useful results.</u>

At a minimum, theory can be defined as a scientific but tentative statement of relationships among diverse phenomena. A quantitative research problem often begins with theory and examines hypothetical relationships within it — a *deductive* process. <u>Qualitative research more often builds theory, moving from observations and open questions to more general conclusions</u> — an *inductive* process. In actual practice, most researchers use elements of both deductive and inductive logic. Both approaches collect and analyze data, draw tentative conclusions, test conclusions, and reinterpret earlier findings based on new evidence. Research across disciplines has at its core a common scientific logic. However, the process of applying the basic logic of scientific inquiry to tangible problems in sexual and reproductive health differs depending on the problem and the theoretical perspective of the researcher.

Frameworks for Research: Paradigms and Theories

Research frameworks range from broad to very specific theoretical approaches that often contain their own vocabulary and logical assumptions. Broad theoretical frameworks, also called *paradigms*, provide researchers with a unified set of concepts, principles, and rules for conducting research. More specific frameworks can be found in substantive theories supported by research findings. A paradigm is a worldview that presents a definition of the social world linked to related sources of information (data) and appropriate ways (methods) to tap these sources (Guba and Lincoln 1994).

Whether consciously or not, every researcher works from some theoretical orientation or paradigm. Perspectives can vary a great deal among researchers who see the world through different cultural, philosophical, or professional lenses. One researcher might seek evidence of the regularity of patterned behavior in trends, rates, and associations. Another might focus on how people understand or interpret what they experience. Both contribute valuable data to describe social behavior but from different paradigmatic perspectives. The questions they ask and the methods they use will be determined to a large extent by their separate paradigms. In the field of sexual and reproductive health, researchers working from a demographic perspective generally operate within a different theoretical orientation or paradigm from researchers

---

Box 2.1
Basic Definitions

Paradigm. A framework that organizes broadly based views. Paradigms "create boundaries within which the search for answers occurs … [and] circumscribe or delimit what is important to examine in a given field of inquiry" (Babbie 1989). A researcher who embraces a feminist paradigm, for example, might conceptualize sexual decision-making through the lens of power differences between sexual partners. Similarly, a researcher studying the same phenomenon from an interpretivist perspective would want to know what sexual decisions mean to men and women in the larger contexts of their lives.

Theory. A "set of interrelated concepts, definitions and propositions that presents a systematic view of events or situations by specifying relations among variables in order to explain and predict the events or situations" (Glanz 1997, 21). Theories "specify the determinants governing the phenomena of interest" (Bandura 1986).

Substantive theories. These organize conclusions about the social world as they emerge from the specific findings of scientific studies. Theories of health behavior change, for example, have been elaborated and refined from the results of numerous studies that document how people perceive health risk and make decisions to alter, or not alter, risky behavior.

Theoretical or conceptual models.
Usually draw on more than one theory to help people understand a problem in a specific setting or context. For example, the Health Belief Model (Rosenstock et al. 1994) incorporates a number of well-tested social-psychological theories to explain and predict health behaviors.

Concepts or constructs. The major components of a theory — its building blocks or key elements. The key concepts of the "Stages of Change" theory (Prochaska et al. 1992), for example, describe individual behavior change in the following stages: precontemplation, contemplation, preparation for action, action, and maintenance of the new behavior.

Variables. Things that can change or differ, quantitatively or qualitatively. Common variables thought to account for differences in health behaviors include: intention, ability or skill, norms, environmental constraints, anticipated outcomes, self-standards, emotion, and self-efficacy (Fishbein 1991).

(Adapted from Glanz et al. 1997, 21-27)

with a social development perspective. Your view of the world — your basic philosophical grounding — influences the problems you study, the sources of data you consider appropriate, the methods you choose to gather your data, and the way you carry out your studies.

In applied research, a paradigm can be an ally — a powerful strategic tool to guide you through the many practical decisions that arise in the design and implementation of your research. We recommend constant awareness of your theoretical position and how it influences the kinds of questions you ask. As you examine your own views of social life, your theoretical perspective is likely to become an increasingly deliberate choice, consistent with the problems you study.

Substantive Theory

Substantive theories are more concrete than the broad theoretical frameworks for research discussed above. Also called operational or working theories, they represent conclusions about the social world that emerge from the specific findings of research studies. Applied research in reproductive health commonly uses substantive theory to define and explain specific behavior in relation to program development and policy. In fact, applied researchers often maximize their ability to explain a phenomenon by combining elements of more than one theory to construct a model. Appendix 1 (see page 207) contains examples of several substantive theories that may be of use in applied studies on sexual and reproductive health.

Putting Theory to Work

In Chapter 1, we endorsed the practice of mixing methods in applied research. In this chapter we will show how choosing research methods is contingent on both practical and theoretical considerations. Methodological decisions are practical strategies tailored to specific problems, but they also reflect the researcher's theoretical orientation to a problem (see Table 2.1, page 28). The qualitative methodology of in-depth interviewing, for example, is a natural outgrowth of an interpretivist paradigm that casts young mothers as experts whose interpretation of their experience can help researchers learn about early childbearing.

If a key theoretical assumption of your work is that individuals have the power to make independent health decisions, then you may decide to use structured, quantitative methods to categorize individual traits and behaviors. On the other hand, if you believe that control of health decisions is variable and dependent upon one's position in social and sexual networks, then it would be important also to use more qualitative methods. We present overviews of three of the most common and important theoretical paradigms related to sexual and reproductive health: *positivism* (a largely quantitative approach), *interpretivism,* and *feminism* (both qualitative approaches). Because qualitative research is a rapidly growing field accompanied by theoretical debate, we will also discuss briefly some of the controversies surrounding the use of methods from these frameworks. In light of trends in the wider field of qualitative research, we advocate a pragmatic approach that recognizes theoretical distinctions but is able to incorporate relevant elements from all three in carefully designed studies.

Finally, because assumptions regarding the quality of research are grounded in one's theoretical orientation, we introduce a set of criteria for judging the rigor of qualitative studies, emphasizing that qualitative and quantitative criteria of excellence are equally important but inherently different.

Quantitative or qualitative?

What is social reality and how do we explain it? The question has stirred debate and polarized social science research between quantitative and qualitative methods. The issue centers on "the capacity of the data, as collected by one method or the other,

Modes of Inquiry: Positioning the Self*

David Bell, M.A., Ed.D.
Center for Community Development

I began my career as a counseling psychologist in my native South Africa, trained to answer questions through standardized tests and psychological instruments. My training was grounded in the empirical, quantitative paradigm. As a doctoral student at the University of Massachusetts, however, I began to realize that my experience working in South Africa's rural communities, townships, and former homelands had shaped my views in different ways. My work in community advocacy and empowerment among the oppressed, the poor, and until recently the disenfranchised, was challenging my traditional notions of research. Answers to my research questions were coming more from my interpretation of people, their behavior, and the words they used to express the realities of their lives, and less from instruments, numbers, and statistical formulas. At first, I felt confused and insecure. Would others see my work as relevant and legitimate if I adopted a more qualitative and interpretivist approach to research?

The uncertainty I felt as a researcher in relation to the people I was supposed to study began to influence the questions I was asking and the methods I was choosing to answer them. Instead of asking questions that emerged from standardized measures and instruments, and relating everything to existing theory, I began exploring everyday life from the perspectives of the people I was studying. I was becoming aware that I could look at research problems differently — I had the power to choose the appropriate methodology for the research question, and I was able to incorporate my personal beliefs and research style at the same time. Research was no longer a clinical and academic act; it was human interaction on a very personal level.

But defining and justifying the critical distinctions between these different approaches was far more difficult than simply selecting new methods and feeling comfortable about the questions. Given the many ways that research can be conducted, how would I justify one methodological choice above another? How could I know what would work best for a particular research problem and provide the most appropriate and relevant information?

As I wrestled with these questions, I turned to a typology that included two useful continua. The first, a subjectivity-objectivity continuum, helped me articulate two related questions: Can the act of research (and the

---

* Based on theoretical models developed in the field of education (Burrell and Morgan 1979; Rossman and Rallis 1998).

actions of the researcher) be impersonal and objective? Or is research a more human act that, by its very nature, is subjective and personal? An affirmative answer to the first question would justify the quantitative studies I had been conducting. It did, however, raise the uneasy question of whether and how objective research affects the very people that the research findings were designed to assist. Was it helping or harming?

The second question, whether research is subjective, also struck a familiar chord with my experience in the former homelands and townships where I had been working. I questioned whether outsiders had any right to use the lives of people in these communities as laboratories for their research. Could my own research lie somewhere between the two poles of the continuum? Could such a midpoint still be respected? Was I one type of researcher in one context and a different type of researcher in another? I saw that the primary stakeholders in the research we were doing were the participants themselves. It was my responsibility as a researcher not only to collect reliable data, but also to enable participants to speak for themselves. I had to be a partner and a listener in the human act of research.

The second continuum that helped me organize my thoughts was a radical change-status quo continuum. This continuum challenged me to think about the social and political implications of my role as a researcher. The questions it raised were: Does my research focus on the underlying unity and cohesiveness of the world (finding information and evidence to explain the status quo)? Or am I really seeking evidence of fundamental and deep-seated structural conflicts and inequities, thereby arguing for radical change? As I considered the purpose of my work in rural South African communities, I concluded that my research would have to do both. On the one hand, participants described many aspects of community life that were strong and good. Although resources were in short supply, people were finding creative ways to help each other and their neighbors. I wanted our research results to reinforce that spirit of self-help and cooperation.

On the other hand, the oppressive consequences of apartheid on people's lives were continuing into the post-apartheid era, and in fact, many women continued to feel oppressed by gender inequities in their own households. How could we document what was happening during this critical transition? We put aside our standardized tools and asked the people, "What does it mean to be oppressed? Describe oppression for us in as many ways as you can." The result was that both women and men began to look more introspectively at their potential for equal participation in their newly won independence. We then asked, "What would need to change in your community to make life more rewarding for everyone? And how can that happen?" Now we were approaching the radical change end of the continuum. People were learning to ask their own questions, analyze the answers, and use the results to plan for change.

Inherent in all of the questions above is the power relationship that exists in almost any form of social inquiry or research. Research can be either empowering or disempowering for both researcher and participants. Placing the power to ask and interpret research questions solely in the hands of the researcher takes the power of understanding problems away from those who are the focus of the research. The phenomenon of power and empowerment is therefore central to the selection of a research methodology. Research that is empowering enables people in their communities to contribute to the process and to interpret the findings. Empowerment research goes a step farther in that it develops the skills and competence of people in communities to formulate their own questions and conduct their own research. Research findings, therefore, should contribute directly to improving the quality of life of the participants.

Examining your intention to empower, or to disregard power, is a critical step for all social researchers. How you position yourself on these continua will ultimately influence the kinds of research you conduct.

subjective ———— objective
radical change ———— status quo

to describe, understand, and explain social phenomena" (Pedersen 1992, 43). Theoretical purists argue that because each methodology reflects a different understanding of research, human behavior, and the nature of social life, the two are incompatible (Greenhalgh 1997). The purist position would require the researcher to choose one or the other approach on the principle that mixing methods violates the assumptions on which either framework is constructed (Patton 1990, 37; Carey 1993, 305).

Our position, on the other hand, like that of many quantitative and qualitative researchers today, chooses pragmatism over "one-sided paradigm allegiance" (Patton 1990, 38). Our purpose in presenting more than one theoretical framework is to help readers understand similarities and differences, strengths and limitations, and the contribution that each can make to sexual and reproductive health research. The methods that emerge from these frameworks "offer a distinct set of strengths and limitations that are markedly different but potentially complementary when combined in a mixed-method research design" (Wolff et al. 1991). Throughout this guide, therefore, we will advocate methodological appropriateness — using theory and related methods to make reasoned decisions "appropriate to the purpose of the study, the questions being investigated, and the resources available" (Patton 1990, 39).

Three theoretical paradigms for sexual and reproductive health

In this section we describe three important theoretical frameworks, or paradigms, that together have generated most of the substantive theory, or knowledge, in the field of sexual and reproductive health today: research based on positivist principles; research that uses an interpretivist approach; and research shaped by a feminist perspective. Given the assumptions of each of these broad theoretical orientations, the positivist perspective is generally,

but not exclusively, associated with quantitative methods, while interpretivist and feminist orientations typically lead to the use of qualitative research strategies* (see Table 2.1, page 28).

Quantitative research from a positivist perspective. Much of what is known today about population and reproductive health can be attributed to research that has developed from quantitative principles in the natural sciences. Quantitative methods have become the norm for describing the state of the world's population — demographic models that project trends in fertility, morbidity, and mortality; epidemiological surveillance techniques to describe patterns of disease, including the proliferation of sexually transmitted infection (STI) and the spread of the HIV/AIDS epidemic; and standardized household surveys that provide statistical data on knowledge, attitudes, and practices related to fertility and reproductive behavior.

A basic assumption of this paradigm is that the goal of science is to develop the most objective methods possible to get the closest approximation of reality. Researchers who work from this perspective explain in quantitative terms how variables interact, shape events, and cause outcomes. They often develop and test these explanations in experimental studies. Multivariate analysis and techniques for statistical prediction are among the

positivism : looking for most objective methods

---

* The social-ecological model is a fourth paradigm that emphasizes the dynamic interaction between biology, social interaction, cultural environment, and physical settings in determining human behavior. Social ecologists investigate a problem at multiple levels of the ecological model. For example, research to examine the linkages between adolescent health and substance use might include observation of physical settings frequented by youth, network analysis of shared behaviors (smoking and drinking) among friendship networks, and separate interviews with adults and young people about acceptable or unacceptable adolescent behavior. In this example, the social ecologist would seek to understand how factors at one level of the ecological model influence those at another level, identifying adaptive mechanisms and points at which intervention is likely to be most feasible and effective at bringing about behavioral change.

Interrogating Data: A Grounded Theory Approach
Susana L. Rance, Ph.D.

Nowadays, I go by the motto "stick close to your data." I read and reread my field notes and transcripts to see what they "tell" me. This approach owes much to the grounded theory method — theory "that is inductively derived from the study of the phenomenon it represents" (Glaser and Strauss 1967).*

In practice, grounded theory typically implies the essential features of qualitative research, including observation from a cultural perspective, building flexibility and iteration into the data collection process, and reflexivity — or examining the influence of one's own attributes and assumptions on the research process. Although I do not follow all the steps prescribed by Glaser and Strauss, I hang on to certain principles that have served me in successive medical ethnographies in Bolivia. First, start with an open mind and leave your research agenda as flexible as possible. Next, rather than taking pre-existing theory as a "given" and bringing it down onto your data, interrogate the data and allow fresh theory to develop systematically from your questions.

Drawing on the grounded theory approach, I have found the following questions to be useful:

- Which particularly vivid expressions – or in vivo codes (Strauss 1987, 33-34) — show me how my research participants represent their own realities?
- How do I order and group these expressions into my own sociologically constructed codes?
- What do I learn in confronting the "messy" record of my own interventions in the field?
- What problems and questions come to mind as I reflect on my research experience?
- What new theories are suggested by these questions, and how can I test their validity in contrasting circumstances and settings?
- Which research methodologies seem most appropriate for exploring these issues further?

As an example, I cite my analysis of interview transcripts from a 1994 study on abortion in peri-urban migrant settlements. Time and again, I found that the same speaker, in the course of an extended interview, would express contradictory views on the subject. One woman who

---

* Although Glaser and Strauss were not the first to advocate an approach in which substantive theory is "discovered" from data, they named the process and described it in terms of both theory and method.

swore abortion was a sin that she would never commit later described her attempts to "lose" a pregnancy "naturally" through a series of self-inflicted procedures. A physician who first condemned abortion as a crime went on to describe it as a social problem whose frequency could be understood in terms of poverty, lack of sex education, and inadequate communication within the family.

From my rereading of these transcripts emerged the question: How could I understand these contradictions? I was unwilling to settle on any one group of expressions as indicative of a speaker's homogenized position. I came to abandon the notion of "attitudes" that had shaped my former research proposal. In commencing a new study on abortion, I started to search for theories and methods that would enable me to deal constructively with difference. Discourse analysis offered me a coherent approach, with its focus on text as a topic for analysis in its own right, rather than as an informative resource (Potter and Wetherell 1987, 34-35). Variability in accounts, instead of being a problem, was embraced as inevitable, fascinating, and illustrative of the different voices a speaker might assume at particular moments, within specific interactions.

Having found my method, I went on to design a study on medical discourses on abortion in Bolivian hospital settings. I followed the methodological recommendations of Cicourel (Cicourel 1973, 64-65) and concentrated on a small number of research subjects observed in a wide variety of interactions. Through following just one willing doctor in each hospital, I was able to register their "changing voices" concerning abortion. I then fed my interpretation of the rationale giving rise to these variations to the entire medical team for their critical comments.

Analysis of these data led me in turn to a further series of questions. What kind of subjects "did abortion," and who "interrupted a pregnancy?" How did (legally allowed) therapeutic interruption of pregnancy come to be registered in medical histories and hospital statistics as treatment of incomplete abortion? How did medical students and professionals confront the conflict between the condemnation of abortion in their embryology classes and the reality of its practice on gynecology wards?

These questions led me into a further year of fieldwork in the medical school. There, I presented students and teachers with real-life hospital stories about abortion, narrated by a series of different speakers. I analyzed their responses and our discussions within the framework of different approaches to medical education. My research, in the end, has come to center on the uneasy relations between sociology and medicine.

The grounded theory approach has remained a constant in my research through years of queries, doubts, and changes. Each time I become intrigued by a new theory, I try to remember to "stick close to my data" and ask: Is this what the texts are really saying? Does the theory still hold? Back to the trying and testing and always, new questions.

classic contributions of this type of research. This framework has evolved largely from a nineteenth-century philosophical approach called positivism, which maintains that reliable knowledge is based on direct observation or manipulation of natural phenomena through empirical, often experimental, means.

Quantitative studies in social science use highly standardized tools with precisely worded questions. Working with representative samples, the interviewer might ask, "How many pregnancies have you had and at what intervals? What contraceptive methods have you used? Who has influenced your decision? Which of the following has led you to discontinue the method you had begun?" In data analysis, answers to open-ended questions are typically classified according to prestructured categories that represent the researcher's theoretical understanding of the problem.

Control of extraneous and competing variables, as defined in this framework, is important in quantitative design. The framework applies rules for incorporating factors from the social environment based on assumptions that are different from other frameworks. Using experimental and quasi-experimental designs, quantitative researchers attempt to distribute evenly the effect of contextual variables through randomization. Their rationale is that context contains hidden determinants, which may affect measurement of causal or associative relationships and bias the outcomes of the study. Control is thus fundamental to quantitative research assumptions because it provides a means to isolate extraneous variables and focus more clearly on the relationships that were highlighted in the research problem.

One viewpoint proposes that all [social scientific] data can in principle be measured or classified; therefore, when we confront nonquantified data, our task is to refine them through analysis so that they are subject to quantification or categorization.

(Selltiz et al. 1976, 460)

Controlling effects also helps researchers to identify and explain in quantitative terms the influence of factors in the study environment on key relationships. For example, if your research problem were to identify factors that predict fertility trends in Peru, you would measure the variable relationships among selected possible determinants of fertility and the relative strengths with which each of these factors can predict the number of births per Peruvian woman. You would control for socio-demographic and other variables that might explain the observed relationships. You would obtain accurate measurements, but since it is impossible to identify, measure, and control every variable that could influence whether a woman will give birth, you would always have unanswered, or partially answered, questions. A versatile investigator might at this point turn to qualitative techniques to explore some of the quantitative findings in greater depth.

In quantitative studies, accuracy, reliability, and relative freedom from bias are critical criteria for judging the quality of findings. The inherent difficulty of ensuring accuracy in any social or behavioral inquiry has led quantitative researchers to stress neutrality, uniformity, objectivity, and replicability. Such goals are consistent with the positivist goal to study phenomena objectively and to express findings in terms of measurable outcomes and relationships. A quantitative strategy emphasizes structure: consistent operational definitions throughout the study, precisely worded questions, and statistical analysis. However, this structure limits the scope of the research by requiring the formulatation of research problems and questions in measurable terms.

Over the years, demographers, epidemiologists, biostatisticians, and other quantitative scientists

Context contains hidden determinants

have met many methodological challenges. Their painstaking efforts to answer difficult questions have resulted in an impressive knowledge base in population and reproductive health. But still missing is a deeper understanding of the circumstances that help to explain why and how people make the decisions they do. Even when working in a quantitative framework, therefore, researchers often turn to other ways of understanding human behavior, specifically the methods of qualitative research (Pedersen 1992), based on different principles and theoretical assumptions.

Qualitative research from an interpretivist perspective. The theoretical framework for most qualitative research emerges from an interpretivist perspective, a paradigm that sees the world as constructed, interpreted, and experienced by people in their interactions with each other and with wider social systems. Research focuses not only on objectively verifiable facts but also on the many subjective meanings that people attach to them. Identifying, sorting, and analyzing those meanings in relation to objective behavior — decisions, actions, practices — are the methodological substance of the interpretivist framework.

Qualitative research is grounded in a philosophical position, which is broadly 'interpretivist' in the sense that it is concerned about how the social world is interpreted, understood, experienced, or produced.

(Mason 1996, 4)

Three key components of this framework, then, are subjective perceptions and understandings, which arise from experience; objective actions or behaviors; and context. Qualitative researchers explore phenomena in the light of related social, cultural, political, and physical environments of the people they are studying – the holistic approach characteristic of the interpretivist perspective. Qualitative analysis also allows the researcher to link findings from the three components to explore the multiple relations among them. For example, a woman usually does not define contraception simply as a means to prevent pregnancy. She interprets its significance in the light of personal and cultural experience and from what other people say and believe about it, including health workers, her partner, her friends, or influential family members. If, as several studies have found, a woman — or the people she listens to — believes that contraceptive pills will "accumulate in her stomach and cause cancer," then that belief will influence her decision to accept or reject the method.

On another level, the social and material contexts in which a woman acts also affect her decisions and behavior. If a woman cannot afford contraceptive pills and the economic environment offers very limited opportunity to generate income, or if isolated living conditions or restrictive social norms make it impossible for her to get to a health clinic for her monthly prescription, these contextual factors will influence both her perceptions and her behaviors. Approaching this problem from an interpretivist perspective, you would take seriously the woman's subjective understanding of oral contraception and would link it to her actions and their potential impacts. Using flexible, in-depth techniques, you would compare your findings with the perspectives and actions of other women, looking for different as well as similar constructions that could explain patterns of behavior. You might also examine the wider context of women's experiences with oral contraception in that culture; for example, barriers to information and service, partner communication concerning family planning, extended family norms, and the influence of fertility on the changing status of women in their extended families.

The kinds of research questions that arise in an interpretivist framework are mainly those that address why, how, and under what circumstances, rather than what and how many. Why has the intrauterine device (IUD) been widely accepted in some countries and rejected in others? Under what circumstances do men in pronatalist societies support child-spacing? Why do some men feel alienated from family planning discussions? How do economically dependent women protect themselves from HIV transmission when their partners are at risk? The same questions can be addressed from a quantitative perspective but in terms of discrete indicators with measurable dimensions. Qualitative methods of participant observation, in-depth interviews, and focus group discussions would elicit data on subjective understandings.

The methods associated with this perspective tend to be those that enable participants to speak freely and to understand the investigator's quest for insight into a phenomenon that the participant has experienced. As subsequent chapters will show, interpretivist methodology seeks information in as natural a context as possible, where the researcher can observe activities and events as they occur and encourage people to respond from their own perspectives and experiences and in their own words. In the IUD example above, the results would be a deeper understanding of motivations, decisions, and circumstances associated with IUD use. They would not answer more descriptive questions concerning extent, patterns, and prediction of use, or measurable indicators of knowledge and attitudes concerning the method — issues that are addressed

in a quantitative framework. The reader should note, however, that a combined methodological strategy in this example would make it possible to use the strengths of each approach while compensating for their limitations.

Qualitative research from a feminist perspective. Like interpretivist scholars, feminist theorists believe that how people interpret their experience is not only a valid, but an essential, focus of research. But until feminist theory was articulated in the 1960s, neither the positivist nor the interpretivist perspectives had taken fully into account the profound influence of power relations in sexual and reproductive health. While critical theorists such as Antonio Gramschi and Michel Foucault have greatly advanced studies of social dynamics of power, grounded in the work of Karl Marx and other critical scholars, feminist scholars have brought this current of thought into the field of gender relations, a field that is consummately important in sexual and reproductive health.[†]

Although feminist research has grown from a commitment to gender equity and increasing equality between men and women, and continues to advance these aims, the feminist perspective addresses power relationships of many kinds, not just those between men and women. It is rapidly restructuring how we design our research, adding concepts and tools to answer numerous important questions we have not before had the means to ask.

Feminist research frameworks are concerned with the gender and power dimensions of social phenomena that shape people's lives. An important premise of feminist theory is that social life and

---

[†] Gender is defined as "the roles that men and women play and the relations that arise out of these roles. They are socially constructed, not physically determined" (Pan American Health Organization 1997).

behavior are constrained in various ways by what is considered acceptable behavior based on gender. Feminist research focuses on the political dimension inherent in understanding these constraints from the standpoints of people in different power and gender positions. The power relationships that maintain boundaries on people's lives often cast women in subordinate positions relative to men, but they apply equally to other forms of power imbalance; for example, those defined by race, economic status, and access to scarce resources.

Recent substantive theories of subordination and domination, constructed within a feminist paradigm, have been instrumental in improving the quality of family planning and reproductive health care delivery (Bruce 1990). Health practitioners and researchers are familiar with the power differential that all too often silences the voices of clients in health care settings. Communications workshops for health providers, as well as efforts to empower women to participate more actively in their health care, have been an outgrowth of studies that identify gender gaps in client-provider relationships. Male involvement in reproductive health decisions is frequently addressed from a gender perspective. For example, how do couples negotiate sexual decisions? How do men learn about fertility, and why do they remain on the margins of many reproductive health programs?

Feminist work sets the stage for other research, other actions, and policy that transcend and transform.

(Olesen 2000, 215)

Box 2.2

The IRRRAG Project: Feminist Perspective in Sexual and Reproductive Health

The International Reproductive Rights Research Action Group (IRRRAG) was founded in 1992 by Rosalind Petchesky on the premise that "until we know more about the local contexts and ways of thinking in which women in their everyday lives negotiate reproductive health and sexual matters, we cannot assume that reproductive and sexual rights are a goal that they seek and therefore one that has universal applicability" (Petchesky and Judd 1998, 1).

One IRRRAG project — part research and part movement for social justice — is an example of how feminist theory has been effectively applied to qualitative research in sexual and reproductive health. Using primarily qualitative methods, IRRRAG researchers talked with women in Egypt, Malaysia, Nigeria, Mexico, Brazil, the Philippines, and the United States about how they conceptualize and act on their sexual and reproductive rights. Feminist and participatory research models guided the project, which focused on two key questions:

1. How do women across diverse countries, cultures, and generations arrive at and negotiate a sense of entitlement with regard to their reproductive and sexual health and well-being?

2. Under what life circumstances and by what terms and strategies do women begin to take charge of their reproductive and sexual bodies? (Petchesky and Judd 1998, 8).

The project was "centrally concerned with issues of moral and political [power] and women's formulation and pursuit of claims to decision-making authority" (Petchesky and Judd 1998, 8). Thus an agenda for action, or social change, was built into the research with the intention to "uncover and enhance the conditions for women [that will enable them to] challenge existing power relations" (Petchesky and Judd 1998, 8).

A distinguishing element in the project was the commitment to feminist research principles and practices, including the use of democratic consensus-building within the international research team. Together, the team built a conceptual framework that highlighted understanding women's beliefs about sexual and reproductive rights and interpreting those insights. The study explored how women formulate and express their ideas about rights and entitlement and how, through both accommodation and resistance, they attempt to negotiate their rights in the contexts of their daily lives.

The IRRRAG researchers discovered that many women do not feel a sense of entitlement to basic human rights on their own behalf until they become mothers. Only when they needed to protect the rights of their children did the women in the study believe they were entitled to any rights at all. The conceptual framework for the study helped to explain this finding as follows: The women's lives were sharply limited by their gender-defined status and roles, that is, by social and cultural expectations for the appropriate behavior (and rights) of women at different ages. As wives and mothers, women in the study were expected to assert and defend their rights to safeguard their children and the well-being of their families. It was less acceptable, however, for a woman to demand her own rights to personal growth, leisure, or sexual pleasure, since these are outside the usual boundaries of women's traditional reproductive and productive family roles.

The IRRRAG study illustrates how a feminist theoretical perspective can be the basis for a research design, incorporating substantive theoretical constructs such as rights, entitlement, accommodation, and resistance. It also demonstrates the practical relevance of theory, since a woman's sense of entitlement can be directly related to sexual and reproductive decisions that shape her life. The finding that women in the IRRRAG study countries often do not believe they are entitled to reproductive rights until they are mothers is critical information for women's advocates. It helps to explain why, despite intensive informational and educational campaigns, many women still cannot accept family planning until they have borne a child.

Feminist theorists point out that women's voices have not been heard in the process of developing and delivering health care to women. Similarly, when we leave men out of sexual and reproductive health programs or research, we are not hearing what they experience and what they think about a host of issues, including sexual relationships, family planning, and protection against infection. As a result, our policy and program perspectives may be too narrow and may neglect questions that are important to men.

The influence of feminist thought and methodology can be found in much of the sexual and reproductive health literature today, often bridging qualitative and quantitative methods while keeping lived experience central to the investigation (Tolman and Szalacha 1999). For example, in development studies, household survey results have highlighted gender differences in relation to other social characteristics such as age, ethnicity, and class. These differences can be further explored with methods that enable people to speak out on issues that are meaningful to them (Caro 1995). Researchers who work from the feminist paradigm tend to select qualitative methods that empower participants who have not previously had a voice in significant debates, like those surrounding international family planning. By alerting us to the potential for bias when researchers do not listen to the voices of certain groups of people, feminist researchers are helping us reformulate how we design and conduct our studies.

Table 2.1 (see page 28) summarizes the logic and language of these three paradigms and outlines major points with a selection of examples from the more comprehensive methodological toolboxes of each theoretical framework. Interested readers are referred to more comprehensive sources such as the *Handbook of Qualitative Research* (Denzin and Lincoln 2000).

Putting It All Together: Qualitative Concepts and Their Relationships

Theoretical components of qualitative reproductive health research include concepts and principles that have evolved — and continue to evolve — under the influence of interpretivist and feminist paradigms. A basic premise of qualitative logic is that since people interpret things, events, and interactions in different ways, they arrive at different understandings, responses, or actions. Public health messages, for example, mean different things to different people because they interpret them differently. To a qualitative researcher, the meanings that people take from an AIDS prevention message, for example, may be attributed to differences in social context, with its profound influence on human thought and behavior. Qualitative researchers are always probing contradictions and inconsistencies in the human condition because it is at this level that we begin to understand the dynamics of human behavior.

Understanding how qualitative research explores these dynamics means becoming familiar with the language that expresses basic qualitative concepts and principles. We have grouped some of the most important concepts to show their relationships:

- **Qualitative research is systematic discovery.** Its purpose is to generate knowledge of social events and processes by understanding what they mean to people, exploring and documenting how people interact with each other and how they interpret and interact with the world around them. It also seeks to elucidate patterns of shared understanding and variability in those patterns.

- **Qualitative researchers value natural settings where the researcher can better understand people's lived experiences.** The natural context of people's lives is a critical component of qualitative design because it influences the perspectives, experiences, and actions of participants in the study. It is the interpersonal and sociocultural fabric that shapes meanings and actions.

- **Researchers express qualitative data in participants' words, in images, and sometimes in numbers.** Language, verbal and nonverbal, has symbolic meaning — expression that may mean one thing to the study participant and a different thing to the interviewer. Qualitative researchers listen carefully to language as participants tell about their experiences without the constraints of externally imposed structure. When we refer to raw data as narrative, we mean participants relating their ideas and experiences in ways that can offer insight into important research concepts and questions.

- **The qualitative research process is flexible, emergent, and iterative.** The study design is never fixed; there is constant interplay between design and discovery. Findings emerge continuously. The investigator is always in touch with the research process, observing how participants respond to the topic and examining data for fresh insights that might lead to altering a technique, modifying questions, or changing direction to pursue new leads. Analysis does not wait until all the data are collected; it begins in the field.

- **Reflexivity — the researcher's critical self-awareness — is a vital process in which you question and observe yourself at the same time you listen to and observe the participant.** With its emphasis on egalitarian relationships, feminist methodology has contributed greatly to this point. In contrast to the detachment required of many quantitative studies, your presence is a vital component of the qualitative research process in two ways. First, you are in a partnership with the participant — working together to explore themes and find answers. Second, as you listen, interpret, and respond to your participant-partner, you are a key research instrument yourself, not only absorbing information but also influencing how it is elicited. Self-examination, documented with other observations in the field notes, is part of the iterative process of interpretation and revision that moves the data collection toward its goal.

Theoretical Models in Practice

Applied qualitative researchers often use substantive theory from the field of health behavior. These behavioral frameworks offer a rich array of concepts and theoretical relationships that can help define qualitative research problems more clearly and guide the research design. If your research is principally concerned with behavior change, we recommend reviewing several frameworks and models and selecting concepts that fit your theoretical perspective on the research problem. For example, many studies in sexual and reproductive health, both qualitative and quantitative, have included concepts from behavioral frameworks that:

- describe cultural models of health and illness to understand "individual and group-level knowledge and beliefs about health threats, transmission dynamics, and behavioral norms"
- identify the social contexts in which beliefs and values are manifested in actions
- identify the conditions that promote or prevent change in risk behaviors, or
- determine the conditions necessary for maintaining individual behavior change

(Trotter 1997, 259-260)

Table 2.1

Three Paradigms for Research in Sexual and Reproductive Health

	Positivist	Interpretivist	Feminist
Basic assumptions	The social world is comprised of observable facts. Reality is objective, independent of the researcher.	The social world is constructed of symbolic meaning observable in human acts, interactions, and language. Reality is subjective and multiple as seen from different perspectives.	The social world is governed by power relations that influence acts and perceptions. Reality is negotiated and differs according to status and power.
Sources of evidence	Facts are revealed through standard scientific processes; are context-free.	Meanings are derived from perceptions, experiences, and actions in relation to social contexts.	Power, control, and contextual factors can be heard in personal accounts that reflect different versions of reality.
Methods	Prestructured data collection, controlled measurement, clinical trials are the norm. Examples: surveys, clinical trials, rating scales, structured observation.	Semi-structured, open questions, and observation enable participants to express thoughts and actions in natural ways. Examples: in-depth interviews, focus group discussions, participant observations, case histories.	Participatory forms of observation and guided conversation enable both marginal and dominant groups to voice opinions and tell their stories. Examples: participatory action techniques, reflexive listening, challenges to political and personal barriers to entrenched positions.

	Positivist	Interpretivist	Feminist
Research intention	Quantitative studies seek explanation, verification, and prediction of human behavior through causal or associative relationships.	Qualitative studies seek discovery, understanding, and insight into the circumstances of human behavior.	Feminist studies seek insight into the influence of gender on human behavior, including differentials in power and control, in an agenda for social change.
Level of participation	Research subjects answer specific, predetermined questions in a structured response format.	Research participants are active partners in data collection and respond to semi-structured questions spontaneously and naturally.	Research participants have relative freedom to direct the data collection process and define follow-up.
Impact on study participants	Impact is neutral. Research subjects may gain new information or insight from the results.	Participants are aware of their engagement in the research process; may gain insight into their own perspectives and behaviors, as well as the topic of the research.	Participation is empowering. Results may lead to a participant-defined action agenda and empowerment to initiate or participate in policy change.

Theory

If you are designing a study that will be of practical use to program managers concerned with reducing HIV risk in a community, you might look for a framework that identifies predictors of risk. Or you might decide to segment a study population on the basis of demographic characteristics suggested in the model. Some qualitative researchers, on the other hand, refer to these models and frameworks only in the analysis and interpretation of their data, comparing themes that emerge from their findings to concepts and relationships in a larger body of theory.

Appendix 1 (page 207) presents summaries of several working behavior change theories that have contributed conceptually to both qualitative and quantitative research in sexual and reproductive health: health beliefs, stages of change, locus of control, and AIDS risk reduction.

Setting Standards for Qualitative Research

At the heart of the debate on research standards is the much used, but often misunderstood, concept of subjectivity. To a quantitative scientist, data are facts that must be isolated as much as possible from the personal, or subjective, values of the researcher; subjectivity can mean distortion. Although the notion of a perfectly objective social science is a widely acknowledged myth, the accuracy of quantitative data often depends on the separation of fact from subjective judgment. Qualitative researchers, on the other hand, defend subjectivity as an important element in the research process. We believe that we perceive the world only partially and there-fore, as researchers, must describe as many aspects of reality as we can and be open to many ways of interpreting the social world. Our access to these multiple worldviews is through the subjective experiences and understandings of study participants. The qualitative researcher's use of self as a reflexive (self-aware) partner in collecting and interpreting

Box 2.3
Checklist for Using Substantive Theory

When applying a theory or model, consider:

- What dimensions of the problem does the theory or model concern?

- Is it specific to the unit of study (e.g., individual behavior, group influences, environmental issues)?

- How does the theory or model explain this portion of your research problem?

- What information does the theory or model suggest that you gather?

- How accurately does the theory or model coincide with your understanding of the problem?

- What aspects of the problem does the theory or model fail to consider?

- In your judgment, how helpful is the theory or model in working with the problem and determining how best to study it?

- What are its limitations?

(Lewis 2000)

information further strengthens the position that subjectivity, applied appropriately and systematically, is a positive element in qualitative science.

Judging quality: the search for trustworthy data

Qualitative and quantitative criteria of excellence are equally important but inherently different (Devers 1999). All of us who design research, or who use research findings, are concerned with quality, but the criteria of evaluation differ in qualitative and quantitative research practice: They are analogous but not interchangeable. Each has its own appropriate and no less rigorous standards. The most widely adopted criteria have been those developed from the positivist framework: Validity, reliability, objectivity, precision, and generalizability are used to judge the rigor of quantitative studies intended to describe, predict, and verify empirical relationships in relatively controlled settings.

On the other hand, qualitative research that aims to explore, discover, and understand cannot use the same criteria to judge research quality and outcomes. Below, we synthesize the work of several qualitative scientists who have articulated standards or criteria for judging qualitative data (Lincoln and Guba 1985; Miles and Huberman 1994; Kirk and Miller 1986). Lincoln and Guba suggest that the fundamental criterion for qualitative reports is trustworthiness. How, they ask, can a researcher be certain that "the findings of an inquiry are worth paying attention to, worth taking account of?" (Lincoln and Guba 1985, 398). In answer, practitioners and consumers of qualitative science ask a new set of questions: How can we know that the data are credible, dependable, confirmable, and transferable? We introduce these concepts below because evaluating the trustworthiness of qualitative data is directly related to the fundamental logic of qualitative theory. In Chapter 6, quality standards are discussed in greater detail in relation to data analysis.

Credibility. In quantitative science, validity is the extent to which a measurement taps the concept it intends to measure. The outcome is accepted as "true" within reasonable limits. Credibility, also called truth value, is the corresponding criterion for qualitative research. Validity assumes correct operational measures for the concepts being studied and, in experimental studies, a potential cause-effect relationship (Yin 1994); credibility focuses on confidence in the truth of the findings, including an accurate understanding of the context:

- Do the findings show a logical relationship to each other, i.e., are they consistent in terms of the explanations they support?
- Are the findings grounded in and substantiated by the narrative data, i.e., is the narrative data sufficiently rich to support the specific findings? Do the findings indicate a need for more data?
- Does the original study population consider reports to be accurate?

(Miles and Huberman 1994)

Dependability. An important test of quantitative reliability is the extent to which findings can be replicated. The goal is not only to obtain the same results in a study (which, given intervening time and change, may not be possible), but to be able to replicate the processes used to obtain these results, even though in different cultural contexts they may be very different (King et al. 1994). For qualitative researchers inquiring into unique constellations of multiple phenomena and meanings, this goal would be meaningless. In other words, the same method is not likely to produce the same results unless the answers are prestructured to conform to definitions imposed by the research design. For qualitative researchers, the methodological parallel to reliability is whether the results are dependable, that the research process is consistent and carried out with careful attention to the rules and conventions of qualitative methodology. We ask ourselves:

- Are the research questions clear and logically connected to the research purpose and design?
- Are there parallels across data sources?
- Do multiple field workers have comparable data collection protocols?

Given the contextual nature of qualitative research, we do not expect to produce exactly the same answers. On the other hand, we do anticipate that if the data are dependable, we will find logically consistent patterns of response that remain reasonably stable over time.

Confirmability. Objectivity is a traditional standard of quality in quantitative data. The term generally implies maintaining distance between the observer and the observed and minimizing any possible influence of the researcher's values on the process of inquiry. Either strategy would be counterproductive in most qualitative studies. From a qualitative perspective, the analogous goal is to confirm, by audits and other methods that will be discussed in Chapters 5 and 6, that the data reflect as accurately as possible the perspectives and experiences of the participants. Confirmability thus means a way of knowing that, even as a co-participant in the inquiry, the researcher has maintained the distinction between personal values and those of the study participants. Applying the concept of reflexivity, qualitative researchers have an obligation to observe and document their own roles in the research process, including assumptions, biases, or reactions that might influence the collection and interpretation of data. Applying reflexivity contributes to the confirmability of the results.

Transferability. Also called extensibility, transferability is the qualitative analogue to the concept of generalizability. Generalizability of the findings to a wider population is a goal of most quantitative studies. Indeed, if every unit in the study sample has an equal chance of being selected, and the sample is large enough to minimize the probability of error, then this goal can be met within certain specified margins. It is a statistically representative sample. Although generalizability by this definition is not relevant to the goals or the methodology of most interpretive work, it is nevertheless important to know "whether the conclusions of a study … [are] transferable to other contexts" (Miles and Huberman 1994, 279). The importance of context in qualitative studies leads some researchers to doubt that results from one context should be transferred to another, while others sometimes appear to apply conclusions from their data too casually. Our position is on middle ground: Lessons learned from qualitative studies can be applied to other contexts if samples have been carefully selected to represent viewpoints and experiences that reflect key issues in the research problem. Our goal is to produce data that are conceptually, not statistically, representative of people in a specific context. Since context is a key influence in any qualitative research, the researcher must account for contextual factors when transferring data from one situation to another. Repeating the study in another population, with similar conclusions, lends credibility to the results and further specifies the circumstances under which the findings will occur. Thus well-documented knowledge might be extended to similar populations, but "the burden of proof lies less with the original investigator than with the person seeking to make an application elsewhere. The original inquirer cannot know the sites to which transferability might be sought, but appliers can" (Lincoln and Guba 1985, 404).

These terms — credibility, dependability, confirmability, and transferability — comprise the standards for evaluating the rigor of qualitative studies that are consistent with the worldview, information sources, and methods of the interpretivist paradigm. In subsequent chapters, we will return to these criteria of quality with further discussion of specific techniques for ensuring the rigor of qualitative studies.

Conclusion

As researchers, we each have a fundamental curiosity about our subject of inquiry. But in designing and implementing the research, we must move beyond ordinary curiosity to a disciplined use of the rules and conventions of our theoretical perspective or paradigm. A great deal has been written from the quantitative point of view that will continue to guide much of our work in sexual and reproductive health. For this book, our theoretical compass is set largely, though not entirely, by the interpretivist and feminist paradigms. We believe that, alone or in combination with use of appropriate quantitative methods, these two theoretical positions can generate qualitative research that addresses many complex issues in sexual and reproductive health, human rights, and gender. In this chapter, we have urged readers to examine their own theoretical perspectives, ask themselves what perspective their work reflects, where their ideas come from, and whether it might be useful to look at a problem through a different lens. It is important to incorporate self-reflection in the research process, to know how one's own worldview influences the questions under investigation. If you understand and use your theoretical perspective as a guide, you will discover new ways to a better understanding of human thought and behavior.

Designing the Study

The design of a naturalistic inquiry (whether research, evaluation, or policy analysis) cannot be given in advance; it must emerge, develop, unfold ...

(Lincoln and Guba 1985, 225)

A well-articulated design is the basis for all research proposals. It presents the rationale for conducting the study in the first place, and it builds a persuasive argument for the methodology you choose for accomplishing your objectives. Design decisions at this stage will demonstrate the value and rigor of your proposed research. They will also show clearly the relationship between your research problem and the conceptual or theoretical framework that will guide your design (see Chapter 2).

Designing the Study

As experienced investigators know, the process of designing research is rarely linear. The steps are interdependent and overlapping, each one challenging the researcher to think ahead to subsequent steps. Qualitative researchers rethink and modify elements of the design even as the data are emerging. However, for the purpose of this discussion, we present important design questions in the following sequence:

- What is the general area of inquiry?
- What is the purpose of the research?
- How is the research problem defined?
- What is the larger conceptual framework?
- What questions will address the research problem?
- What methods will best address the research questions?
- Who should participate?
- What ethical standards will assure the protection of study participants?
- How should the data be collected?
- How will data collectors be trained and monitored?
- How will the data be analyzed?
- How will the results be disseminated?

Written answers to these questions should provide your initial design strategy with sufficient detail by which others can judge the relevance and rigor of your proposed research. Such documentation often becomes the basis for proposals submitted to donors for funding. (See Appendix 3, page 212 for an example of a study design.) Donors looking for evidence that the design is appropriate to the purpose of the study often have their own criteria for judging quality and relevance (see Appendix 9, page 229).

Establishing an Area of Inquiry

Most applied researchers are drawn to an area of inquiry out of personal interest or experience, a desire to help solve a problem, or perhaps in response to a request from a donor. The choice is rooted in values and expectations that the inquiry will in some way benefit society. In sexual and reproductive health, areas of inquiry might be the quality of prenatal care in a health service, the introduction of a new method to protect against infection, the prevalence of HIV in a low-risk population, or perhaps an alarmingly high rate of adolescent abortion. It is not unusual to develop a cluster of different studies in one substantive area, employing combinations of qualitative and quantitative methods, but all focusing on a single broad domain.

Stating the Research Problem and Purpose

As you narrow your focus to a more manageable field, you begin to define the broad area in terms of specific issues that will form the core of the study. If the area of inquiry is quality of prenatal care, the research problem might be to explore women's perceptions of the care they receive at a clinic, the nature and consequences of client-provider interaction, or women's decisions whether or not to seek prenatal care. If the area of study is the introduction of a new method of protection, the purpose of the research might be an assessment of women's and men's perceptions of the need, efficacy, and safety of the method or of the sociocultural factors that may influence its use in the community. To some extent, these questions can be addressed by quantitative methods, but exploring how and why places the problem in an interpretivist framework, which will offer theoretical direction for later decisions. Any of the above examples suggest that the design should enable the researcher to understand and interpret the situation from participants' varied points of view.

A research problem may also come from earlier studies, perhaps a query as to why or under what circumstances a finding has occurred. For example, a household survey carried out in Haiti at the height of the AIDS epidemic revealed that women reported significantly lower risk behavior than men but greater fear of acquiring HIV (Adrien and Cayemittes 1991). Subsequent qualitative research addressed the gap between risk status and fear of AIDS, exploring in greater depth women's perceptions of their own vulnerability (Ulin et al. 1995). Or, an initial research problem may be generated by a donor organization interested in a particular issue, such as how to allocate limited resources in a country to reduce unwanted pregnancy or maternal mortality.

Literature review helps to make a case for the importance of the problem, to build it into a conceptual framework, and to avoid duplication of effort. When you state the problem and purpose of your research, you usually are describing a gap in scientific knowledge, a puzzle to put together, or a mystery to solve. Referring to previous research adds clarity to the problem by placing it in a larger empirical context. It is useful to know the extent to which quantitative research has examined the problem and to identify questions that other quantitative methods studies have left unanswered. Are earlier studies consistent or inconsistent? Qualitative researchers frequently welcome divergent findings because they suggest multiple and sometimes contradictory dimensions of a problem that qualitative methodology can address.

In applied research, we usually extend the statement of purpose to potential utilization of the results; for example, to help improve access to, and quality of, prenatal care or to help lower the rate of sexually transmitted infection (STI) in a population. Even at this early stage of design it is important to think ahead to the results, or the kinds of information that you will want to report and to the potential recipients who will use it. Therefore, an important resource for research questions may be policy-makers and program managers who need to know how to make programs more accessible, health care more effective, or services more acceptable. In designing a qualitative study of contraceptive use in Mali, we asked local family planning managers to share some of their concerns. Their interest in the involvement of husbands in family planning decisions led to a modification of the research problem, with results that ultimately played an important role in the analysis and dissemination.

It is important to note that a single researcher might view a problem from different perspectives at different times, depending on the information needed. From a quantitative perspective, the researcher might wish to describe the scope of a problem or test a hypothesis concerning its occurrence. Using a qualitative perspective, one might shift focus to understanding why the problem occurs or how it is perceived. From a feminist perspective, the researcher might introduce the concept of power as a determinant of an individual's or group's position on an issue. In most areas of inquiry in sexual and reproductive health, more than one perspective is useful for understanding a problem to the fullest extent possible.

Conceptualizing the Problem in a Larger Framework

One way to keep your design centered on the research problem is to take the time to develop a conceptual framework. A conceptual framework is a set of related ideas behind the research design. It may be a simple list of concepts and their possible associations or a more elaborate schematic diagram of key influences, presumed relationships, and possible outcomes of the research problem (see Figure 3.1, page 42). Motivated by a compelling problem or some critical gap in knowledge, most researchers begin a study with at least a tentative notion of what factors may be important and how they might fit together in a logical scheme. And as pointed out previously, a literature review can identify findings from previous research that will suggest ways of conceptualizing the current problem.

Proposing Qualitative Research to WHO

Iqbal Shah, Ph.D.
World Health Organization

Since its inception in 1972, the Special Programme of Research, Development and Research Training in Human Reproduction (HRP) at the World Health Organization (WHO) has supported focused, in-depth social science research on issues related to family planning and, later, reproductive health. From 1985 to 2000, HRP launched major research initiatives on: (1) contraceptive use dynamics; (2) acceptability of condoms; (3) determinants and consequences of abortion; (4) sexual behavior and reproductive health; (5) role of men in reproductive health; (6) adolescent sexual and reproductive health; and, most recently, (7) quality of care in reproductive health. HRP has received and reviewed, cumulatively, over 1,000 submissions and supported projects ranging from small qualitative studies to intervention projects with semi-experimental designs. A large number of these have included qualitative research methods, especially focus group discussions (FGDs).

Increasingly HRP receives proposals for studies that intend to apply a battery of qualitative techniques, including body mapping, freelisting, in-depth interviews, case studies, and FGDs. Whereas these techniques can be enriching, little attention is being paid to the rationale and need for each one, or how the data arising from a mix of methods will be integrated, analyzed, or interpreted.

HRP's policy is to seek proposals of good scientific quality that incorporate a study design appropriate to the stated objectives. Many proposals describe use of a combination of cross-sectional surveys and FGDs. While some qualitative research submissions have been of high caliber, many others have been weak, particularly when proposing FGDs. Based on many years of experience reviewing such proposals, I would like to offer some insights on avoiding common mistakes in such proposals.

Inappropriate use. The single fatal flaw in any proposal is to set forth incorrect research methods to meet the stated objectives. We have received submissions proposing use of FGDs to measure the prevalence and incidence of contraceptive use or violence, or to collect individuals' personal information and experience; for example, relating to sexual behavior. These proposals were not approved because FGDs are not suitable to measure prevalence or incidence. On the other hand, proposals that have suggested using FGDs to ascertain normative patterns, to develop a survey instrument, or to explain or expand on survey findings have frequently been approved. Also reviewed favorably are FGD proposals to understand community norms and attitudes toward specific reproductive health issues.

Design concerns. Researchers frequently make mistakes related to the composition and number of FGDs, selection of participants, the focus group guide, and the conduct of FGDs. For example, one basic requirement of FGDs is that of homogeneity; you do not mix men and women in the same group, or adolescents and older women, etc. And it is inappropriate to extend the norms of quantitative research sampling to this technique. Nevertheless, we receive proposals that suggest holding enough FGDs to represent all age, socioeconomic, gender, religious, and ethnic groups.

Investigators may have a poor understanding of the appropriate number of groups to hold — we have seen proposals that ranged from one or two to over 400 focus groups per study. Clearly, the rationale for an optimum number of FGDs was neither understood nor provided. Successful researchers suggest six to eight FGDs, and understand that one must reduce or increase the number to avoid redundancy and to seek new information on substantive issues. Researchers often omit justification for the number of participants in each FGD. The majority of researchers suggest 8 to 10 members per group, which is normally appropriate, but we see proposals ranging from two to 50.

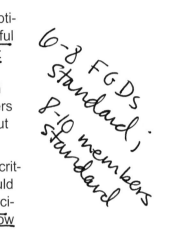

6-8 FGDs Standard; 8-10 members standard

Investigators frequently fail to provide enough information about other critical aspects of their studies. Sometimes they imply that reviewers should just trust them. Necessary information is often missing about how participants will be selected, where and how FGDs will be conducted, and how information will be recorded, compiled, and analyzed. In addition, concerns around confidentiality, informed consent, and storage and access to information are not always discussed. The FGD guide is rarely provided. This lack of information delays the proposal review as investigators are asked to provide supplemental information and assure reviewers that the structure of the questions is appropriate for a FGD.

A less common, but equally serious pitfall is for investigators to propose using statistical techniques to analyze the results of FGDs; for example, chi-square or t-tests, with some going as far as to suggest multivariate analysis.

Other precautions. Having now supported a number of scientifically sound qualitative research proposals, HRP has also accumulated experience on implementation and analysis. The implementation of FGDs does not usually present major difficulties, but some exceptions include holding mixed groups or allowing one or a few participants to dominate the group discussions. However, major challenges exist in the analysis and interpretation of focus group data. Most researchers find the amount of information they have collected overwhelming, and often do not develop or follow a codebook or an analysis plan. The interpretation of FGD data is not always straightforward, and we receive reports from investigators who have reflected FGD findings with means, medians, and percentages. Finally, most researchers find it very difficult to summarize qualitative information in a succinct and meaningful manner.

Features for success:

- Articulate a clear and convincing rationale for the choice of the method of study, irrespective of the type of method (qualitative or quantitative or both).
- Provide complete details of the procedures to be used, including a draft questionnaire or guide, ethical considerations around informed consent and confidentiality, data management, and field procedures.
- Pay attention to the analysis and interpretation of data and to how information collected using more than one methodological approach, irrespective of the type, will be integrated.
- Include training of the staff and moderator for the conduct of FGD, collection and coding of information, and analysis.

See World Health Organization 2000 in the references list. For further information about submitting research proposals to WHO, contact: Dr. Iqbal Shah, Department of Reproductive Health and Research, World Health Organization, 1211 Geneva 27, Switzerland.

Most qualitative researchers start with a set of thoughtfully defined concepts and tentative associations as they design the research and begin to work with study participants. As the study progresses, concepts and their relationships become clearer, articulated in the voices of the participants. In many cases, the elements of the framework are discovered during the study rather than anticipated at the design stage. Thus, some studies conclude with a schematic diagram that shows graphically how concepts interrelate.

A conceptual framework does more than help outline research questions. It also provides a context in which others will be able to understand the research. Evidence-based findings contribute to theoretical generalizations, which in turn can be useful to colleagues developing new research. Whether a simple list of concepts or a more elaborate schematic diagram, your framework will be the springboard from which you will both launch your investigation and communicate what you are studying.

For example, one study (Koo and Woodsong 1997) drew on both qualitative and quantitative methods to investigate the dynamics and meaning of unintended pregnancy in a sample of women and their sexual partners. The researchers' purpose was to develop and test measures of pregnancy intendedness, focusing on contextual influences on decision-making. To conceptualize the dynamics of unplanned pregnancy, they constructed the model in Figure 3.1 (see page 42).

This model contains several clusters of variables:

- **Environment** — Influences in the social, economic, and interpersonal environment that affect contraceptive choice.
- **Individual factors** — Characteristics, motivations, experiences, and gender images of women, their partners, and significant older family members.

- **Pregnancy intentions** — Couples' conscious or unconscious attitudes that influence contraceptive behavior.
- **Contraceptive use** — The "gate" by which sexually active couples enter or avoid pregnancy: method choice, consistency and correctness of use, and non-use.
- **Contraceptive method**s — Method characteristics and access.
- **Pregnancy** — The occurrence of a pregnancy, classified as (a) successful avoidance and (b) pregnancy intended or unintended.
- **Near-term outcomes** — Whether the pregnancy results in birth or abortion, and if a birth, whether the woman receives assistance with child care and support, whether she can return to work, and the effect of the birth on family and social relationships.

The conceptual framework enabled the researchers to consider many different facets of the problem and possible relationships among them in order to identify appropriate qualitative and quantitative research strategies. The framework also proved useful in presenting the proposal to a funding agency in that funders could visualize quickly core concepts and interrelationships to be studied. Preliminary hypotheses, developed from the conceptual framework, further clarified goals and expectations of the research. However, from a qualitative perspective, the reviewers understood that the hypotheses were illustrations only, and that working hypotheses would be developed from the results of focus group discussions in the first round of data collection.

As this example demonstrates, a conceptual framework is a tentative mapping of the research domain. The example also illustrates the iterative process of qualitative design. The researchers used their framework as a guide, continually examining assumptions and methods in the light of new evidence. As new constructs and new relationships

Figure 3.1.

Conceptual Framework: The Dynamics and Meaning of Unintended Pregnancy

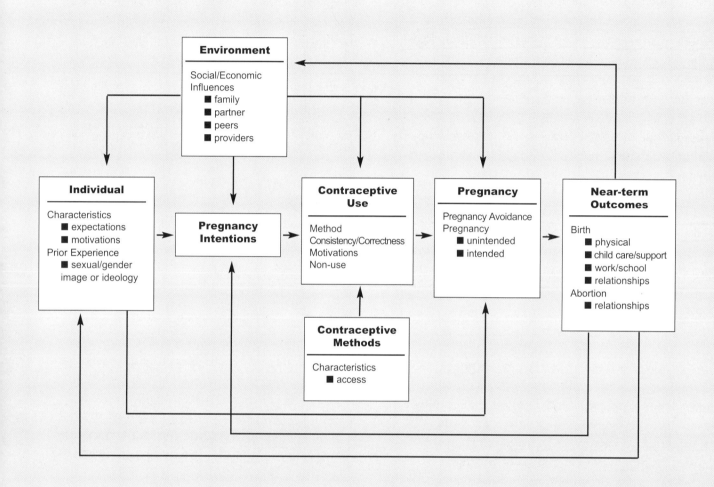

(Koo and Woodsong 1997)

emerged, the structure of the framework changed. For example, research questions related to pregnancy intentions suggested an open-ended, exploratory approach — how or by what process and under what circumstances do couples arrive at decisions to space pregnancies? But the researchers also recognized that questions concerning the parameters of method choice — source of supply, frequency and consistency of use or non-use — could be better answered in a survey design. From survey data, they then compiled personal profiles of a subsample of participants' experiences with contraceptive methods. The profiles helped them construct a qualitative instrument that they used to explore the decisions, relationships, and meanings of these choices in qualitative interviews with the subsample. In this way, qualitative and quantitative data were analyzed separately for some components of the framework, yet fully integrated in others.

Asking Qualitative Research Questions

As the previous example demonstrates, a thoughtfully constructed conceptual framework can be a valuable compass to help keep your work oriented to the central research problem while ensuring flexibility and credible results.

A carefully defined research problem is an invitation to examine the issue with more specific research questions. There are different kinds of qualitative questions, as outlined in Table 3.1 (see page 44). The research problem will determine whether your design should focus on people's experiences, actions, and behaviors; on their opinions and values; on their feelings or emotional responses; or on what they know or believe to be true in certain situations. Most qualitative studies combine two or more. Note that some of the questions in Table 3.1 could be asked from either a qualitative or a quantitative perspective.

A quantitative interviewer might suggest several topics and ask the respondent to rate their importance in a discussion with an adolescent son. However, qualitative questions give participants more freedom to structure their answers as they wish. For example, as a researcher in reproductive health, you might want to know what a family planning program can do to reduce rates of unwanted pregnancy in an adolescent population. Stated this broadly, you can do little except speculate on a possible solution.

First, you need to break the big question into specific, researchable questions:

- What are actual rates and trends in adolescent pregnancy?
- What services do local family planning clinics offer young people?
- At what age do adolescents become sexually active?
- What are contraceptive use rates among teenagers?

Much of this information can be obtained from records, surveys, and other quantitative sources. It is valuable information for describing the extent of the problem, constructing the context, and understanding the problem of unwanted pregnancy in this population.

As you continue to explore the problem, however, you probably will want to know where adolescents themselves stand on this question. An interpretivist perspective framework can guide you in articulating additional, specific questions:

Table 3.1

Types of Qualitative Research Questions

Type of Question	Purpose	Examples
Experience/behavior questions	Intended to elicit descriptions of experiences, behaviors, actions, activities; what a person has done, seen, heard, or thought.	If I were present when you talk to your adolescent son about AIDS, what would I hear? How did you introduce your partner to the idea of using a condom as well as the IUD?
Opinion/value questions	Aimed at how people interpret specific events or issues; answers reflect a <u>decision-making process</u> and may reveal goals, opinions, norms, intentions, desires, and values.	What do you think about a girl your age getting pregnant? In the reorganization of this health service, what programs do you think should have highest priority? In your opinion, who should have the final say in decisions about how many children to have?
Feeling questions	Probes emotional responses to experiences. Typically spontaneous, often not the result of a decision, often nonrational. May emerge in responses to other kinds of questions.	How did you feel when you learned you were HIV positive? How do women react to situations where they fear physical violence?
Knowledge questions	Intended to discover what people consider factual information — what people think is true. Interviewer records but does not correct misinformation, except at the end of the interview.	Tell me about some different kinds of family planning you know. If a man and woman have just had unprotected sex, is there anything they can do to avoid a pregnancy? What are some ways that a person can get the AIDS virus?

(Adapted from Timyan 1991)

- How have adolescents experienced reproductive health services?
- How have young people understood the information they have received about sex and sexual health?
- How do young couples negotiate sexual protection?
- What do early sexual relationships mean to adolescents in terms of costs and benefits?
- What has happened when adolescents have tried to reduce their risk of pregnancy or STIs?

Using a feminist perspective, on the other hand, you might decide to examine the meaning of negotiation in relation to the balance of power in the relationship and the ability of adolescents to participate in decisions affecting their health.

Questions like these call for a qualitative approach, because in different ways they ask *why* adolescent pregnancy in this community is so high. They expand and elaborate on the original research question — how to reduce adolescent pregnancy — by addressing some of the underlying dynamics of adolescent sexual experience. They also have the potential to elicit a range of information, including knowledge, experience, opinions, and feelings, as well as their social context — types of questions that are summarized in Table 3.1.

However specific such questions seem in the beginning, later data collection may uncover material that leads to new and more insightful questions, which in turn may suggest yet more ways to understand and articulate the nature of adolescent pregnancy. What do clinic personnel believe is their responsibility to young people who want contraceptive advice? To what extent do young women discuss pregnancy and disease prevention with their partners? Such is the iterative nature of qualitative research at the level of problem definition. Even after the data collection begins, you may find that you continue to refine and build on your research questions in the light of new insights.

A source of research questions not to be overlooked are stakeholders in the project, individuals and groups who understand the context of the problem and whose own goals will be served by the results of the research. In the example from Mali cited earlier (see page 37), the researchers had not been aware that service providers were worried that so many women were coming to the family planning clinic in secret. Asking practioners "What information would help you provide better service?" can generate new questions that will lead to more relevant and useful conclusions.

Leaders of women's advocacy groups can also be a valuable source of collaboration if your research problem is consistent with their agenda for women. In our experience, advocacy organizations often lack the resources to conduct research and are eager to share their own knowledge as insiders to develop mutually rewarding research questions.

When you take your research questions to the field, remember that in the iterative process of qualitative inquiry, your design work may not be finished. Qualitative research problems are often deeply stratified, composed of layers of meaning that have not been accessible to other methods in the past. Thus it may take several iterations before the experienced researcher is satisfied with a set of research questions that will tap the underlying dimensions of the problem. The natural evolution of a qualitative research question is a growth process in which a basic question (e.g., "Why are people not coming to this clinic?") can continue to generate new and more refined questions. On the other hand, the tendency of good research questions to grow and multiply must not imply design without form. Vigilance is needed to ensure that emerging research questions retain an internal consistency and clear relationship to the basic problem or purpose of the research.

Table 3.2 illustrates how an initial set of questions can emerge from a single broad research problem. Questions from the dual method study in this example suggest that participants will come from at least three groups: sexually active women, sexually active men, and reproductive health care providers. Discussion of these topics may lead to additional questions that would explore further the implications of participants' comments. Understanding the problem — how to introduce dual method use — might be further enriched by using quantitative techniques.

Selecting Data Collection Methods

Once your research problem has become a set of questions, you are ready to put them to work. Using your conceptual framework as a guide, the challenge now is to match the research questions with the methods and techniques that can yield the richest information. Table 3.3 (see page 64) compares the characteristics, strengths, and weaknesses of four types of data collection, from the least structured, qualitative format to a more structured, typically quantitative design. Researchers sometimes combine these types to address different dimensions of a research problem. However, in this field guide, we focus mainly on techniques for asking qualitative questions in an open-ended format.

Since the scope of this guide cannot adequately cover all qualitative techniques, we focus on three major methodological strategies: observation, including study of existing documents; in-depth interview; and focus group discussion. Each is discussed in more detail in Chapter 4. Observing, interviewing, and managing group discussion, aided by careful note-taking and transcription, are basic methods of qualitative science. Once you master the principles and skills of observation and interaction, and learn to use documentary materials to understand human behavior, you will have a valuable set of tools that can be adapted to numerous research problems and circumstances.

Be aware as you design your study that the methods you choose in the beginning may not be the only ones you will use. Even with the study underway, a qualitative researcher must have the flexibility to modify the design, to pursue new leads, to add new questions, or to turn to other subgroups in the population for different perspectives. For example, pilot data from a focus group may reveal that people are reluctant to disclose their views on certain topics in front of others, or they are not accustomed to expressing opinions on controversial issues. You then may decide that individual interviews or one of the projective techniques discussed in Chapter 4 will be a more comfortable and rewarding approach.

We urge readers to use the suggested readings and internet resources (see page 247) to explore the many possibilities for gathering qualitative data. We also encourage you to devise your own techniques, adapting the strategic frameworks presented in Chapter 2 to new research problems and contexts. Many of the innovative techniques reported in qualitative literature today have come from the creative improvisation of researchers seeking better ways to help participants express their perspectives on, and experiences with, sensitive topics. These field-driven techniques have included information-generating strategies such as asking young people to photograph significant moments in their lives and training HIV-positive women to interview each other. In both examples, analysis is enhanced by the interpretations of the study participants.

Individual interviews or focus groups?

Whether to interview participants individually or in groups is a common design question not always easily answered. *In-depth individual interviews establish a one-to-one relationship between interviewer and respondent, while participants in group interviews relate to each other as well as to the interviewer.* In an in-depth interview, information comes from the thoughtful reflection of one person aided by

Table 3.2

From Research Problem to Research Question:
A Qualitative Study of Dual Method Use

Research Problem

To assess the feasibility of introducing dual method use (DMU)* among couples at risk of pregnancy and STI/HIV.

Research Questions

◼ How and to what extent do women perceive themselves to be at risk of pregnancy and STI/HIV?

◼ How do women view DMU?

• What experiences have women had with the simultaneous use of condoms and another method?

• What do they know about DMU?

• How do they describe negative and positive aspects of DMU?

• How do they perceive others' experiences with DMU?

• To what extent will women accept DMU?

• Under what circumstances do women believe DMU is an appropriate choice?

• If a woman believes DMU is appropriate and effective, why might she not use it?

• Whose decision does she believe it is to use two methods?

◼ How do men view DMU?

• What do men believe is the purpose of using two methods?

• Under what circumstances do they believe couples should or should not rely on two methods?

• What do they see as the partner's role in promoting or discouraging DMU?

◼ What are providers' opinions of DMU?

• How do providers describe their current practice regarding recommendation of DMU to couples?

• Under what circumstances do providers believe DMU is indicated and not indicated?

• What obstacles do providers identify in promoting DMU?

• How do they think providers can circumvent these obstacles?

---

* Dual method use is defined as use of condoms with another contraceptive method.

exchange with the interviewer — one person's point of view. In focus groups, information comes from interaction among members of the group — several points of view.

Highly sensitive topics such as sexual behavior or domestic violence may argue for an individual interview format with maximum privacy and intimacy. However, if study participants are already accustomed to informal exchange on the topic among themselves — for example, discussion of disease prevention among commercial sex workers — then the investigator might choose a focus group. Ask the question: sensitive to whom? Questions that would cause embarrassment in a group of middle-class women might be handled easily by women whose livelihood depends on sexual services at enormous risk to their own health and well-being. In our study of family planning decision-making in Mali, many of the participants were covert users of contraception, often in defiance of the pronatalist wishes of husbands and elders. Individual interviews were the only option for encouraging these women to share their experiences while protecting their secret. Researchers encounter similar constraints in studies of women who have broken the law, for example by seeking abortion, and resolve the problem of disclosure by interviewing them individually in maximum privacy.

When the research problem focuses on cultural norms, attitudes, or reactions of a group to some aspect of their environment, the group discussion can be a rewarding technique. What attitudes toward family planning prevail in a traditional Islamic community? What factors are likely to encourage parents' support of a new program for adolescent sexual health, or discourage young people's participation? How do women negotiate protection for STIs and HIV/AIDS? Questions such as these focus on group norms, rather than individual behavior. In each example, a group of people committed to the issue will probably enjoy an opportunity to express their opinions, hear other people's

views, challenge one another, and participate in studying a topic of compelling interest. By stimulating interest in a common problem and listening to the views of others, participation can also motivate people to initiate change. As they wrestle with questions posed by the moderator (and sometimes by others in the group), participants' comments and debate among themselves will reveal the wider perspectives of their community, revealing clues to the context, or the social environment, in which individuals make decisions that affect their lives. Spontaneous exchange among participants will also reveal nuances in the language of ideas — what terms people use and the frameworks they commonly construct for understanding their worlds.

Mixing Methods

Since no single research method can tap all dimensions of a complex research problem, *it is often valuable to combine two or more methods, drawing conclusions from a synthesis of the results.* Multiple method use, also called triangulation, unquestionably results in a broader perspective on the problem and often more persuasive findings for policy-makers. Similar results from two or more methods could increase the credibility of the findings, whereas dissimilar results might raise questions about alternative interpretations.

FGDs can reveal something about social context / social environment

It is important to note that different results from one method do not necessarily invalidate the results of another. Given that reality is defined in many ways and in many contexts, different data collection tools may reveal a variety of perspectives, different ways that people conceptualize and evaluate the same situation. Like a photographer attempting to capture a perfect likeness, the careful researcher considers the research problem from different angles, using quantitative or qualitative methods or integrating both in various combinations.

In the past ten years, increasing numbers of researchers have discovered the benefits of studying a problem from more than one theoretical perspective (Tashakkori and Teddlie 1998; Knodel 1997; Obermeyer 1997). Their research reports demonstrate that combining qualitative and quantitative strategies in a single study can result in a more powerful design than either used alone. For example, a study of condom acceptability in a population at risk of STI/HIV transmission might include a structured survey of knowledge, attitudes, and practices regarding condom use (a quantitative component), in addition to in-depth interviews with a subset of the survey population (a qualitative component) and observation in pharmacies where condoms are sold (both quantitative and qualitative). Each technique would yield different but complementary results, and together they would give you a more complete picture than one approach alone.

In applied sexual and reproductive health research, there are few problems that do not have the potential for qualitative and quantitative inquiry. While investigating the incidence of maternal mortality in a population (a quantitative problem), the

Let us be done with the arguments of [qualitative versus quantitative methods] ... and get on with the business of attacking our problems with the widest array of conceptual and methodological tools that we possess and they demand.

(Trow 1957, 35)

researcher might also ask why women are not seeking prenatal care or how they conceptualize pregnancy in relation to health and disease. Similarly, in a study of popular beliefs concerning maternal morbidity (an appropriate topic for a qualitative study), it would be useful also to know the extent to which self-diagnosis is related to help-seeking behavior, a relationship that could be measured with multivariate quantitative techniques.

In a study of the lactational amenorrhea method (LAM) of contraception, a statistically representative survey enabled researchers to generalize information about LAM beliefs and practices to a larger population of childbearing women in Bolivia (Bender et al. 1990). In the same study, an equally rigorous qualitative component led to important insight on women's understanding of the link between breastfeeding and LAM.

In a different application of mixed methods, a team of investigators sought to develop a valid and reliable instrument that could help monitor the prevalence and nature of domestic violence against women (Smith, Earp, and DeVellis 1995; Smith, Tessaro, and Earp 1995). Their first concern was to reconceptualize violence by exploring the meanings that battered women attach to the particular physical and psychological violence that they experienced. Data came from transcripts of focus groups in which women were encouraged to talk to each other about what battering meant to them. From these meanings, the researchers developed a conceptual framework that replaced the traditional concept of violent acts as discrete events (number, frequency, and behavioral characteristics) with a continuous concept that captured battered women's sense of perpetual vulnerability. From the qualitative transcripts, the researchers then identified

Combining Methods to Understand Women's Positions in Their Households

Sri Moertiningsih Adioetomo
Demographic Institute, Faculty of Economics
University of Indonesia, Jakarta

The research literature indicates that lowering fertility increases women's labor force participation. Women who use contraception generally spend fewer years pregnant or rearing children and therefore have more time to work for income. Since the literature also suggests that working for income is associated with greater household autonomy, we decided to examine the assumption that working women actually have greater bargaining power in household decisions than women who are not formally employed.

To test this relationship, we conducted a secondary analysis* of the 1993 Indonesia Family Life Survey (IFLS), a survey of 7,000 households in 13 provinces of Indonesia. Using logistic regressions, we found that family planning only partially explains women's work status. Completing high school, husband's low income, and urban residence were stronger predictors. And the link between work status and household autonomy was even less clear.

Although the IFLS is a rich data set for many purposes, it does not contain information about women's autonomy — that is, the extent to which a woman's daily household activities and economic decisions are free from her husband's control. Even if the survey questionnaire had included questions about household decision-making, we could see that a structured questionnaire would not elicit the sensitive information we needed to understand women's domestic situations. To overcome this limitation, we decided to conduct in-depth interviews with women and separate interviews with their husbands, choosing a small sample of couples from the area where the IFLS was conducted. We selected eight couples from West Java and eight from North Sumatra for a total of thirty-two in-depth interviews. Purposive sampling took into account socioeconomic variations, culture and religion, and urban and rural residence. We were rewarded with a richer understanding of the relationship between family planning, labor force participation and women's household autonomy in Indonesia.

---

* Our study was a collaboration between the staff of the Demographic Institute at the Faculty of Economics, University of Indonesia, and the Women's Studies Project of Family Health International and took place from 1997 to 1998 (Adioetomo and Eggleston 1998).

As a quantitative methodologist, I found it unnatural at first to combine two such different methodologies in one study. Instead of specifying the variables and their relationships in advance of data collection, our understanding of key influences on autonomy emerged as we reviewed data from the interviews. However, our quantitative framework helped us to focus the problem for the interviews and to develop our semi-structured interview guides. In the interviews, we listened to women and men describing what family planning meant to them. Then we asked them to tell us in their own words how women and men make decisions in their households.

Women told us that family planning had indeed benefited their lives because with fewer children, they had more time to themselves. However, they did not make the connection between lower fertility and the opportunity to work for income — regardless of whether they used family planning, they felt free to work outside the home if they wished. Nor did they think that family planning determined their influence in household decisions and their use of family income for basic expenses. Couples felt that family planning had freed women's time for activities other than child care. Having smaller families also helped them stretch their limited resources to ensure that their children will have the food, health care, and education they need. The qualitative research enabled us to conclude that family planning and women's employment are both elements of a common household survival strategy, which includes women's and men's joint participation in household decisions. Hearing couples talk about their lives enabled me to understand in a new way the association between family planning, working for pay, and household autonomy.

Box 3.1
Common Ways to Mix Methodologies

If you understand the basic principles and techniques of qualitative and quantitative strategies, you will discover useful ways to combine them:

■ A qualitative phase (e.g., focus group discussions) that precedes a quantitative phase (e.g., household survey) can provide information for generating hypotheses and designing the instrument, as well as to identify language meaningful to the study population.

■ Quantitative data can provide useful background information for designing a qualitative study.

■ Quantitative data on study participants (e.g., socio-demographic data and sexual and reproductive histories) can help to interpret qualitative results or highlight important subgroup differences.

■ A qualitative phase can occur at the end of quantitative data collection and help to interpret quantitative findings.

■ Qualitative and quantitative techniques can be used independently to examine a problem from different perspectives.

■ Qualitative (open-ended) questions can be included in a quantitative instrument to collect limited data on issues that cannot be answered in the structured format.

■ Qualitative exit interviews can be conducted with a sample of quantitative survey participants to check the external validity or comprehensiveness of the measures.

potential scale items that seemed to highlight women's continuous perception of susceptibility to danger, loss of power, and loss of control in relationships with male partners. These items became the basis for construction of the Women's Experiences with Battering (WEB) Scale, a valid and concise measure for studying relations between battering and health or health behavior, estimates of prevalence, and evaluation of the impact of interventions on battered women's situations.

In either qualitative or quantitative study design, written material such as clinic reports, letters, newspapers, and advertising also can be combined with other sources of data. Documentary evidence offers valuable insight into the context of relationships, decisions, and actions, sometimes helping to explain or expand on data gathered with other methods. Chapter 4 will discuss documentary methods in greater detail.

A practical strategy for mixed-method design

Much has been written in support of mixed methodology, but the reader is often left to manage the technical task of combining very different techniques in a coherent design. Once you have established the strategic relevance of two or more methods to the research questions, you will need to decide how to coordinate them. For this purpose, we advocate the Priority-Sequence Model (see Figure 3.2, page 54), an approach that integrates the "complementary strengths of different methods through a division of labor ... within the same overall project" (Morgan 1998, 366). The division of labor requires two basic decisions, one that assigns *priority* and one that determines *sequence*.

The four-cell model represents four basic designs in which "(a) the *principal method* is either qualitative or quantitative (priority) and (b) the *complementary* method occurs as a preliminary or a follow-up stage to the primary method (sequence)" (Morgan

1998, 367). In each cell of the model, the primary method is abbreviated in capital letters and the complementary method in lowercase letters; arrows indicate their sequence in the design. Thus the model shows four types of design:

1. A principally quantitative study that begins with a smaller qualitative study. The qualitative component might be participant observation or focus group discussions to develop the content of a survey questionnaire. A Demographic and Health Survey (DHS), for example, might use the results of exploratory work to ensure that the survey instrument covers important topics in language familiar to the respondents. In clinical trials, a preliminary qualitative phase could provide valuable information on the trial population and the likely acceptability of the contraceptive method to be tested.

2. A principally qualitative study that begins with a complementary quantitative study. A preliminary survey, for example, might guide selection of study sites and help to define the sample. Qualitative research frequently begins with a review of secondary data from the national DHS, census, and other population surveys in order to relate the research problem to a larger demographic context. Quantitative findings may highlight important issues that raise questions to explore with qualitative methods.

3. A principally quantitative study with a complementary qualitative study as a follow-up. An important purpose of the qualitative phase in this design is to help interpret the results of the quantitative study. The qualitative component may or may not be part of the initial study design. For example, a national survey of AIDS knowledge, attitudes, and practices turned up the finding that the majority of respondents understood the basics of prevention but chose not to protect themselves. The researchers then decided to explore this finding by inviting survey respondents to participate in focus groups to discuss what AIDS transmission and protection meant to them and to others in their community. Similarly, quantitative researchers sometimes build into their designs a plan for analysis that includes a small qualitative study at the end in which individuals from the study population discuss and help interpret selected findings.

4. A principally qualitative study with a complementary quantitative study as a follow-up. In this design, the quantitative phase may be a valuable way to test the extent to which qualitative findings are generalizable in a larger population. Or one might want to look at qualitative data on attitudes toward STIs from a different perspective by using standardized rating scales in a subsample of the study population. For example, a qualitative study of STI risk among adolescents identified fear of infection, embarrassment, and age as important constructs in attitudes regarding protection. In a follow-up study, the researcher constructed scale items from comments of the adolescent participants; then, having validated the scales and confirmed their reliability, they applied scale analysis techniques to study quantitatively the dimensions, fear, and embarrassment in relation to age. Construction of the WEB Scale, cited previously, is another example of this type of integration.

In some mixed-method studies, qualitative and quantitative components may be equally important. Different methods of data collection may occur simultaneously, guided by complementary objectives. In analysis, the researcher might draw on both at the same time to address the central problem. Or analysis of data from one method might serve to illuminate data from the other.

Mixing different qualitative techniques is also useful but only if the data collection and methods of analysis are carefully matched to the research questions. For example, a study of adolescent sexuality in Malawi combined in-depth interviews, participant observation, and focus group discussions. The

Figure 3.2
Priority-Sequence Model: Decisions for Integrating Methods

Quantitative	Qualitative
1. Qualitative Preliminary qual → **QUANT** Smaller qualitative study helps guide the data collection in a principally quantitative study. ■ Can generate hypotheses, develop content for questionnaires and interventions, etc. *Example:* Focus groups shape culturally sensitive versions of a new health promotion campaign.	**2. Quantitative Preliminary** quant → **QUAL** Smaller quantitative study helps guide the data collection in a principally qualitative study. ■ Can guide purposive sampling, establish preliminary results to pursue in depth, etc. *Example:* A survey of different units in a hospital locates sites for more extensive ethnographic data collection.
3. Qualitative Follow-up **QUANT** → qual Smaller qualitative study helps evaluate and interpret results from a principally quantitative study. ■ Can provide interpretations for poorly understood results, help explain outliers, etc. *Example:* In-depth interviews explain why one clinic generates higher levels of patient satisfaction.	**4. Quantitative Follow-up** **QUAL** → quant Smaller quantitative study helps evaluate and interpret results from a principally qualitative study. ■ Can generalize results to different samples, test elements of emergent theories, etc. *Example:* A statewide survey of a school-based health program pursues earlier results from a case study.

(Morgan 1998, 368)

purpose was to examine the social and information networks of adolescent girls: how they learn about sexuality, how they perceive the risk of HIV infection, their experience with sex, and the skills they learn to avoid infection. The authors reported that "focus group discussion elicited more socially correct answers and produced good data on social norms but not very good data on deviations from those norms. By contrast, in-depth, one-on-one interviews were necessary to elicit good data on actual knowledge and experience. ..." Using more than one qualitative research method "not only broadens the quality of information that can be obtained about sexuality and reproductive health issues in a community, it also opens the way to finding culturally acceptable ways of disseminating information inside your community with the support of and benefit to all its members" (Helitzer-Allen et al. 1994, 81).

Integrating Qualitative and Quantitative Methods for Problem-Solving in Research

Deborah Bender, Ph.D.
School of Public Health, University of North Carolina at Chapel Hill

In Bolivia, where breastfeeding initiation is almost universal and duration continues for as long as two years, we conducted a study to understand women's knowledge and preferences related to breastfeeding as a means of child-spacing. Our ultimate purpose was to garner information that could assist in developing guidelines for the promotion of the lactational amenorrhea method (LAM) of contraception at the community level (Bender et al. 1990). In this study, we wanted to examine the statistical inter-relationships among infant feeding practices, contraceptive use, and lactational amenorrhea in a representative sample of childbearing women. But at the same time, we wanted to know more about how women understand the link between breastfeeding and LAM.

A total of 416 women having a child under 18 months of age, living in a peri-urban community of Santa Cruz, responded to our survey. From survey data, we learned that 60 percent had heard of LAM, although only 40 percent were aware that this protection lasts for only part of an extended breastfeeding period. Bivariate analysis also revealed that formal education was directly related to correct knowledge of the duration of LAM protection. Even among women who had completed primary education or more, only 45 percent correctly reported the duration of LAM's protection from pregnancy.

These findings raised questions concerning the rationale that led so many women to believe that breastfeeding could offer indefinite protection from pregnancy. Therefore, we invited 63 women who were outside the survey sample but lived in the same communities to participate in focus groups. The purpose of the focus group discussions was to explore in greater depth women's knowledge of breastfeeding as a method of contraception.

Although focus group participants were somewhat older than survey respondents, educational levels were similar, with approximately 60 percent of women finishing eighth grade or less. On the question of LAM protection, we found even less consensus among focus group participants than in the survey. Women in six out of eight focus groups said they had heard that breastfeeding can prevent pregnancy and believed it to be true. However, most participants believed breastfeeding protected only some women and that lactational infertility was dependent on an individual's physical constitution. This belief, that a woman's fertility is related to her individual physiology, had not surfaced in the survey but is frequently reported anecdotally in Bolivia. According to traditional beliefs, a woman's constitution is an indicator of her health and marks her as either strong or weak. Many people believe that a strong woman has more blood than a weak woman and, therefore, can easily have many children without harming her own health.

Other focus group participants mentioned that they had heard breast-feeding could help prevent pregnancy but did not believe it. Note the lack of consensus in the women's responses:

> *Well, if you are nursing and your period doesn't return and you nursed your child for a year or two you are protected during that time.*

> *Yes, I have heard this, but I have also seen friends who are nursing become pregnant.*

> *It's a lie, because I became pregnant while nursing.*

> *Not all women have the same make-up or ovulation [sic]. Some people ovulate before menstruation, and there are others who ovulate after menstruation returns. In my case, I ovulate before. The women who ovulate before and are breastfeeding become pregnant.*

> *I have heard that it protects you for only 6 months.*

To elicit more detail on the meaning to participants of postpartum anovulation, we used a simple probe: "Why, what is happening?" Some women had no response, while others made various guesses.

As the focus group facilitator probed beyond the more superficial survey responses, it became apparent that women were making contraceptive decisions with little substantive knowledge of how breastfeeding relates to pregnancy.

Posing similar questions in two formats — the survey and the focus group discussions — allowed us to probe for depth of meaning in narrative responses as well as to understand the distribution of beliefs and practices by women's educational levels. It enabled us to hear some of the deeply held convictions that influence women's contraceptive decisions. Using both forced choice and open-ended methods for similar questions also gave us a set of checks on data reliability and validity.

Selecting a Sampling Strategy

In decisions about whom to interview, researchers are typically guided by the paradigm, or theoretical framework, they have chosen for a study. The interpretive perspective views ordinary people as experts by virtue of the experiences and ideas they can share and their willingness to help you explore the research problem. As always in the iterative process of qualitative research, selection criteria may change as the study progresses, allowing the researcher to follow new leads with information from new sources (Rubin and Rubin 1995).

Generalization versus insight

A typical goal of quantitative research is to generalize findings to larger populations, achieving a high degree of reliability. To minimize sampling error, every case in a sampling frame must have an equal probability of selection. The purpose of most qualitative studies, on the other hand, is to produce information-rich data from a sample chosen for its ability to speak to the research issue (Patton 1990, 169). Qualitative research emphasizes depth more than breadth, insight rather than generalization, illuminating the meaning of human behavior. Although qualitative researchers commonly use numbers and frequencies to record observations, conceptual rather than numerical considerations determine sample selection. The challenge for the qualitative researcher is, therefore, to select participants who will be able to provide the most meaningful information on the topic. The extent to which results may be relevant to other populations will be enhanced by careful documentation of the conceptual links between research problem, sample selection process, and emerging data.

Selection: theoretical or a priori?

In qualitative design, there are two basic approaches to selecting participants; each places more emphasis on the level of experience or insight of potential respondents than on their random selection. One of these approaches, called *theoretical sampling*, is particularly appropriate when the main purpose of data collection is to generate substantive theory (Strauss and Corbin 1990). Beginning with a small number of individuals or groups, the researcher asks, "Given what I am learning, what information do I need next and where — or in what groups — will I find it?" (Flick 1998, 65). In other words, theoretical sampling is continuous and gradual, guided by data collection, analysis, and interpretation as theory builds. (See discussion of grounded theory on page 19.)

A priori sampling is the approach more familiar to applied researchers in sexual and reproductive health. Based on your research problem and purpose, you define in advance of data collection the characteristics and structure of the sample. If your purpose is to understand the sexual attitudes and behaviors of adolescents in a community, you will select participants from this group as well as other individuals whose opinions on adolescent sexuality or whose actual experiences with young people give them special insight into your area of inquiry. If different perspectives and behaviors are known to prevail in the population, then you would choose participants who differ in these respects. At this point you will also decide the numbers of participants in each category and the background characteristics that will help you interpret their responses.

Note that *a priori* selection does not preclude sampling additions and changes as the study progresses. The most important consideration in qualitative sampling is the richness, or the explanatory value, of the data. In the above example, you might discover that young people with conservative religious views perceive sexual norms differently from their peers with a different religious orientation. The next step could be to invite a sample of religious leaders in the community to help you explore religious influences in adolescent sexual decision-making.

Study Design

Sample size

When a goal of the study is to generalize findings from a sample to a larger population, as in many quantitative designs, a representative sample size can be calculated from a formula. In qualitative studies, optimum size is less clear. The investigator is guided by the degree to which incoming data adequately answer the research questions — an ambiguous rule at best. But if sample size depends on completeness of the data (Rubin and Rubin 1995, 73), how do you know when data are complete? If the research problem is a simple one, it is possible that one individual could provide the whole answer.* In practice, however, most research design is not that simple. Generally, you collect data from as many groups or individuals as necessary to answer the research questions. When little new information is coming from your observations, interviews, or focus group discussions, you can be reasonably confident that you have saturated that source of information to the point of redundancy (Glaser and Strauss 1967).

In most funded research, such indeterminate measures as saturation and redundancy are likely to be impractical for budgeting, and the length of time it might take to reach that point unacceptable to donors. Qualitative researchers might begin with "minimum samples based on expected reasonable

> *The validity, meaningfulness, and insights generated from qualitative inquiry have more to do with the information-richness of the cases selected and the observational/analytical capabilities of the researcher than with sample size.*
>
> (Patton 1990, 185)

coverage … given the purpose of the study and stakeholder interests" (Patton 1990, 186). Once in the field, you will make a decision as to whether you need to expand your sample. Altering the subgroup composition in your design is justified in qualitative research if doing so will enrich your findings.

The qualitative researcher tries to collect information representative of the *range* of experiences, perspectives, and behaviors relevant to the research question. In contrast, quantitative approaches are more likely to result in samples that represent the *distribution* of these variables. The important thing to remember is that *"the logic of purposeful sampling is different from the logic of probability sampling"* (Patton 1990, 185). Small, purposive samples are ideally suited to qualitative inquiry. A large, random sample could not accomplish the objectives of an in-depth study, any more than a small, nonrandom sample could accurately represent a large population. For the qualitative researcher, it is crucial to describe, justify, and explain small sample selection so that others can judge its strengths and weaknesses. "Exercising care not to overgeneralize from purposeful samples, while maximizing to the full the advantages of in-depth, purposeful sampling, will do much to alleviate concerns about small sample size" (Patton 1990, 186).

---

* In case-study design, the sample may be a single case or multiple cases, where the case represents a unique event or an example of a complex phenomenon for in-depth study (Yin 1994). Case study is not included in this field guide.

Recruiting participants

Study participants are drawn from a community, any of its institutions (clinics, schools, workplaces, bars, brothels), or wherever there are people willing to share knowledge and experience related to the research topics. In some studies, researchers visit sites where potential participants gather, chat informally with people, and select an initial sample based on the apparent readiness of individuals to address the research issues. In other studies, clinic records or membership lists serve as a sampling frame, particularly when individuals in the frame share a common characteristic of interest to the research. As in all sampling strategies, decisions must also be made regarding other selection criteria, such as age or marital status. In our study of new contraceptive users in Mali, researchers worked with clinic personnel to identify every married woman who had come to the clinic to begin family planning for the first time. But since this study used a longitudinal design, the invitation to participate was extended only to women who were geographically accessible for follow-up interviews.

In community-based studies you may want to enlist the help of residents to identify and invite eligible individuals to participate. If so, select such recruiters carefully to avoid possible coercion or alienation of important subgroups. Incorporating local people into the field team at this point is especially useful in unfamiliar cultures or where there are language barriers. It is important to orient helpers to the purpose of the study, rehearsing with them how to introduce it, how to invite participation, and how to assure potential participants of confidentiality and freedom to decline.

Sample selection techniques

Selecting a sample for a qualitative study is not haphazard, but neither is it bound by rigid rules of reproducibility. It should be systematic but flexible, guided by clear research questions as articulated in your theoretical framework. Since the purpose of qualitative design is to explore in depth, the investigator carefully selects cases that can typify or shed light on the object of study. Therefore, to identify and gain access to those who can teach you the most about your topic, it follows that sampling methods will generally be based on purpose rather than on statistical probability of selection. In qualitative sampling, *purposiveness* is a strategic approach, not a single technique. It means selecting participants for their ability to provide rich information. *Purposive sampling should never be confused with sampling for convenience.* The latter, motivated primarily by ease of access to respondents, may be economical, but it does not necessarily reflect the purpose of the study, and it may weaken significantly the quality of the data.

There are many purposive strategies, each linked to the purpose of the study as expressed in the initial research question. Following one such typology (Patton 1990), we describe several strategies that in our experience have been useful tools for qualitative sampling decisions. Although we present these techniques separately, readers should be aware that many studies combine more than one.

purposive sampling ≠ convenience sampling

Extreme sampling. Extreme, or deviant, sampling selects extreme cases in order to highlight and understand conditions or characteristics of more typical situations. For example, a study of reproductive health provider effectiveness selected two clinics known for high levels of client satisfaction and two with a poor reputation in the local community. By observing services and interviewing clients with experience in each setting, the investigators were able to identify and prioritize qualities that favored optimum utilization and those that discouraged it. In using extreme cases, the investigator must take care not to distort reality by making the unusual seem to be the norm. The purpose is not to generalize to all clinics but to magnify certain characteristics.

Intensity sampling. Intensity sampling focuses on excellent, but not necessarily extreme, examples of the phenomenon. Samples are small and rich in information but not unusual, such as in the case of people with particular experience in the topic or clinics that provide services relevant to the research problem. In a case-study design, the sample may be a single case or multiple cases, or a unique or exemplary case for in-depth study (Yin 1994). In Bolivia (Paulson 1996) and Jamaica (Barnett et al. 1996), researchers selected women-centered reproductive health services in order to demonstrate how health delivery can be sensitive to the particular needs of women. In any small exploratory sample, intensive exploration of selected issues with a few well-informed people or groups can add interesting, insightful and reality-based perspectives and information.

Homogeneous samples. Whether to emphasize similarities or differences in selecting a sample again depends on the purpose of the study. People in homogeneous samples have basically similar characteristics. This type of sample is appropriate if you are studying one or more groups in depth; for example, exploring the impact of an AIDS prevention program on male truckers at risk of HIV. Preliminary study may be necessary to establish the criteria that determine risk. By limiting sample selection to individuals who meet these criteria, you are better able to focus on a central issue that is relevant to all of them. Focus groups typically use this approach, stimulating people with a common identity to discuss their shared experiences.

Heterogeneous samples. Heterogeneous samples, on the other hand, may be useful for studying issues that cut across individual or program variation. Qualitative investigators sampling from a diverse population may want to highlight variation in some complex phenomenon; for example, different perspectives on whether and how to intervene in the practice of female genital cutting. Or they may be looking for common themes that emerge even in the presence of other differences. A study of rural, urban, and suburban family planning clinics serving different socioeconomic groups revealed the common perception that providers were unwilling to discuss emergency contraception. The discovery of similar experiences, behaviors, or perceptions in an otherwise heterogeneous group may warrant further in-depth study in separate homogeneous samples.

Typical cases. Often in operations research or evaluation it is useful to describe a typical case, program, or participant that serves as a profile for understanding the principal features of a group of programs or a class of individuals. The researcher may sample a typical case as illustrative or as a unit of analysis. Program planners and policy-makers may be more interested in data on typical facilities, not services that are extremely good or extremely poor. What constitutes typical is a subjective judgment, but key informants who are especially familiar with the general category can likely identify examples that are average — not extreme in any sense related to the study.

Snowball sampling. Snowball sampling is a technique for locating informants by asking others to identify individuals or groups with special understanding of a phenomenon. The investigator asks each participant to suggest others with similar ability to address the issues, asking "Who knows a lot about … ?" "Where can I find good examples of what you're talking about?" Thus the "snowball" grows as it rolls, collecting an information-rich pool of resources for exploring the research question. Since informants with special expertise can likely identify other knowledgeable people, this technique can be a valuable one when the researcher does not know the field. It is also useful when individuals with the knowledge or experience to provide rich data are difficult to reach, such as secluded women, people whose behavior or lifestyle deviates from social norms, or anyone fearful of public exposure. When such individuals are willing to trust the researcher, it is especially critical to protect their privacy and confidentiality.

Opportunistic sampling. Since qualitative strategies can change in response to findings as they emerge in the field, you may need to select additional study participants — making an "on-the-spot decision to take advantage of unforeseen opportunities after fieldwork has begun" (Patton 1990, 179). In our study of new users of contraception in Mali, we discovered that a small group of women had been using family planning for several years. We took advantage of this opportunity to look at contraceptive norms of experienced users, women who had successfully negotiated their way around cultural barriers in order to space or limit their pregnancies. This modification meant drawing a purposive sample of women who were coming to the clinic to renew their family planning methods.

"When you encourage people to talk to you openly, you incur serious ethical obligations to them."

(Rubin and Rubin 1995, 93)

Ethical Decisions for the Protection of Study Participants

Your ability to conduct a study while respecting research ethics will be linked closely to your research design. All human research should begin with the informed consent of participants, but how it is implemented depends on the nature of the research and the type and degree of risk that participation entails. At its most basic, informed consent means that study participants understand:

- possible risks and benefits
- voluntary participation
- assurances of confidentiality
- the purpose of the research
- how they were chosen to participate
- data collection procedures
- whom to contact with questions and concerns

It is important to remember that *potential harm to study participants is not just physical but can be psychological, social, economic, or professional.* In fact, physical wounds may heal more quickly than wounds to a person's reputation or sense of security (Williamson 1995). In culturally sensitive studies of sexual and reproductive health, your ethical responsibility goes beyond the simple statement of informed consent. Moreover, many of the topics that commonly arise in reproductive health research are likely to elicit delicate material — secret experiences, wishes, fears, even confessions — that the participant wants only the interviewer to hear. Avoiding deception, asking permission to record what they say, being willing to turn off the tape recorder, and being honest about the intended use of the research are all part of your responsibility to your participants, along with ensuring that they come to no emotional, physical, professional, or financial harm because they agreed to speak with you (Rubin and Rubin 1995). The common practice of coding participants to protect personal identity can be explained as further assurance of confidentiality. Researchers should also make sure they are not under any legal constraints; for example, requirements to report certain kinds of illegal behavior. If they are, they must inform participants of these legal obligations.

Risk to participants

What kind of harm might come to a participant in a reproductive health study? In strongly patriarchal societies, subordinate women may be especially at risk in studies of contraception, abortion, female genital cutting, domestic violence, or any reproductive decision that might conflict with norms of behavior. Clandestine contraceptive users in Mali feared rejection or divorce if their husbands discovered their pills. Women in Haiti feared physical abuse if they demanded that HIV-infected partners use condoms. Brazilian adolescents suffering the consequences of unsafe abortion might have been arrested if discovered. Providers who reveal actions by their superiors that compromise service quality may endanger their jobs. Your first responsibility to your study participant is to assess the possibility that simply talking with you may pose a risk and to protect her from harm, even if it means changing the interview site or omitting material that might jeopardize the participant's safety. Ethical considerations related to specific methods are discussed in Chapter 4.

The signed consent form — do you need it?

How will participants indicate their consent? Most written study designs are expected to answer this question in detail. The signed consent form is a hallowed tradition of institutional review boards (IRBs)[†] everywhere, but in some cases oral informed consent may be a more appropriate format. Examples are studies in which a breach in confidentiality could have profound repercussions for the participant, such as clandestine users of contraception, men who have sex with men, women who have undergone unsafe abortion, or unmarried adolescent clients of a family planning clinic. For a study of adolescent women admitted to a hospital with complications of abortion, an IRB ruled that the parental consent requirement for participation in the study was inappropriate, since it could put the participant at greater risk than the study itself.

U.S. federal regulations (45 *CFR* 46) include several different sets of potential waivers:

- waiver of documentation of informed consent (i.e., no signature needed)
- waiver of particular items from the list of required elements for informed consent
- waiver of informed consent (usually only used for things like chart review studies or lab studies using stored specimens)
- waiver of parental consent for minors

U.S. IRBs are constrained in the extent to which they can grant each of these types of waivers.

[†] Institutional Review Boards (IRBs), or Protection of Human Subjects Committees, are mandated by governments and research institutions to protect participants in research by reviewing proposals for compliance with internationally recognized guidelines.

Most IRBs can be expected to waive the signature requirement if:

(1) the only record linking the subject and the research is the consent document;

(2) the principal risk would be potential harm resulting from breach of confidentiality; and

(3) the research presents no more than minimal risk of harm to subjects and involves no procedures for which written consent is normally required (Williamson 1995).

As a substitute for signed consent, the interviewer may be asked to sign a statement for each participant confirming that the participant has read (or heard) and understood the statement and has given oral consent. However, regardless of the mechanism for obtaining consent, the study design should include a description of possible risk that could result from participation in the study, as well as the statement of informed consent as it will be presented to the participant. Protecting human subjects should also include a referral plan or other response to possible harm should it actually occur in the course of the study. (See Appendix 2, page 210 for examples of consent forms used in qualitative studies of reproductive health.)

Collecting Data

Designing the data collection process means making basic decisions about how you will build trust in the community, understand the cultural context, and create relationships with participants. Your design should include a plan for introducing the study to the community or site, enlisting local field assistance, creating a comfortable and secure environment for interviews or focus groups, and managing the data. How you will train and monitor field staff are also part of the design. These are discussed in Chapter 5.

Designing the study also raises critical decisions about the kinds of data you will collect and how to do it in a way that best matches the purpose and flow of the research. Whether your data will come principally from observation or from interviewing or group discussion (see Chapter 4), plan the study in such a way that you will be able to alter or modify the process as new information and questions emerge.

An important decision at this point concerns the degree of structure in the questions you will ask participants. Although open-ended questioning is a basic tool in qualitative research, questions can be asked in many different ways. You will need to decide at the design stage how much structure is appropriate for your purpose (Patton 1990). Alternative structures are shown in Table 3.3 (see page 64).

Table 3.3

Structural Differences in Qualitative Data Collection

Type of Interview	Characteristics	Strengths	Weaknesses
Informal conversational interview	Questions emerge from the immediate context and are asked in the natural course of things; there is no predetermination of question topics or wording.	Increases the salience and relevance of questions; interviews are built on and emerge from observations; interview can be matched to individuals and circumstances.	Different information collected from different people with different questions; less systematic and comprehensive if certain questions do not arise naturally; data organization and analysis can be quite difficult.
Interview guide approach	Topics and issues to be covered are specified in advance in outline form; interviewer decides sequence and wording of questions in the course of the interview.	The outline increases the comprehensiveness of the data and makes data collection somewhat systematic for each respondent; logical gaps in data can be anticipated and closed; interviews remain fairly conversational and situational.	Important and salient topics may be inadvertently omitted; interviewer flexibility in sequencing and wording questions can result in substantially different responses from different perspectives, thus reducing the comparability of responses.
Standardized open-ended interview	The exact wording and sequence of questions are determined in advance; respondents are asked the same basic questions in the same order; questions are worded in a completely open-ended format.	Respondents answer the same questions, thus increasing comparability of responses; data are complete for each person on the topics addressed in the interview; reduces interviewer effects and bias when several interviewers are used; permits evaluation users to see and review the instrumentation used in the evaluation; facilitates organization and analysis of the data.	Little flexibility in relating the interview to particular individuals and circumstances; standardized wording of questions may constrain and limit naturalness and relevance of questions and answers.
Closed, fixed response interview	Questions and response categories are determined in advance; responses are fixed; respondent chooses from among these fixed responses.	Data analysis is simple; responses can be directly compared and easily aggregated; many questions can be asked in a short time.	Respondents must fit their experiences and feelings into the researcher's categories; may be perceived as impersonal, irrelevant, and mechanistic; can distort what respondents really mean or experience by so completely limiting their response choices.

(Adapted from Patton 1990, 288-289)

The first alternative, an informal conversation with little or no preparation and sequencing of questions, is appropriate if your purpose is to explore a topic on which you have very little information. You do not know exactly what questions you will ask until prompted by clues from the participants and the study environment. It is well suited to some participant observation studies because questions emerge naturally from what you are seeing and hearing (Patton 1990). Thus one question or observation leads to another as you build your understanding of the situation. However, the flexibility of this kind of questioning also tends to make it time-consuming. Moreover, it assumes a great deal of experience on the part of the interviewer and may increase the difficulty of the analysis. For less-experienced observers and for most in-depth interviews and focus group discussions, we recommend the more structured, but still open-ended, format of the interview guide approach or the standardized interview.

The second option, a topic guide or outline, helps you to focus the interview or group discussion without prestructuring the questions. You decide in advance the areas you want to explore but not the wording or the sequence of the questions. The chief advantage of this technique is that data collection is systematic but gives you the flexibility to adapt questions to participants and circumstances. It is a commonly used tool for gathering comprehensive information on specific research questions in a relaxed, conversational style. The resulting data are less comparable than in a standardized open-ended interview, but they may be more responsive to the way that participants naturally construct a situation. (Construction of topic guides is discussed in Chapter 4.)

A third strategy, asking a predetermined set of open-ended questions, is the most standardized approach to qualitative data collection. If you choose this type of questioning, you lose flexibility but gain comparability and more straightforward analysis. It is especially useful for comparative studies when it is important to maximize common features while remaining sensitive to cross-cultural differences among the study groups (Knodel 1994). This format also lends itself to studies that are highly focused; for example, a program evaluation in which you want to interview a number of different service providers who have little time to spend on the interview (Patton 1990). Structured questions may be a good strategy if you have several different interviewers or focus group moderators with varying experience and different interviewing styles.

Analyzing the Data

Chapter 6 presents in detail the steps in analyzing qualitative data. However, there are certain aspects of data analysis that will need careful consideration as you design your study. Specifically, you should determine in the design phase:

- who will conduct the analysis
- what level of detail will be needed to respond to your research questions
- whether analysis will be computer-assisted or manual

If a computer will be used, decide in advance on a qualitative package for text analysis. If using mixed qualitative and quantitative methods, you will want to have a clear plan of analysis for each and a strategy for interpreting the results in an integrated discussion.

Qualitative analysis can be a deeply personal and subjective exercise. For this reason, some qualitative researchers decide from the outset of a study to use a team approach to analysis, involving data collectors as well as researchers more removed from daily field activities. The process of examining, negotiating, and incorporating multiple perspectives on data can strengthen their final interpretation. If using a team approach, it is especially useful to anticipate the analysis process at the beginning:

• Will all team members read and work on all the data, or will specific team members be responsible for different aspects of the investigation?

• Will team members work separately and then meet to share and reconcile their findings, or will analysis be conducted in group meetings?

• How will differences of opinion be resolved?

For more information, see the Field Perspective, "Training Field Staff in Data Analysis," page 124.)

 If only one person will conduct analysis, it is important to review the data as they are collected. If not actually collecting data, the principal investigator or analyst must at least have access to interim data in order to identify areas for clarification or further probing.

Another decision to make at the design stage is the form your data will take. The purpose of your qualitative study will imply a certain level of detail. For example, you may be able to explore broadly the different personal, relational, and institutional barriers to use of dual protection from pregnancy

and STIs by summarizing preliminary information from other observations or from interviews or group discussions. On the other hand, if you want to use qualitative data to design interventions that increase individuals' skills in negotiating dual protection, you will want to know exactly how people do and do not express themselves in such intimate circumstances. Fully transcribed tapes of interviews, in addition to notes about nonverbal or body language, would be more appropriate. If you are embarking on a mixed-method study, you will also need to decide in advance how you are going to handle the data from different methods and coordinate the findings in an integrated discussion.

Finally, the level of detail you anticipate and, to a lesser degree, the number of people involved in analysis, will influence decisions about the use of computers. Manual analysis is sufficient when your goal is to map out broad categories of information or when the volume of data is small. As the analysis becomes more complex (i.e., examining the nuances of language or comparing responses between a number of subgroups) and as the volume of data increases, a computer can greatly assist the analysis process. Again, if the analysts themselves will not be keying in data or operating analysis software programs, give some thought to how the data will be moved from field notes to data files to analysis procedures. Some software packages have special features to assist a team approach. (Specific advantages and disadvantages of different types of software packages are discussed in Chapter 6.)

Disseminating Results

In order for study results to be accessible to and used by others, you will need to build into your design a plan for dissemination, with a corresponding budget. Your study purpose has direct implications concerning how and for whom you will write your findings, as well as for your own role in their dissemination. (See Chapters 7 and 8 for a fuller discussion.) Likewise, as you focus your research questions, consider the eventual audiences for your findings and plan the length and detail of your report or presentation accordingly. When you sit down to write, "you begin a systematic inquiry of what you already know, what you need to know, and what you are looking for" (Wolcott 1990, 22). In short, outlining your study purpose and design can be done at the same time you develop a tentative table of contents for your final report. This approach will sharpen your focus and help you sequence your material.

Conclusion

A well-organized research design is a strong argument for the relevance and integrity of the research. However, qualitative design is always a work in progress. While a sound written design at the outset of your project gives you and your reviewers a frame of reference, it is a plan rather than a contract. It systematically details the problem driving the research and the strategy for solving it, but it remains flexible to change, as repeated questioning and analysis in the field lead you to new questions and new ways to delve deeper. Such flexibility, ill advised in most quantitative research, is a necessary feature of qualitative methodology. The researcher's ability — indeed, obligation — to examine data as they arrive, to throw out invalid assumptions, to restate questions, and to shape the design as the study progresses will ultimately contribute to the vitality and credibility of the results.

CHAPTER 4

Collecting Qualitative Data:
The Science and the Art

*Every interview is an interpersonal drama
with a developing plot.*

(Pool, cited in Holstein and Gubrium 1999, 112)

Three primary methods form the bedrock of qualitative data collection: observation, in-depth interview, and group discussion. We distinguish *method*, a systematic approach to data collection, from *technique*, the art of asking, listening, and interpreting. Each of these three methods applies special tools and techniques for gathering data — the "basic units or building blocks of information" (Rossman and Rallis 1998, 5). Qualitative

Collecting Qualitative Data: The Science and the Art

research methods differ with respect to the relationship between the data collector and the participant. Observation varies from nonreactive (unobtrusive) techniques, where the observer's intent is to be unnoticed, to more interactive (participant) techniques for observing a social process. Many techniques of in-depth interviewing and group discussion are designed to help study participants collaborate more actively with the researcher, generating rich, detailed data through expression of their own views and experiences.

This chapter describes the qualitative researcher as observer, interviewer, and group moderator. For each approach to research, we offer a variety of techniques, but our selection is not exhaustive. As you become more experienced in qualitative research, you will discover many more techniques of creative listening and learning. Working from an interpretivist or feminist perspective, you will focus on different issues, uncover new sources of data, and find more ways to enable people to tell their stories. But wherever you go, the basic principles of observing and interacting with individuals and groups will be the foundation on which you build your practice.

Observation

Observation is the oldest and most basic source of human knowledge, from casual understanding of the everyday world to its use as a systematic tool of social science. It is hard to imagine any field research, qualitative or quantitative, without an element of observation. Data collection does not begin and end with an interview. Interviewers and focus group moderators are also observers, noting body language, facial expression, and other nonverbal clues to subtle meanings. Qualitative researchers, particularly, must be acutely aware of context, observing the ebb and flow of activity around the study site. A chance conversation, an unexpected event, a spontaneous gathering — all may contain clues to understanding participants' expressions and meanings in the more formal interviews and discussions.

Depending on the purpose of your research, you will have to choose whether you are going to observe from an *outsider's* or an *insider's* perspective — or somewhere in between. Outside observers maintain distance in order to view events from their own perspectives. Inside observers reduce distance by joining activities and interacting with people in order to view events through participants' eyes and ears. Each approach has its place among the tools of scientific observation. As a researcher, it is unlikely that you can ever be a true insider, but you can get insiders' perspectives from study participants. Your own perspective as an outsider enables you to listen, question, and interpret what they share with you. In this chapter, we present these two ways to observe separately. But in practice, most field observation involves skillful interplay of both. With experience, you will learn to gauge the proper distance between yourself and your participants, knowing when to step back and when to join in.

Experienced observers use both qualitative and quantitative techniques, with qualitative observations differing from quantitative primarily in their focus on process rather than numbers. For example, counting the numbers of clients in different health center clinics could reveal variation in clinic use. However, it would not capture the qualitative interaction between clients and providers in the same clinics, a finding which might help explain different patterns of clinic attendance. Regardless of how and what you observe, observations become data only when they are guided by theory and conducted according to the rules and conventions of scientific inquiry.

Nonreactive techniques: observer as outsider

One strategy for observation is to remain on the fringe, watching people and events as unobtrusively as possible, observing without participating. Following the early work of Eugene Webb (Webb et al. 1966), we have adopted the term nonreactive to describe techniques in which the researcher collects data without interacting or reacting visibly to participants' activity. Choose this technique if you want to see how something happens rather than how other people perceive it happening, gathering your own impressions by direct observation instead of through the eyes and ears of study participants.

Program evaluation and operations research often combine nonreactive observation with other measures — for example, in quality of care studies — to observe firsthand the client experience, including the dynamics of interaction between client and provider. In such a setting, you might want to know how clients are received and how long they wait, who directs conversations, how information is offered, how questions are asked and answered, and whether providers initiate counseling on certain topics such as sexually transmitted infection (STI) protection, emergency contraception, or side effects.

Nonreactive observation is sometimes used to validate interview data or other information reported by study participants. For example, family planning counselors may have told interviewers that they always provide clients with information on a range of method choices — an insider perspective. Direct observation — the outsider perspective — could confirm their reports by the presence of a variety of contraceptives in half-empty boxes and colorful family planning posters on the walls, as well as actual counseling on the methods. However, several days of observation might reveal that, in practice, providers usually mention only one method to clients and have only that one in the supply closet. In the case of contrary evidence, the challenge to the qualitative researcher is to discover the reason for the apparent contradiction; for example, through in-depth interviews with clients and providers.

The quality of your data will depend on your ability to watch and listen without interrupting the natural flow of activity. Observers almost always have some effect on the study situation because, unless hidden behind a one-way vision mirror, as in some laboratory-controlled studies, their presence is noticeable. To minimize distortion of the observed behavior, an observer might be introduced simply as someone who is learning about health care in that area, taking a position behind the client-provider pair and observing silently from the sidelines. Longer, rather than shorter, periods of observation are usually more effective because, as people become accustomed to the observer's presence, they return more easily to their natural interaction.

In most observation sites — a busy pharmacy, an active community center, a clinic full of people waiting for attention — the din of activity can be distracting. Beginning with a prepared list of things for which to watch will help you focus your attention. The list may be as simple or as detailed as you wish, but it should be incorporated into your notes

and revised at the end of each observation period. What you see and hear will almost always lead to new insights and new questions about relationships and events in the setting. Although taking notes on what you observe is essential, it is important to do so as unobtrusively as possible. Frantic scribbling of verbatim conversations and flipping notebook pages will only remind people that they are being observed and raise anxiety about your intentions. To minimize note-taking, some observers use checklists with space for short, abbreviated comments. Others jot occasional notes on small cards, taking mental notes as much as possible. As soon as possible after each observation period, summarize your notes, incorporate mental notes and impressions, and reflect on what they have revealed about the research problem. Add interpretations, or tentative conclusions, to your notes and formulate new points to observe in the next session.

Documentary research

When observing human behavior, it is almost impossible not to intrude in some way. We include documentary research, also known as content analysis, under nonreactive methods because it is the only totally unobtrusive way to observe a culture. It also offers other interpretations of the phenomena you are studying and, in some cases, an historical perspective that is available only through writings from the past.

In documentary research, the material you are examining has been collected by others for other purposes, yet it can tell you a lot about how people think and behave in natural settings with no outsider influence. Large databases, such as epidemiological surveys or a country's Demographic and Health Survey (DHS), provide a wealth of information from which to learn about a study population. Documentary sources appropriate for research in sexual and reproductive health also include hospital and clinic records, health education materials, newspaper stories, radio and television shows, magazine advertising, billboards, school materials (for example, health education curricula), religious writings, sermons, personal journals, diaries, and popular songs. Qualitative researchers also use this method for secondary analysis of transcriptions from interviews or focus group discussions conducted in the past.

Topics in sexual and reproductive health that might be addressed through documentary data collection include: knowledge and attitudes related to fertility or STIs, government policy on HIV/AIDS as presented in the press, violence in advertising, gender bias in radio and television drama, or differences in health information given to different social groups as documented in clinic records. For example, an AIDS activist in Kenya gathered information on adolescents' concerns about HIV/AIDS through their letters to an AIDS advice column for young people in a local newspaper (Kimani 1990).

Documentary methods are similar to other qualitative data analysis. If you were studying gender bias in a series of radio comedies, you would start with an operational definition of gender bias and identify types of dialogue or situations that might contain bias toward men or women. Following the classic questions in communications research, you would focus on "Who says what, to whom, how, and with what effect" (Babbie 1998, 309). Creating a file of newspaper stories or taping and transcribing the radio series would enable you to code emerging themes and analyze the text, using rules of analysis like those for transcripts from interviews and focus group discussions, as covered in Chapter 6.

As a secondary source of data, existing documents can add immeasurably to the researcher's understanding of the context of the research. Popular norms, cultural values and beliefs, and people's hopes, fears, and triumphs all can be found in materials they have created to express different aspects of their lives. However, like all research, documentary analysis has its limitations. Questions of credibility arise if one person interprets the data without benefit of multiple coders. Are the criteria selected by the researcher valid representations of the key concepts in the present analysis? The same words or behaviors may have had different meanings at the time the document was created. Moreover, one can never be certain that the material reflects the views of a wider group, not just the voice of one author. The best strategies for ensuring rigor in documentary analysis are first, to keep a meticulous record of the analysis process, noting how you arrive at your interpretations and conclusions, and second, to work with multiple reviewers who conduct independent analyses and compare their results.

Participant observation

Participant observation brings the researcher into direct interaction with people and their activities. As defined by anthropologist H. Russell Bernard (Bernard 1995, 136), participant observation "involves getting close to people and making them feel comfortable enough with your presence that you can observe and record information about their lives." As the foundation of cultural anthropology, this method has many uses in different domains of social science. "The thing to remember

Ethical Dilemmas in Development Research: An Anthropologist's Perspective

Nancy Stark, R.N., Ph.D.
Bowman Gray School of Medicine, Wake Forest University

Anthropologists disagree about the extent to which social scientists should become involved in the decisions and choices of people they study. The notion of cultural relativity is central to anthropological research. Embracing local viewpoints is considered essential if one is to accurately understand and represent a society. Yet anthropologists have always had to contend with ethical dilemmas in the field, at times witnessing what they might consider discrimination, cruelty, unfair practices, and even crime. In each situation they must decide how to respond. In general, the anthropologist in the role of participant observer attempts to be transparent, participates in the culture, and observes but does not attempt to lead or initiate change.

More recently, some applied anthropologists have challenged the notion of cultural relativity. The contradiction between the principle of cultural relativity and the role of the researcher as a change agent has been especially apparent in international development, where applied research often accompanies interventions to improve health care and reduce mortality.

When the researcher is also a nurse or a physician, there is the added complexity that the study community may expect the medically trained researcher to respond with medicine, technical advice, information, and care. The researcher is therefore caught between the standards of her academic discipline for rigorous research and the ethical responsibility of her caring profession to help people in need.

As a registered nurse with a background in obstetric nursing, I had the opportunity to conduct fieldwork for my Ph.D. in cultural anthropology through the International Centre for Diarrhoeal Disease Research (ICDDR, B) in Bangladesh from 1989 to 1990. In an effort to reduce maternal and neonatal mortality, the center had recently implemented a program in which nurse midwives were trained to respond to obstetrical emergencies. Since my research addressed decision-making among families who would have access to these nurse midwives, my fieldwork included observation of deliveries. The question of how I might respond in an obstetrical emergency became a key issue that affected both my research practice and the expectations of the international staff at the centre.

In order to understand how families make decisions about obstetrical complications (when to call for assistance, whom to call first, who makes the decision that care is needed) families needed to make those decisions without interruption. However, my own ethical code as a health professional and the views of my colleagues at the ICDDR, B compelled me to decide that I would intervene if necessary. At the very least, I planned to notify the nurse midwife in emergencies should the family resist seeking care in a timely manner or fail to call for help. I also decided that I would take action only in the most dire circumstances. When the first delivery I observed presented a complication, I was surprised, in retrospect, at how I reacted.

A lay midwife had invited me to be present at a birth. Childbirth in the village is a very private matter — to protect the mother and child from spirits that come through the wind to cause birthing complications, the windows and doors of the house are kept shut during childbirth, and the laboring woman is expected not to cry out, so that others will not know that a child is being born. Thus the family did not invite me; in fact, the mother of the woman who was having her first child was not pleased that I had come with my research assistant.

As the woman's labor progressed, I observed without comment the midwife's technique. Even lay midwives in the ICDDR, B communities have received training in safe delivery techniques,* but I saw little sign of any such instruction and worried that a complication could result from unsafe practice. Labor seemed to be progressing normally until prior to the birth, I noticed meconium staining in the amniotic fluid. Without hesitation, I put down my notebook and pen and attempted to clear the baby's mouth as he was delivered. My action brought a cry from the lay midwife to "Stop! You could kill the baby!" I did stop, still concerned that the infant might aspirate meconium. But the baby cried spontaneously, and all was well.

I, in contrast, was exhausted from the ordeal. Now that the infant was breathing normally and crying, my concerns turned to how I might have damaged a fledgling relationship with the lay midwife, an individual central to the success of my research. I was concerned about the mother's reaction and how her experience might affect community attitudes toward me, possibly undermining my ability to conduct the research. Finally, I worried about my relationship with the ICDDR, B, the institution that had made my research possible. It occurred to me that if something were to go wrong during a delivery, I risked being held responsible by everyone.

---

* The instruction included techniques such as wearing gloves when performing vaginal exams, avoiding cervical massage or pulling the umbilical cord, and cutting the cord with the sterile razor provided in a safe birth kit that is routinely supplied to the pregnant woman by a community health worker.

I overcame those worries and attended other deliveries. As time passed, I became more familiar with delivery customs in the village and with the lay midwife, and I no longer felt the need to intervene. As I became more comfortable with the village culture, my attitude about the need to act softened, and my stress subsided.

These are a few of the lessons and insights that I gained from this experience:

- The researcher must (or perhaps will, in spite of herself) be true to a personal ethical standard.

- Belief systems can change. What is considered an ethical dilemma at the beginning of research may not be considered a problem later.

- Multiple cultures frequently converge in applied social science research, and all must be respected — the researcher's culture, the culture of the supporting institution, and the culture under study.

- Prior to initiating a research project, it is important to anticipate, as much as possible, the ethical challenges that may arise and to discuss them with others who have conducted similar research. What worked for them? What failed? And why?

- And finally, be ready for surprises.

about participation," Bernard reminds us, "is that it belongs to everyone, positivists and interpretivists alike. … Whether your data consist of numbers or words, participant observation lets you in the door so you can do research" (Bernard 1995, 137).

Unlike nonreactive observation — in which you must be as unobtrusive as possible — in participant observation, you will ask yourself: How can I get close to people? Will they share their lives, their thoughts, their activities with an outsider? In this more interactive approach, your responsibility is to stimulate conversation and behavior that will let you enter the culture as a guest of its members. In initiating the observation, your challenge will be to adapt your interactive style to the cultural style of the participants. For example, you would approach young schoolgirls differently from the way you might introduce yourself to commercial sex workers on the street. Experienced observers learn to present themselves in whatever way will put study participants at ease while simultaneously stimulating their interest in interacting with the observer. In some participant observation studies, the observer has adopted the lifestyle of the people observed, such as driving a taxi or working in a restaurant in order to study taxi cab drivers or waiters. In reproductive health research, the observer is more likely to remain an outsider on the inside, maintaining identity as a researcher but spending enough time in the cultural setting to know and understand people in the natural course of their lives.

The techniques for entering a culture are as many and varied as cultural variations themselves. The map-making exercise in Box 4.1 illustrates how, by starting with an activity that arouses curiosity, you can soon have a willing group of informants who want to participate because they find what you are doing interesting. *The common goal is to enable people to accept you and interact naturally with you for sustained periods of time.* As they get used to your presence, they will act almost as if you were not there (Gans, cited in Bernard 1995, 136). Once

Box 4.1
Using Participant Observation to Introduce a Study

At the start of a multisite HIV behavior change project, a team of qualitative researchers set out to conduct some geographic mapping exercises to learn about the social networks that would be targeted for an intervention. Researchers used this activity as an opportunity for community members to become familiar with the team, as well as for collecting the map data needed to begin the study.

After courtesy calls on community leaders, the researchers began to spend casual time in the communities, drawing their maps. Inevitably, they were approached by curious individuals. This enabled the researchers to start conversations and inquire informally about what they had observed in the course of their map-making.

As they became more interested in the maps, the community members began to offer advice and supply additional information. These interactions in turn led to informal invitations to share a drink or snack in a local eating place, which then offered more opportunities for observation.

Thus, as a component of a large research project, participant observation resulted in: maps pertinent to social networks, which were then validated by the research community; introduction of the field staff to the community; identification of key informants, gatekeepers, and stakeholders; and the beginning of community trust and a foundation for community participation in the research project.

(Woodsong 2001)

accepted, you must continue to balance insider and outsider perspectives as you watch and listen to what unfolds. With practice, you will respond naturally and flexibly to fluctuations in the research environment, always alert to unexpected events that could reveal important information on the cultural dynamics of the group.

To illustrate this process, imagine that you are going to study how women make health decisions for themselves and their families. Following preliminary introductions in the community, as described in Chapter 5, you obtain permission to join a local mother's club. The group meets weekly to socialize and discuss their concerns as young mothers. At the first meeting you attend, you explain why you want to join them as an observer, sharing your concern for issues the women believe are important. Until the women know and trust you, you probably do more listening than active participating. Remember that you are there as an observer, not masquerading as a mother in the group. As the women become comfortable with your presence, you might begin to ask a few questions or steer discussion toward topics related to their health decisions. Participating will give way to listening, with occasional questions to explore interesting leads. Be open also to questions the women might have about you and be willing to reciprocate by sharing some of your own experience. However, avoid becoming an authority in their eyes. Emphasis on common experiences, values, questions, and concerns will help to minimize the effect of your presence on the views expressed by the group.

Between the club's weekly meetings, you might arrange individual visits with some of the members at their homes, or informal visits to other places the women gather, such as a church group or local health center waiting area. A process similar to snowball sampling can enable you to reach out farther into women's networks. As you become known and accepted as a visiting member of the community, you will be an increasingly effective observer. Over time, you will piece together data from many conversations, noticing how they converge around certain recognizable themes or, on the other hand, where conflicting messages suggest new directions to explore. In contrast to an interview, the participant observer's commitment to the study group is likely to be more intimate and sustained over a longer period. For understanding sequences and connections of events that contribute to health decisions, participant observation can be a powerful tool (Bogdewic 1992).

In the above scenario, the researcher is a woman, but there are equally rich opportunities for men to conduct participant observation. Examples are studies of AIDS awareness among male assembly-line workers, HIV risk-behavior of truckers driving long-distance routes through countries with a high prevalence of infection, and attitudes of migrant farm workers toward contraceptive use. Although on sensitive topics, participant observers of the same sex may be able to put participants more quickly at ease, same-sex research is not always a necessity. There are numerous studies in which an observer has gained the confidence of both men and women in the study site, with skillful integration of different gender perspectives in the analysis.

Ability to communicate in the local idiom is a valuable asset but often not an option in cross-cultural observation. Although an experienced local assistant can help you to offset a language gap and offer cultural, as well as linguistic, interpretation, the non-native-speaking foreigner must realize that one is observing the scene through the eyes and ears of another person whose perspective is likely to be very different. (Use of field assistants is discussed in more detail in Chapter 5.)

Using Qualitative Research to Understand How Providers Spend Their Time

Barbara Janowitz, Ph.D.
Family Health International

Qualitative research offers important methods for use in cost analysis that go far beyond poring over figures provided by the finance division of a reproductive health program. To analyze reproductive health program costs, we concentrate on how resources are used to provide services. One of the most important resources is labor. If programs are to understand whether their workers are being used efficiently and whether there is a way to reduce costs, then programs need to find out what workers are doing.

To study how workers use their time, FHI has used participant observation, or activity sampling (also known as time and motion studies). We started using this methodology is 1993 during a cost study in Bangladesh (Janowitz et al. 1997). In one component of that study, we accompanied workers to the field and noted how they spent their time, including traveling to the field, traveling between households, and talking with clients. In addition, we used a checklist to note the activities that providers carried out with clients. Our results showed that the costs of expanding family planning services to households could be greatly reduced if fieldworkers increased their level of effort. In addition, our findings indicated that interactions with clients often involved no more than the dispensing of pills or condoms when these were needed. But when they were not, little effort was being made to counsel women about the potential benefits to them of using family planning.

In similar studies, we have observed staff members at clinics that provided reproductive health services. Instead of measuring the duration of each activity, we used a technique called activity sampling. This involves obtaining information about exactly what a staff person is doing during a defined sample of time. Using a beeper that went off every three or five minutes, we noted on a checklist what activity the person was engaged in at that moment. Activities were grouped into categories that included client contact time, client-related activities, general administration, tea/coffee/lunch breaks, and unproductive time. The latter included such things as coming to the clinic late or leaving early, talking with friends in person or on the phone, or simply waiting for clients to arrive at the clinic.

We used this information to determine whether providers might in fact have time to expand their interactions with clients in order to increase the quality of their services. If they could do this without reducing the number of clients that they saw, then there would be no cost to the clinic in terms of a reduced number of women obtaining services. We found that on an average day, providers had a considerable amount of time that they could be using to expand their contact time with clients. This time was mainly clustered very early in the morning or in the late afternoon, in large part because providers arrived late and left early. We concluded that it could be difficult to get providers to be at the clinic for a full day and for them to be busy during late afternoon hours.

Our findings generate a number of other questions about how services are organized. More qualitative research would help:

■ to better understand what providers actually want from their jobs;

■ to learn why they arrange their schedules as they do;

■ to determine what interventions would work to change time allocation;

■ to find out how clients feel about waiting times in the current model of service provision; and

■ to ascertain whether clients might prefer to get services at some other time than mid-morning if it meant they would not have to wait.

Mystery client technique

In some situations, the presence of an observer may cause participants to alter their usual behavior and, consciously or unconsciously, create what they believe to be a favorable impression. At such times, researchers sometimes turn to a mystery client technique — a special form of participant observation that may combine qualitative and quantitative data collection. It has been used particularly in client-provider studies where the presence of an observer might significantly change the provider's customary behavior. Simulated clients, trained to act out roles that reflect real-life experiences, present themselves to actual health providers in the natural setting. These actors may be professional data collectors or local people from the service area. After each encounter, they typically record their experience on a structured form and report their observations to researchers in in-depth interviews. For this kind of research, an observation checklist is an important tool because it enables the observer to assess the same factors in different settings.

A study in Nepal used the mystery client technique to examine interactions between clients and staff of family planning clinics (Schuler et al. 1985). The simulated clients asked for guidance in choosing a method, including available alternatives and potential risks and side effects. The researchers found that providers' responses depended on their perceptions of clients' social and economic status, with lower-class participants receiving little information and brusque or rude treatment. Mystery client observation has also been used to compare information provided over the counter in different pharmacies, where the simulated customer asks for

I want to understand the world from your point of view, I want to know what you know in the way you know it. I want to understand the meaning of your experience, to walk in your shoes, to feel things as you feel them, to explain things as you explain them. Will you become my teacher and help me understand?

(Spradley 1979)

contraceptive advice. Another application of this technique is in studies that explore family planning providers' attitudes toward adolescents, wherein the mystery clients are young people who present themselves to the clinic as sexually active adolescents seeking family planning services.

Note that in the above examples, the provider is unaware of the real identity and purpose of the visitor. We caution readers that the deceptive nature of this technique has raised serious ethical questions about its use. Some researchers have addressed this issue by obtaining informed consent from both staff and supervisors to use the technique at unannounced times over a period of several months. Nevertheless, a decision to use the mystery client technique should be made only after careful reflection on the purpose and ethical implications of doing so.

Key informants in participant observation

Ethnographers have always relied on key informants to help them make sense of their observations and interactions in unfamiliar cultures. Key informants are individuals with special knowledge, status, or communication skills, who are willing to share what they know with the researcher (Gilchrist 1992). Although all qualitative research participants are asked to share their knowledge and perspectives, a key informant usually has a different relationship to the researcher, providing information, introductions and interpretation, often on a day-to-day basis, as well as access to observations that an outsider would not normally have. You should expect to have more personal involvement with a key informant who becomes your trusted advisor and guide to the culture. While your relationship to interview and focus group participants is one of rapport, key informants are likely to become your friends. Why should a qualitative researcher develop a special relationship with a few people instead of regarding all study participants as equal collaborators? Pragmatic limits constrain the researcher (Gilchrist 1992). One cannot be in all places at all times, observing everything and interviewing everyone. A personal relationship with a key informant, developed over time, helps to ensure more efficient access to rich information.

For example, you might begin a study of gender influence on HIV risk with participant observation in a community known to have a high prevalence of STI/HIV infection. As you get to know people in the community, perhaps two or three stand out because they are particularly interested in the problem and are knowledgeable and articulate on topics concerning sexual risk. When you introduce yourself around the community, people often refer to such individuals as the ones who "know what's going on." You visit with each of them and find them willing to share what they know and take you to people and places that will help you understand gender relationships in relation to sexual risk in this community. These will be your key informants. They might explain cultural norms that govern partner relationships, including the meaning of sexual behavior that seems to deviate from the norm. They will comment on your interpretation of conversations with others in the community and help you synthesize pieces of information from different sources. They might introduce you to other potential key informants, such as a youth leader, a member of a women's advocacy organization, or a prominent commercial sex worker.

As in all qualitative data gathering, it is important to formulate a basic set of questions to start the process. Although these questions could be written, they should be incorporated casually into conversations with key informants. Accompanied by your key informant, you might start with a tour of the facility or workplace you plan to study, or a community or neighborhood where potential participants gather. Initial questions might be as general as: Who comes here? What do they do? To whom do they talk? As you begin to make connections, your questions will become more focused on specific issues related to the purpose and context of the study: Why do certain things happen? How do people deal with a new event or a stressful situation? In this way, a key informant can orient you to the study population in their natural environment.

Although we advocate use of key informants in most studies, quantitative as well as qualitative, we caution that there are limits to the information that most informants can provide. Key informants are not infallible. A trusted informant may be reluctant to admit not knowing something, or try to please you by telling you what he or she thinks you want to hear. Key informants also may have their own biased interpretations, especially if they come from different ethnic, religious, or socioeconomic groups than the study population. Just as you look at a situation from different methodological perspectives, it is wise to have more than one key informant so that you are not dependent on the interpretations of one person. Contradictions or new ideas can then be raised and discussed with other informants until you have consensus on an issue or perhaps decide to look elsewhere for different insight.

Be sensitive also to comments made by community members about your close interactions with key informants and take steps to correct misperceptions. Always ask yourself how any key informant will affect your acceptance in the wider group. While an informant may have much to offer, giving a single person extra attention could have negative consequences, engendering jealousy or other issues in the group under study. Thus it is always important to weigh the risks and benefits of developing a particularly close relationship with any individual in the study setting.

Making the most of field notes

The importance of good field notes — clear, detailed, and descriptive — cannot be overemphasized. New field observers often make the mistake of writing notes that are vague and imply judgment: "The unpleasant young woman who came into the clinic was loud and impatient." Using descriptive terms can eliminate vagueness and reduce obvious bias: "The woman who appeared to be in her early twenties approached the clinic supervisor and claimed in a loud voice that she had been waiting for three hours to see the nurse. The receptionist asked her to take a seat and told her the nurse would be with her shortly. The woman shook her head forcefully and replied in a loud voice that she had been told the same thing twice already." The second note presents a more vivid picture of the scene without the overlay of observer judgment. In this case, it would be equally important to include observation of objective facts such as the actual time the woman had been waiting, the number of staff on duty, and the number and behavior of others who were also waiting. Notes on comfort, noise level, lighting, decor, posters, health information, and other descriptions of the scene will help you analyze later the observed behavior in relation to the context. The extra effort to capture the moment in detail will provide you with rich observational data that will be meaningful when you review your large accumulation of field notes.

The journalist's query — who, what, when, where, why, and how — is also a useful guide to recording field observations. Make a practice of recording conversations and events as soon as possible after they happen and set aside time every day to complete your notes. Start each note with the date, time, location, and a brief sentence about the purpose or circumstance of the observation. State clearly the ages, sex, and number of people you have observed or conversed with. Recall conversations, record thoughts and impressions, develop working hypotheses, plan next steps and revisit and

revise what you have written on previous days. As you record observations, keep asking new questions, interpreting and reinterpreting what you have seen and heard. If you are also using audiotapes, summaries of the transcriptions can be entered into your notes. Gradually, interpretations take the shape of tentative conclusions, which add structure to what you are observing. This running account will help you organize your search more efficiently, building from concrete instances to more general understanding.

As we pointed out earlier, participant observation can begin from any theoretical perspective. It is important, therefore, to be keenly aware of your own orientation as an outsider and interpreter of the scene, documenting the distinction between what you see and what it means to you. Similarly, the observer's awareness of self in relation to the field of observation is critical to record. Qualitative researchers must frequently ask themselves two common reflexive questions, "What effect am I having on this scene?" and "How is what I observe affecting me, the observer?" Experienced participant observers learn to recognize the subtle interplay between the observer and the observed and to make it part of the record as they interpret what they see and hear.

As your field notes grow, it may become increasingly difficult to keep them organized. In Chapter 6, we discuss techniques of coding text in large data sets, a process that can help the participant observer, as well as the interviewer, begin to analyze and interpret raw data while still in the field.

Managing bias and maximizing rigor

Participant observation by definition entails subjective interpretation and therefore the potential for bias. However, there are a number of things you can do to keep subjectivity in control and maximize the rigor of observation data. While for participant observation it is important to become part of the group, be aware of the boundaries that distinguish your role as observer-researcher. For example, young staff conducting work in an HIV surveillance study were chosen in part because their youthfulness would facilitate the blending-in process and help build rapport with the young research participants. However, since their work would include observation of drinking and sexual behavior in bars, they benefited from careful guidance by supervisors on the limits of their participation (Woodsong 2001).

Another strategy for enhancing the rigor of a participant observer study is the careful documentation we have discussed above. At the end of a long day in the field, it is an easy pitfall not to document what you have observed. But neglecting this important step risks losing what you may have learned, or valuable information could remain only in the mind of the observer and not become available to the rest of the team. Lost data can have serious consequences in potential misinterpretation of other data and lead to erroneous or incomplete conclusions. It also leaves you vulnerable to claims that your research may not be reliable. By creating an audit trail (see Chapter 6), your observations and conclusions will be documented in such a way that other researchers will be able to reconstruct the process that has led you to your results (Denzin and Lincoln 1994, 230). Participating in the creation of an audit trail can also be a valuable learning experience for members of the research team.

The general way of approaching the reliability problem [in qualitative research] is to ... conduct research as if someone were always looking over your shoulder.

(Yin 1994, 37)

Other techniques to maximize the rigor of observation data include comparisons among multiple observers or multiple coders and verifying results with additional observations or semi-structured interviews with other informants. However, as we emphasize further in Chapter 6, discrepant findings do not necessarily mean methodological weakness; they may be a reflection of multiple realities, contradictory but valid perspectives and experiences in the study population.

In-depth Interviews

In-depth interviews are typically an exchange between one interviewer and one respondent. Although interviewing style is usually informal, guided by a few broad topics rather than a detailed questionnaire, there are many ways you can create structure without compromising the open exchange that is the hallmark of most qualitative techniques. This kind of intensive, one-on-one interviewing has been called a *conversational partnership* (Rubin and Rubin 1995, 10), *conversation with a purpose* (Burgess 1984, 102), and a *social encounter* (Holstein and Gubrium 1999, 106). These terms reflect the uniquely interactive nature of qualitative interviewing, differentiating it from the standardized survey interview. In most survey research the interviewee is expected mainly to respond to structured questions. Qualitative researchers encourage study participants to take a more active role in determining the flow of the discussion. Interviewer and participant are collaborators, "working together to achieve the shared goal of understanding" (Rubin and Rubin 1995, 11). In a relaxed and comfortable setting, the conversation generates empirical data by enabling participants to talk freely about their lives (Holstein and Gubrium 1999, 105). A qualitative interview should not be a mechanical reading of standardized questions; collecting information-rich data requires mental agility, sensitivity, and always, practice.

Framing qualitative questions

Whether in individual interviews or group discussions, qualitative questions are informal, nonjudgmental, and open. Speak clearly but casually, avoiding any suggestion that one answer might be more desirable than another. Inexperienced interviewers often use words that inadvertently suggest answers. Asking, "Do you believe all those things you have heard about emergency contraception?" suggests they really are not true. Asking participants simply to comment on the information they have received so far about emergency contraception (EC) is a more open invitation to express a candid opinion. Sometimes interviewers ask a yes or no question with an immediate follow-up question for more detail, but in general, it is advisable to avoid dichotomous wording and emphasize open-ended questions that encourage participants to interpret questions themselves.

Although we refer to qualitative interviews as conversations, most interviews and focus group discussions follow a pattern comprised of three kinds of questions: *main questions*, *follow-up questions*, and *probes* (Rubin and Rubin 1995; Patton 1990). The pattern is flexible but helps the interviewer or moderator cover the topics in sufficient depth to make the most of the rich information that participants can offer.

As Table 4.1 illustrates, the pattern begins with a clear idea of the topic, or the direction you want the question to take. Since you will already have explained in a general way the purpose of the interview, the topic does not have to be repeated to the participant with each question. Main questions

come from the themes and subthemes of the research problem. They introduce topics to be discussed in the form of questions. If one theme of a program evaluation is client perception of services, you might begin by asking, "What has been your experience with this health center?" Or for a study of women's vulnerability to HIV/AIDS, "How do you manage to protect yourself from infection?" Main questions are open enough to encourage spontaneous response but specific enough to keep the dialogue focused. If the discussion moves too far from the topic, you may want to repeat the main question, perhaps in a different way, to get back on track. On the other hand, be aware that "getting off track" may be a clue to a different way of looking at the problem or an idea you might want to pursue or return to later in the interview.

Main question. Your main questions should reflect the logical flow you anticipate in the conversation, moving from easy and least threatening questions to more complex and interesting issues as you build rapport. However, as experienced interviewers know, this sequence may be logical only to the researcher. Participants often answer a main question before you have asked it. You must then decide quickly whether to continue with that topic or suggest coming back to it later. Or the participant may reconstruct the meaning of the question in a different way, requiring your flexibility to keep the discussion focused while encouraging participant perspectives and experiences. Interviewers and moderators often ask the most important — and perhaps more difficult — questions more than once, from different angles and at different points in the interview. Through experience, you will learn how to move around among the main questions, pursuing each to its logical conclusion while not neglecting questions or new ideas.

Table 4.1

Levels of Interview Questions in a Qualitative Study of Emergency Contraception (EC)

Qualitative interviews typically begin with a few broad questions, then move to more specific questions, following participants' clues and encouraging depth and detail. The direction and pattern of movement can vary, depending on how the participant responds to the issues.

Topics	Main Questions	Follow-up Questions	Probes
Knowledge	Can you tell me what you know about EC?	What have you heard from others? In your opinion, are these things true?	Anything else about EC?
Source of information	Where did you hear about EC?	How did you happen to be discussing it? What did this person say about it? Who else is talking about EC these days?	Tell me more about that. Can you give me some examples?
Experience	Do you know anyone who has used EC? Have you used EC yourself?	Why did you decide to use it? What was using it like for you? Were you glad or sorry you had tried it? What made you glad or sorry?	Who influenced your decision? Why did you decide that way?
Opinion	What do you think are the advantages and disadvantages of EC?	How could EC help or harm someone like yourself? How do you think others would react to your use of EC? Do you think women you know would want EC to be available? Why or why not? Would you want EC to be available for yourself? Why or why not?	What are some ways EC could help or harm a person? What about your husband/partner/mother-in-law? What would women say if it were offered to them? What about men? What are some reasons that people you know might not want to use EC?

Follow-up question. A follow-up question moves the interview or discussion to a deeper level by asking for more detail. Follow-up questions are a natural part of any conversation. They suggest to the speaker that the listener is interested enough in what has just been said to want more information. To some extent, you can anticipate follow-up questions in advance, but even in a standardized open-ended format, you can not know exactly what they will be until participants respond to the main questions. In the example in Table 4.1, a participant might have answered the first question by saying, "Well, I hear emergency contraception can prevent pregnancy." You would then ask for detail on what the person has heard and whether she or he knows it as fact (a knowledge question).

Probe. A probe is a kind of follow-up question that takes the discussion into still deeper territory, with or without specific reference to the topic. For example, the interviewer might say, "Please tell me more about that" or "Then what happened?" or "I don't think I know what you mean — can you explain?" As you gain experience, you use these conversational devices naturally. They tell the participant that you are listening closely and that what is said is important. They also indicate to the participant the level of detail you want and enable you to clarify points or pursue new ideas in a conversational manner. Note, however, the importance of maintaining a comfortable balance between too much detail and not enough. Insufficient probing could suggest boredom, but aggressive probing might be intrusive (Rubin and Rubin 1995). Through experience and careful listening, you will know how to probe sensitively and when to stop.

Stages of the interview

A particularly versatile format for in-depth interviews and focus groups in applied sexual and reproductive health research is the semi-structured approach introduced in Chapter 3. Interviewers typically use a written set of flexibly worded topics

or questions that keep the conversation guided and on track but without imposing boundaries on the participant's style and expression.

Rubin and Rubin (Rubin and Rubin 1995, 129-139) describe this type of in-depth interview in a series of stages:

- creating natural involvement
- encouraging conversational competence
- showing understanding
- getting facts and basic description
- asking difficult questions
- toning down the emotional level
- closing while maintaining contact

Although these stages are presented here for in-depth interviews, they are easily adapted to focus group discussions.

Creating natural involvement. Beginning with an informal chat is a good way to set the stage for the relaxed atmosphere you want to create for the interview. It helps to be able to comment on events or situations that are familiar and important to the respondent. If possible, link the purpose of the interview to some common experience; for example, "A young man in my office passed away with AIDS the other day. It has been hard for all of us who knew him." Sharing experience is a way of expressing the bond that you hope will develop into the conversational partnership that will generate the information you seek. Women interviewing women, or men interviewing men, may find common ground in gender; for example, in family relationships, childbearing, job-seeking, or other experiences in the context of being a woman or a man. Expression of concern about the widespread prevalence of a common problem like adolescent pregnancy or AIDS may also be a springboard to the conversational partnership.

Early in the introduction, it is important to explain clearly what the study is about and why the respondent has been asked to participate. This is a good time to clarify the rights and responsibilities of participation and to obtain the individual's informed consent to continue. As you begin to develop rapport, you will move into a more formal introduction, explaining who you are and what you want to know. The respondent meanwhile will be assessing you, trying to decide what you really want and whether you can be trusted. It is important to show that you are genuinely interested, that you do not come with a judgmental attitude, and that you will honor his or her confidentiality and trust.

Encouraging conversational competence. In the first few minutes of the interview encounter, you set the tone for the conversation that follows. People often agree to participate in an interview but are insecure, or skeptical that they would have anything to offer. The interviewer's job is to give participants the sense that their opinions and experiences are important to the study. Starting with easy, nonthreatening questions allows them to feel sure about what they know and pleased to have an appreciative ear. Participants familiar with survey interviews may instantly adopt a compliant role, offering impersonal, monosyllabic answers to questions. It is therefore critical to dispel as quickly as possible the notion of passivity or subordination to the interviewer.

As you develop your own qualitative style, the language you use should help to establish you as a partner rather than an interrogator. "I'm hoping you will help me understand how women make choices about pregnancy." "I'd like to explore with you what it means to be the mother of a large family." "When it comes to housing and feeding the family, we men have a lot of responsibility. Let's talk a little about …" "I know that as a mother-in-law you care very much about how your grandchildren are raised. I'd like to know how you feel

about …" Whether or not you agree with the participant's views, your manner should reflect great interest and compassion. As they come to trust you and the confidentiality of the interview, participants will welcome a sympathetic listener; they will become more personally invested in the topic and will move with you to deeper levels of their experience. The interviewer-partner does not coax answers from the respondent but enters actively into the discussion in a way that explores incompletely articulated thoughts and encourages new directions (Holstein and Gubrium 1999, 115).

Showing understanding. As the interview progresses, you can encourage openness and depth by showing that you understand and empathize with what the respondent is telling you. When a mother of six in a very poor village was telling the interviewer how hard it was to have so many children, the interviewer responded, "Yes, I can imagine life is very hard for you right now. How do you keep your children looking so healthy?" The question builds rapport by showing that the interviewer understands and by reinforcing the respondent's competence in her role as a mother. Emotional support comes through in a sympathetic tone of voice, responsive facial expression, murmurs, and gestures — all of which suggest acceptance of the person. It is not necessary to relate one's own personal experiences or to approve of what the individual has done. Your role is to put the conversational partner at ease to share life experiences without fear.

Getting facts and basic descriptions. Once the partnership is established and conversation flows easily, you are getting into the heart of the interview. Now you can encourage longer answers by asking the partner to tell you about an incident or describe a typical encounter related to the topic of the research, following it up with simple, direct questions. At this stage of the interview you focus on descriptive material, holding delicate or emotionally charged questions for later.

A topic to introduce at this stage might be how a young person gets answers to questions about sexual relationships. An adolescent will probably talk about conversations held with friends or questions asked of health providers, which will lead into details of the questions and perhaps reveal personal concerns about sexual matters. The exchange may prompt the interviewer to explore possible gaps in adolescents' understanding of health services or contradictions between the information young people want and the answers that providers are prepared to give. As a skilled listener, the interviewer will be alert to clues that the participant is ready to move to more sensitive levels of discussion.

Asking difficult questions. Save your most difficult questions until you sense that your conversational partnership is relaxed and trusting. Be aware not only of your partner's stage in the process but of your own comfort with the relationship and your readiness to raise issues that may take considerable skill to manage. Researchers in reproductive and sexual health must frequently discuss topics that lie outside normal discourse with strangers. In varying degrees, open discussion of sex is taboo in virtually all cultures; women, especially, may be socialized to strict norms of sexual privacy. As you enter this stage of the interview, it is important to respect the fact that you may be violating certain expectations of behavior and to be especially sensitive to the effect of the conversation on your participant. Remember that important questions can be asked and repeated at different points in the interview. Repeating a difficult question later in a different way gives the participant a chance to think about it and offers you an opportunity to ask it from different angles.

When the research problem requires you to ask very difficult questions, there are ways to soften their impact. You may need to remind your respondent that the interview is confidential, that no names will be recorded, and that identification will not

be revealed. It also helps to acknowledge the sensitivity of the topic with a simple comment like, "I know this is a hard thing to discuss — I really appreciate your sharing."

Another way to show responsiveness and empathy is to use familiar words and expressions in the conversation — an advantage of the informal style of qualitative interviewing. Telling a story or showing a picture that illustrates the topic is a way of depersonalizing a difficult area without sacrificing spontaneity. When you ask respondents to talk about an issue through fictitious characters, you are allowing them to control the extent to which they disclose information about themselves. If necessary for the research, the interviewer might ask if the picture or story is like anything in their own lives, but qualitative interviewers who have used this technique usually find that the respondent shifts spontaneously from the impersonal third person to the first person expression of self.

Hesitation may not mean embarrassment, but rather difficulty understanding the question. It can also mean that the respondent, especially if a woman, has never been asked her opinion on any topic. We have found that women in some societies are so unaccustomed to being consulted on matters of fertility that it may take several interviews before they are able to participate as partners in the interview conversation.

Toning down the emotional level. When participants have been open with you on sensitive or embarrassing topics, they may begin to feel uncomfortably exposed. As the interviewer, you may need to help restore the sense of privacy that enabled them to share their lives with you in the first place. Again, you can simply remind them of the confidentiality of the information. When toning down the emotional level of the conversation, the researcher can turn the interview around and ask if the participant has questions to ask — or answers

Clandestine Contraceptive Use: A Prospective Study

Sarah Castle, Ph.D.
London School of Hygiene and Tropical Medicine

Although family planning has been available in Africa since the 1960s, many couples today are becoming acquainted with it for the first time. In Bamako, Mali, only about 16 percent of married women use a modern contraceptive method, and the discontinuation rate is high. In order to understand the experiences of new contraceptive users, the Centre d'Etudes et de Recherche sur la Population pour le Développement (CERPOD), with Family Health International, conducted a prospective study of 55 first-time contraceptive users in Bamako (Castle et al. 1999). Three in-depth interviews were conducted over a period of 18 months with each participant who remained in the study.

When the study was designed, the theme of clandestine use was not high on the research agenda. However, it became clear in the first round of interviews that a high proportion of women, 17 out of 55, were using contraception without their husbands' knowledge. All but seven of these women had attempted unsuccessfully to discuss family planning with their husbands before resorting to secret use. A feature of qualitative research is that it allows a certain degree of flexibility in the research content and methodology. Therefore, once we discovered this phenomenon, we were able to modify the interview guide to explore it in greater depth in the second and third interviews.

The use of repeated in-depth interviews, conducted at a location of the participant's choice, enabled interviewers and participants to develop relationships of rapport and trust. It also enabled the research team to follow the family planning process over time, to build on information as it emerged, and to test our interpretation of what contraceptive use meant for these women. The topic guide for each subsequent interview with each woman thus reflected the discussion of the previous interview.

In round two, three of the 17 original clandestine users' husbands had found out about their use. Two had directly told their husbands. One husband had spotted his wife's appointment card but had not commented on it. Thus, although spousal communication has now become a key theme in family planning research, this study indicates that there may sometimes be nonverbal communication about family planning use. These two women, who guessed that their husbands were likely eventually to accept their action, left clues that would present their decisions as a fait accompli.

However, most of the women feared dire consequences of divorce or physical violence if they were discovered. We asked why they thought their husbands and others in the family were opposed to family planning. The most common response was that the husband simply wanted many children. Three believed their husbands' objections were related to their understanding that the Islamic religion opposed the practice of family planning. Two women said their husbands were afraid family planning would make them unfaithful. Several clandestine users related their secrecy to their perception that they had been neglected or treated unfairly by their husbands, and they did not want to risk obligations in an unstable union.

All the women had confided in someone, most often a sister-in-law. Informal support groups for family planning seemed to exist among younger members of the family, illustrating how within households typified by the dynamics of cooperative conflict, allegiances are formed among those with vested interests. Because many of the clandestine users interviewed lived in extended families in which young women's time and movements were monitored and controlled by older female marital relatives, they had to employ cunning strategies to deceive not only their spouses, but also their older marital kin.

As the study progressed and the women's experiences unfolded, their strategies to obtain contraception and to maintain secrecy became central themes. The transcribed texts were coded and analysed using the computer software *Ethnograph*. Clandestine use became a main (parent) code during the overall analysis, while aspects of clandestine use, such as type of method, techniques to ensure secrecy, social consequences of discovery, etc., became subcategories (child) codes.

A major methodological problem in this study was the number of study participants who could not be found for the second and third interviews — seven of the original 17 clandestine users. Given the secret nature of their behavior, this was perhaps to be expected. In most cases, they had given fictitious addresses at the time of the first interview, which was conducted at the clinic. Fear of discovery may have made them unwilling to participate in the research, although some clandestine users remarked that the discretion and sensitivity shown by the interviewers encouraged them to continue. Nevertheless, we cannot say whether there are fundamental differences between the clandestine users who dropped out and the women who were using contraception openly. The study did indicate that among those who remained in the study, a higher proportion of clandestine users had stopped using contraception by the end of the study period compared with overt users. Methodologically, the high drop-out rates did present some problems that could only be resolved by not generalizing the results to all women in the study. The study methodology points to the importance of flexible research methods, careful interviewer training, and recognizing the limitations of results from small samples.

to other questions. By this time, most participants will have identified themselves as partners and be able and eager to add clarifying information.

But sometimes it is difficult to move away from interview conversations that have stirred up strong emotions. If the conversation is upsetting to the participant, you can decide to change the topic or discontinue the interview. Another alternative is to allow participants to ventilate their feelings until they become calmer or until you can shift naturally to a more neutral topic. A risk that qualitative interviewers often face is that they may learn more than participants want them to hear (Alty and Rodham 1998). The more comfortable the respondent is with you, the more easily she or he will disclose information not meant to be shared. You may hear such off-the-record comments after the interview or focus group has ended. The interviewer's ethical response to material that seems to go beyond the participant's original informed consent is either to interrupt the conversation at that point or to ask the participant whether those remarks can be included in the transcript. It might be important to have these comments in your personal notes to help you understand the meaning of broader issues. However, if the participant does not want them shared, your ethical obligation is to indicate clearly in your notes that they should never be quoted in full or described in publications.

To some extent, we can predict topics that are potentially embarrassing or disturbing: sexual intimacy, deviant or prohibited sexual practices, abortion, infidelity, domestic violence, and contraception that may be in conflict with religious or other cultural beliefs. Other topics may evoke painful emotion; for example, loss of children. Or a topic may have political sensitivity that you as an outsider

have not guessed. In short, you need to be always on the alert for change in the tone of the interview conversation which could suggest that you are entering a vulnerable area. Rather than risk further discomfort for your respondent, avoid the question if it is not essential to the purpose of the research. If what you need to know is whether infidelity is a common experience for women in the community, it is not necessary to probe the marital relations of your conversational partner. If you ask her about women in general, she is free to illustrate her response with her own experience only if she wishes to do so.

On the other hand, there is another important but often overlooked ethical question that qualitative researchers must be prepared to answer: *What is the responsibility of the interviewer when a study participant asks for help?* Even if violence is not the topic of the research, questioning women on contraceptive decisions may suddenly lead to personal accounts of an abusive relationship. The interviewer must be prepared for such unanticipated disclosures, balancing the requirements of the interview with ethical responsibility for the well-being of the participant. In one country where we experienced this scenario, we were able to refer vulnerable women to a local intervention program for battered wives by handing all participants a card at the end of the interview with the name, address, and phone number of a women's counseling center. Other problems to note include a participant's fear of having an STI or disclosing recent untreated complications of an unsafe abortion. In such situations, the interviewer's ethical responsibility is to refer the person to a sympathetic health practitioner. Not all problems will have such convenient solutions, but interviewers should be prepared to identify distress and respond with empathy and appropriate referral.

Closing while maintaining contact. Once the participant has accepted the role of conversational partner, it can be difficult to terminate the conversation. You will need to express thanks for the time taken to share valuable information, perhaps reiterating the confidentiality of the record. In case you need to return later to ask the participant to confirm or elaborate on a statement, it is wise to ask permission to call on the person again to verify contact information. Although the interview has ended, informal conversation usually continues. Be alert to casual banter because it may contain unexpected clues or new leads to answering the research question. Unless participants indicate that parting comments are off the record, make notes on your observations at the moment or as soon as possible.

Focus Groups

A focus group is the use of group interaction to produce data and insights that would be less accessible without the interaction found in a group (Morgan 1988, 12). The key phrase here is group interaction. Unlike simple group interviews in which several people may be interviewed at once for convenience, focus groups depend as much on the exchange of ideas among participants as they do on answers to specific questions from the interviewer. The interviewer, in fact, is called a moderator, underscoring the role of guide and facilitator in the group process.

Moderating a focus group has much in common with in-depth interviewing. Introducing topics with main questions, asking more specific follow-up questions to elicit more detailed information, and probing the meaning of responses are as important in focus group discussions as they are in individual interviews. The reader is referred to the in-depth interview section of this chapter.

A focus group is the use of group interaction to produce data and insights that would be less accessible without the interaction found in a group.

(Morgan 1988, 12)

The methodology of focused group interviews was first developed for social science during World War II by sociologists studying military morale and the impact of propaganda materials on public opinion (Merton et al. 1956). Later, sociologist Harold Blumer used focus groups in a series of drug studies, remarking that "A small number of … individuals who are acute observers and who are well-informed … brought together as a discussion and resource group, is more valuable many times over than a representative sample" (Blumer 1969, 41). Focus group discussion has also proved a useful tool for marketers studying consumer opinion on commercial products.

In recent years, focus group methodology has been applied increasingly to research in population and health. Its use by researchers and consultants in these areas has shed new light on people's understanding of fertility and HIV risk, health decision-making, gender perspectives in family planning, and the influence of gender on sexual decisions. On the other hand, indiscriminate use of focus groups by researchers with little experience in qualitative methods sometimes creates confusion about how and when focus groups should be used. In fact, in some circles their popularity has made focus groups seem synonymous with qualitative research. In practice, focus group discussions are only one of a growing number of qualitative methods, valuable in situations where the most rewarding data will come from interaction in a group (Morgan 1988).

As discussed in Chapter 3, there are relatively clear indicators for choosing a focus group over an individual in-depth interview. Groups can be highly effective sources of data for studies that focus on social norms, expectations, values, and beliefs. Especially rich topics for focus groups are those that stimulate people to share their own ideas and debate the views of others. Focus group discussions thrive on controversial topics. However, it is critical to the quality of the data that participants be well grounded in the topic, either through personal experience or a vested interest arising from a particular role or position. For example, a study of the acceptability of a new microbicide in a population at high risk of STI might suggest recruiting commercial sex workers who could speak from their experience of using the product with their clients. Or, if the purpose of the research is to explore the feasibility of community-based reproductive health education for young people, it would be useful to hear not only from adolescents, but from parents, teachers, and religious, political, and other community leaders whose views on adolescent sexual behavior could influence the program.

Composition and size of focus groups

Most focus groups are relatively homogeneous, composed of people who are similar with respect to characteristics related to the topic. A family planning study might start with people of childbearing age. But it soon could become apparent that women feel uncomfortable speaking with men about reproductive issues. Or younger women are sometimes reluctant to express their views in the presence of older women. Mothers may be unwilling to listen to women who have not borne children. *Both sex and age often become defining variables when assigning people to discussion groups.* Similar constraints may divide members of different ethnic groups, rural residents from urban, educated people from nonliterate, professional, and technical workers from manual workers. Or it may be important to the research design to segment participants for the sake of stratification in analysis, the ability to compare and contrast the views of different subsets of the population (see Chapter 6). As the study progresses, you may find it advisable to expand the sample if emerging data suggest tapping new or different sources of information.

For most purposes, groups of eight to ten participants are sufficient to stimulate good but manageable discussion for the moderator, who must keep the discussion focused while encouraging everyone to take part. The smaller the group, the less likely that discussion will express wider norms, values, or opinions. On the other hand, a large group is not only difficult to manage but may provide incomplete data if reticent members defer to their more voluble peers.

While you hope that everyone in the group will contribute freely and openly, it is important to select individuals who will not dominate the discussion or inhibit the participation of others. If the study design calls for the opinions of people in positions of authority — the company manager, a hospital director, or an official of the community — consider including them in individual interviews or as key informants rather than as focus group participants. Alternatively, you might decide to invite these authorities, or a subset of them, to take part in separate focus groups.

Should focus group participants be strangers or friends? Writers on focus group methodology often emphasize the importance of anonymity among participants, on the premise that one can speak more freely with strangers than with people one knows and will meet again. However, in many settings, especially in developing countries, it is neither feasible nor advisable to expect a group of strangers to participate in a discussion. It may be difficult to find participants who are not already acquainted. In some cultures women, and sometimes men, are uncomfortable sharing their perspectives with people they do not know. The investigator will base this decision on local norms of interaction. Under no circumstances should you allow observers or interested bystanders to listen to the discussion.

How many groups?

The rule of thumb in deciding how many focus groups to form is to conduct at least two for each defining demographic variable. For instance, if the groups are divided only by sex, four groups may be sufficient. In practice, focus groups are seldom divided on only one variable, and the necessary number of groups quickly multiplies. If two age categories (younger and older) are added, the number jumps to eight. Adding an education variable with three categories will bring you to 24 groups. And if you decide to conduct the study in three locales — rural, urban, and peri-urban — there will now be 72 discussion groups, an unwieldy sample size for most field studies. The lesson many qualitative researchers have learned is that you have to balance the number of variable subsets (sex, age, residence) against the resources (time, money, personnel) available for transcribing, translating, coding, and analyzing the data. This equation takes you back to the study design. If you have more groups than you can handle, the chances are that your study design is too complex for the resources at your disposal. It may be necessary to revisit the study objectives and focus them more tightly. Remember that establishing a comfortable balance between number of groups and available resources should take place at the level of design, not once you are in the field.

A normal rate for focus group data collection is one group per day, including transcription. A two-hour discussion is likely to generate 25 to 40 pages of transcript. In the above example, 72 discussions could yield as many as 2,880 pages to code and perhaps translate by the end of the study. Simple arithmetic demonstrates the importance of selecting criteria carefully to include variables essential to sound design while keeping the size of the data set within limits established by the research.

Collecting background information

A brief profile on each participant can provide valuable information for later analysis and presentation of the findings. Knowing something about the individuals whose comments are recorded on the transcript will help you describe your sample, interpret what participants have said, and analyze emerging themes in the light of contextual differences and similarities. Background information can also enliven reports by highlighting the people behind the findings ("A 30-year-old factory worker and mother of six commented that …"). If included in a focus group study, this information should be brief and clearly related to the research problem, such socio-demographic characteristics as age, education, occupation, marital status, or family size. In sexual and reproductive health research, qualitative investigators sometimes use information from the sexual and reproductive history to help them understand their data — age at first pregnancy, use of contraception, number of pregnancies and live births, desired number of children, and so forth.

The rules in collecting background data for focus group analysis are simple:

- keep it relevant
- keep it short
- keep it confidential

If socio-demographic or other data will enhance your analysis, it can be collected with participants' informed consent before the discussion begins. It is important to keep the background form simple; one page or less of easy, short-answer questions is usually sufficient to record a few relevant facts. Participants may provide the data by completing the forms themselves or responding orally to a researcher. This is not a group exercise; it is done individually to preserve confidentiality and anonymity. The forms are identified only by codes

Research versus Support: Focus Group Participants Living with HIV/AIDS

Michele G. Shedlin, Ph.D.
Sociomedical Resource Associates

Focus group discussions (FGDs) offer an opportunity for individuals to exchange ideas and validate personal experiences. This interaction is one of the methodological goals of FGDs, but it can also benefit the participants, who enjoy the opportunity to be heard and valued. However, it is crucial first, that facilitators anticipate potential problems that could arise from discussion of sensitive topics, and second, that they have the skills to prevent, control, or process such problems effectively.

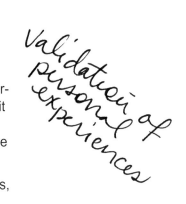

Validation of personal experiences

Whether discussing their own experiences or their perceptions of others, raising stressful topics such as risk behaviors, illness, dying, and loss can trigger powerful emotional reactions. Facilitators need guidelines to help them respond sensitively and appropriately to these situations. They also need to know when it is appropriate to continue the discussion or terminate it. At issue is the dilemma that can arise when the need for scientific rigor and systematic data collection are not possible without compromising the well-being of the group or an individual.

Because focus group participants must be willing to share their experiences and perspectives openly with the researcher and the group, an experienced facilitator will be aware of the following possibilities:

■ Emotional distress can emerge from the discussion at any point.

■ Some or all participants may have prior experience with group sessions for support or education, and these — rather than research — may be their only points of reference for group discussions.

■ When people are experiencing the stress of chronic illness, mutual empathy and support are a natural aspect of any group process.

■ When a group responds spontaneously to the emotional needs of any member, the facilitator's first priority is to the well-being of all of the participants; the second priority is to the research objectives.

Twenty years of work with marginalized people have brought me in close touch with the urban poor, the incarcerated, people living with HIV/AIDS, and affected individuals. To help focus group facilitators understand and resolve potential contradictions between the emotional needs of the group and the objectives of the research, I have developed the following guidelines:

Data Collection

(1) Establish ground rules for discussion, especially that people respect and listen to one another.

(2) When introducing the session, stress the purpose of the discussion, which is to *teach the researchers*. Remind participants that they are the experts and the reason for their recruitment is to share their knowledge and experience. Explain clearly that it may be tempting to become a support group, but that if possible, they should maintain their roles as teachers and advisors. This acknowledgment of the possibility clarifies the participant role and encourages both focus and thoughtfulness. Reinforcement of their role as teachers is always empowering, a role not previously experienced by many participants.

(3) Be aware of body language as well as what people are saying. Participants give nonverbal signals of distress, which often can be handled in a supportive way by the facilitator before the group intervenes. This may save a participant from experiencing (unwanted) temporary loss of control and from the embarrassment of tears or outbursts, and helps them to continue to participate.

(4) If an individual is not able to continue, acknowledge their distress and give them a quiet moment to regain composure; ask them what they need and what they would like to do. Most often the individual wants to continue and the group supports this verbally and nonverbally.

(5) If the person is not able to continue, either: a) allow group members to provide support and encouragement and continue; or b) allow the group to provide support, and the facilitator acknowledges the member's need and group's response and ends the session.

(6) You should have three major concerns:

- that the person in distress has appropriate support and a referral if necessary;

- that the experience is processed with the group so that the participants are not discouraged or frustrated, and their supportive reaction is validated as the most important issue; and

- that if the individual and group want to continue, the research focus has not been lost and the collection of valid data is still possible.

(7) If you decide that the research focus has been lost, thank the group for what they have accomplished and minimize the early termination. The session should not end abruptly, but be allowed to have appropriate closure with discussion that may or may not be relevant to the research but is necessary for the participants.

(8) To respond appropriately to emotional distress, you must be thoroughly informed on HIV/AIDS issues and should have access to a list of the local referral services available. Ideally, you should have familiarity and access to a local HIV/AIDS service agency or point person wherever the research is being implemented.

(9) Unless you have appropriate professional training and credentials, and prior permission from the facility or program within which the discussion is taking place, the support group mode should never become the objective of the session.

Responsible focus group research with persons living with or affected by HIV/AIDS adds an important way to gather the qualitative data that inform our response to the epidemic. The focus group method also can be an interesting and positive experience for participants. I believe the researcher's highest priority when conducting focus groups should be to see that all participants have a positive experience and do not leave the session in distress or frustration. Our research objectives should always be secondary to participants' well-being. With good planning, it is possible to ensure that both participants and researchers are satisfied with their collaboration.

that correspond to code numbers worn by the individual participants during the discussion. Completed forms are securely stored, accessible only to the researchers and their assistants. Of course, the researcher will respect the preference of any participant who wishes not to be so identified. However, in our experience, most participants like their coded tags. They are a reminder that a system is in place to protect the anonymity of anything they say. Sometimes participants refer to each other by the numbers they are wearing, even when they know each other by name ("I agree with 8 that..."). In the following pages, we will describe how participant code numbers can be used by note-takers and entered into the transcript for analysis.

Conducting the discussion

As we have seen earlier in this chapter, qualitative interviewing requires a high level of interpersonal skill in developing conversational partners. Similarly, the special task of the focus group moderator is to create a group of conversational partners, listening with nonjudgmental interest while keeping the discussion focused and moving (see Appendix 3, page 212). Whether individual interview or group discussion, the responsive interviewer or moderator shows interest, curiosity, empathy, and encouragement, but also must be flexible, creative, and able to tailor questions and comments to the unique responses of each person. A topic guide, discussed later in this chapter, is an important tool for keeping the discussion centered while encouraging participants to speak naturally and spontaneously. As in the in-depth interview, a topic as sensitive as reproductive health is likely to be more acceptable to members of a focus group if the moderator is the same sex as the participants. If women are not accustomed to expressing their views to men, even the most skilled male moderator may inhibit discussion. Other characteristics will depend on the topic of discussion and cultural norms that prescribe who can discuss what with whom. Similarly, respondents in developing countries who have had little opportunity to know Westerners may be uncomfortable with an American or European interviewer. An effective partnership may therefore depend on cultural similarity and the ability of researchers and participants to understand each other's language and perspectives.

The moderator and note-taker team[†]

To ensure accurate data and to facilitate analysis, focus group discussions usually are taped. While videotaping would capture more nonverbal expression, participants may find the camera more intrusive than a simple tape recorder. For sensitive data collection, we therefore recommend audiocassettes. However, over-reliance on the tape recorder is a common pitfall with negative consequences when technology fails. The most efficient organization is a team of two trained moderators, one to guide the discussion and the other to monitor the tape recorder while recording as much of the discussion as possible. Although verbatim text from transcripts will be of great value in the analysis, notes on the discussion are also important. The skilled field researcher learns to take good notes unobtrusively and quickly expand them after the interview, regardless of whether the discussion has been taped. In case of an inaudible recording, a power failure, or lost tapes, the researcher will have recorded on paper enough of the discussion to preserve the raw data. In addition to copious notes on the verbal process, the note-taker also enters observations which will enrich the transcript with nonverbal messages that have a bearing on the discussion. For example, notes might state that "Participant A appeared angry and left the group" or that "The group seemed much amused by this remark."

[†]Adapted from Hogle et al. 1994.

If background information has been collected, it is usually the note-taker's responsibility to assure that data identification codes correspond to codes worn by participants. The note-taker follows the discussion carefully, indicating the number or letter for each speaker. The code and the first few words of each comment are usually enough to identify the speaker when the note-taker's observations are transferred later to the transcript. It is not essential to identify every comment, and in fast-paced discussions, it is often impossible. However, to the extent you are able to identify who said what, you will have a richer analysis and a livelier presentation, because comments from the transcript can be amplified with information about the speaker. (Integrating participants' comments and characteristics into the report is discussed in Chapter 7.)

With the note-taker playing the role of recorder and observer, the moderator is responsible for creating a comfortable climate for open exchange, encouraging participation, and guiding the discussion. As participants enter, the moderator seats them in an informal circle with the note-taker seated just outside the circle to avoid distracting the group. The tape recorder is placed where it can easily record the discussion but with as little distraction to participants as possible.

The moderator welcomes the group and introduces herself or himself and the note-taker, explaining the role of each. The moderator also explains the purpose of the tape recorder: to enable the researchers to capture ideas that emerge from the discussion and not identify the speakers by name. Participants are assured that written reports will not include names and that tapes will not be shared outside the research team. In the process of administering informed consent, remind participants of the

group's responsibility to guard the confidentiality of the discussion. Partici-pants should also understand that there are no right and wrong answers and that all opinions are welcome.

It is important for participants to understand the goals of the discussion. However, "clarifying goals does not necessarily mean revealing ... the questions under study. Clarifying goals does mean communicating to participants what you want to know from them" (Basch 1987, 416). Indeed, in an overly informed group, members may obligingly supply the answers they think you want to hear, regardless of their truth. Once there is general understanding of the topic and procedure, the moderator may then ask participants to introduce themselves, although if anonymity in the group is important, introductions can be replaced with informal conversation and nonthreatening questions to put the group at ease and encourage them to talk among themselves.

The moderator then asks participants to accept ground rules, such as speaking one at a time, not interrupting each other, and speaking clearly and slowly so the tape can pick up the words. Participants should be asked to suggest additional ground rules, which will reinforce the idea that their contributions are a valuable part of the research process. The moderator encourages participants to speak freely, addressing questions any way they want, while at the same time reminding them that discussions sometimes wander off track and may need to be refocused. This can be a difficult course to steer but may be greatly facilitated by a well-designed — yet flexible — topic guide, as discussed later in this chapter.

Following this warm-up period, the first topic is introduced. The moderator should observe the group closely, watching for signs that some participants might merely be agreeing with others rather than voicing opinions of their own. Other signs of potential problems in the group process are participants who are unenthusiastic, aloof, confused, overly positive or excessively negative; are highly critical of others; or attempt to control the discussion with their own points of view. Early identification makes it easier to respond effectively to these problems. For example, a domineering participant might be seated next to the moderator, or the group might be reminded that ground rules include respectful listening.

Ending the discussion

At the end of the discussion, the moderator may ask the participants to summarize what they have said, adding any additional comments they want to include. Or, the moderator might supply the summary, beginning with, "Since we are almost out of time, I will try to summarize what you have told me." The summary is a chance to clarify issues and give the group a sense of work accomplished. Participants are able to restate points and correct any misunderstanding of the moderator. The tape recorder is then turned off. Most groups conclude with light refreshments, which can be organized by local assistants.

Some researchers include a debriefing with participants at the close of the discussion, inviting feedback on the discussion experience. Did they feel included? Were they comfortable with the topics? Do they think the topics were fully explored? Were there topics or questions which should have been discussed but were not? Can they think of how the discussion should have been conducted differently? Debriefings can be useful not only for evaluating and revising the discussion protocol, but also for additional context in analysis of the data. They are also an important learning resource for the field team.

The question of reimbursement to participants frequently arises in focus group research. Should participants be reimbursed for the time they contribute to discussing the research questions? Projects that pay focus group participants sometimes come under criticism for raising expectations that future researchers may not be able to meet. A compromise is to offer each participant a modest gift that expresses the researchers' appreciation without setting an unrealistic precedent. A rule of thumb on this issue is to take local customs and expectations into consideration. If people have come to expect payment, then it is appropriate to pay them according to the local scale.

Appendix 4 (see page 215) elaborates on the steps in managing a focus group discussion. These steps can also help guide your preparation of a budget. Appendix 5 (see page 217) shows an example of costs to consider when proposing a focus group study, from the planning stage to interpretation of the data and final presentations.

Structured Data Collection Techniques

It is often the case that individuals or groups will be able to organize and articulate their thoughts more easily if they have a concrete reference point. There are a number of ways to add this kind of structure to interviews and focus groups without compromising flexibility and spontaneity. Centering a question on an image or task adds a tangible dimension to an otherwise abstract issue. It also helps to frame potentially uncomfortable issues in a less personal context. The interview or focus group guide might start a topic with a statement of presumed fact: "We have heard that women are not going to the clinic for prenatal care. Can you comment on that?" or "A woman in another village told us that she had been beaten several times by her husband. Are you familiar with such a problem in your own community?" This indirect structure is likely to elicit a more open response than "Why did you not attend the antenatal clinic?" or "Have you ever experienced domestic abuse?"

The following techniques for adding structure to data collection can be used with almost any qualitative method, particularly when you are interested in helping a group to center on specific research issues, as in focus group discussions and participatory action research.

Freelisting and pile sorts

An old technique with application to qualitative research in reproductive health is *freelisting*, combined with *pilesorting*, in which participants are asked to make a list of all instances of some phenomenon. Items on the categories list are then transferred to cards that participants sort into piles according to their own criteria and labels. This approach is based on the principle that people make sense of their worlds by grouping their observations and experiences in classes known as *domains*. A cultural domain is "a set of items or things that are all of the same type or category" (Schensul, Schensul, and LeCompte 1999). How people assign items to domains indicates to the researcher how they interpret the meanings of these items in their own lives. For example, if you are interested in popular perceptions of STI, you might ask participants in a study to list all the diseases and symptoms they can think of and organize them in groups according to common characteristics. The common denominators they use can tell you a great deal about the meanings people attach to STI symptoms. You may discover that people classify symptoms according to traditional notions of cause and effect, attributing some to supernatural causes, while others sort the cards into piles that represent biomedical or environmental explanations.

To take this example a step farther, you might want to explore possible links between cultural definitions and choice of provider. You could ask participants to group the items in help-seeking categories, including different types of healers as well as peer consultation, self-help, or no action at all. Whether individual or group data collection, this technique lends itself well to qualitative exploration, because in probing the logic behind assignment of items to categories, the researcher may uncover reasons for popular perceptions and behaviors that may not otherwise be apparent. The lists that participants create are, themselves, an important linguistic tool if they provide insight into cultural expression on topics related to sexual and reproductive health.

Most participants enjoy sorting items into categories and then talking about their decisions. The process itself can be interesting and the outcome motivating, as people begin to reinterpret familiar experiences in new ways.

Photo narrative

The interviewer may present a visual aid such as a poster or photograph and ask participants to talk about what it means to them. In a study of Latina women's perceptions of the quality of prenatal care, participants were shown photographic prompts — pictures taken in a clinic setting with staff and client actors (Bender and Harbour 2001). An interviewer asked participants to describe each photograph, including how the woman in the photo was feeling. She then asked the participant if the photograph reminded her of any experience she had had and, if so, to tell the story of that experience. As these researchers point out, photographic prompts allow the participant to talk about herself in the third person, projecting experiences and opinions that may not be socially desirable onto the subject in the photograph.

Also known as *photo voice* (Bender and Castro 2000; Wang 1999; Wang and Burris 1997), the photo narrative technique is well suited to feminist inquiry because as documentary evidence, it has the potential to give "voice" to people on the margins of society. Researchers have put cameras into the hands of women, enabling them to capture scenes that reflect their own lives and to communicate their perceptions and experiences more effectively than by words alone. The photographic record empowered the women to enter into critical dialogue on issues that affected their everyday lives and to present their concerns directly to policymakers.

Storytelling

Another way to introduce structure is by telling a story — fictitious but designed to include issues at the heart of the research problem. A focus group study of sexual decision-making and HIV/AIDS risk in Haiti presented the topic through the story of an imaginary young woman, Joujou, who believed she was at great risk of acquiring HIV from her partner, René (Ulin et al. 1995). Issues to be explored were embedded in a culturally familiar context of women's economic dependence and sexual subordination. When she discovers that René has other sexual partners, Joujou must decide how to protect herself. The interviewer then opens the discussion to the group, inviting their ideas and suggestions, while prompting them to think beyond their initial reactions with such questions as "How do you think René would react to that?" or "How can Joujou support herself and her children if she leaves him?" Participants in both men's and women's groups quickly recognized Joujou's dilemma and entered into vigorous discussion of alternatives and their consequences for women's lives. As in Bender and Harbour's photo narrative study, storytelling relieved the pressure of self-disclosure by asking people to comment on the problems and decisions of another person, albeit like themselves.

It is important to note that, used in focus groups, these techniques elicit participants' perceptions of cultural norms, views, and behaviors of people like themselves and are not a dependable record of case-based behavior. As discussion builds, speakers frequently identify with the photo or story actors, switching easily from third person to first person narrative. Nevertheless, in most instances only the individual interview and similar techniques, with or without additional structure, can adequately capture individual perceptions and behavior.

won't capture indiv. behav. → only interviews

Exploring the Birth-Weight Paradox with a Photo Narrative Technique

Deborah Bender, Ph.D. and Dina Castro, M.P.H., Ph.D.
School of Public Health, University of North Carolina at Chapel Hill

In the United States, prenatal care is positively associated with improved birth outcomes, particularly the reduction of low birth weight. However, birth weights of Mexican-born Latinos tend to be higher than those of Latinos born in the United States. This relationship is surprising, since recently arrived Latino immigrants are less likely to have received timely or adequate prenatal care (Scribner and Dwyer 1989). The birth-weight paradox has remained constant regardless of the mother's age, marital status or educational attainment (Cobas et al. 1996).

The idea of resilience offers a conceptual framework for studying the birth-weight paradox. Resilience has been defined as a universal capacity that allows a person, group, or community to prevent, minimize, or overcome the damaging effects of adversity (Rutter 1993). Gaining understanding of what generates resilience offers an opportunity to develop initiatives that will help people to be less vulnerable in the face of adversity (Werner 1993).

We wanted to know why birth outcomes to newly arrived Latinas were better than those of their U.S.-born counterparts. Through focus groups and photo narratives, we explored topics related to pregnancy, prenatal care, and social support with Latina women, using their pregnancy experiences to probe for their perceptions of which factors are protective — give them resilience — and which pose a risk to their health status.

After the focus group discussion, women were invited to assist in the collection of data by serving as community photographers. Their two-week assignment was to take pictures of people, places, and things they considered important to their health and well-being (Williams 1984). Each woman selected six to eight photographs to illustrate her personal story, which she elaborated in an individual, in-depth interview. For each photograph, the woman described a) who was in the picture; b) what was happening; and c) why the picture was important to her.

The following themes of resilience and risk were identified through analysis of the focus groups and photo narratives transcripts:

- access to health care services and self-care during pregnancy
- strong family relationships, especially with one's mother
- aspirations for a better life in the United States
- education for one's children
- dreams of eventual return to Mexico
- unanticipated hardships of life in the United States, particularly related to language barriers

Data Collection

Examples of the concerns expressed by the women are presented below:

Catalina delayed initiation of prenatal care due to the pressure of work. She felt that the quality of care was compromised by language differences. She explained:

Well, when I arrived [at the hospital] here they began to treat me a little badly. I don't speak English, but I speak a little. Then, when they saw that I could speak some English, they began to treat me better because I was trying to communicate with them.

Maintaining strong family relationships was a theme expressed repeatedly by the women. Angélica was pregnant with her first child in this country. Her sister was nearby, but she still found it necessary to call her mother in Mexico to discuss her fears. Her mother reassured her that her pregnancy was normal. Angelica explained:

A mother always listens; a mother always helps; a father protects you. Here, no. Here, nobody protects you; nobody listens, nobody pampers you.

One woman's photograph of a telephone hanging on an otherwise blank wall spoke to the importance of regular phone contact with absent family members. The photographer, Carmen, explained her selection:

The telephone is very important for communication. You can communicate with your family [in Mexico]. It is not considered a luxury in this country, but a necessity. It is not like in my country; here the lines go to everywhere.

Carmen also described a photograph of herself with her language teacher and talked of the importance of learning English to be able to manage one's own daily life.

Knowing English you can solve problems that happen to you better. Before, my husband had to go with me to the doctor, the dentist, the bank, and the post office. He was losing time from work. Now, I do not have to depend so much on him.

When the women spoke of returning to Mexico, some of their words hinted that their dreams might not be realized. Opportunities for work and economic gain in the United States seem to take priority. Luisa already knew that her husband had little intention of returning.

When I ask my husband "When are we going back to Mexico?" he answers "I am not going to put myself in the position of working in Mexico, having to resign myself to earn 200 pesos per week while here I earn that money in a day."

Although economic opportunity in the United States has enabled the families of the women who participated in the focus groups to create a better life, each woman spoke of unanticipated difficulties. Elena took a photograph showing the wrought iron staircase in an otherwise dark apartment entrance. Three women are ascending the stairs; the viewer sees only their backs. She explained that although living conditions are better in the United States than in Mexico, there are risks here, too. In Mexico, everyone knew every one else; it was safe. In the United States, women were afraid to go out. She summarized:

Here, we live in a cage of gold, but it never stops being a prison.

Elena's eloquent but simple words describe the paradox of life in the United States for Latino immigrants.

When we asked the women to take photographs of people, places, and things that were important to them, we hoped they would select themes that could be classified as related to resilience or risk. In fact, the photographic choices of the women were exquisite, their stories poignant. The women were able to articulate clearly how the people or objects they had photographed were important in their lives. It was apparent that the factors they identified had contributed, negatively or positively, to how the women evaluated their health in pregnancy. Spontaneously, they selected themes related to demographic characteristics and medical and behavioral risks that are recognized to have an impact on health status during pregnancy.

Body mapping

Body mapping is a projective technique in which participants draw maps of the human body. It is particularly useful in studies of people's perceptions of reproductive anatomy and physiology, fertility awareness, and other reproductive health issues. It may also be a more comfortable means of expression for participants who are reticent to speak openly about sexual matters. As a visual representation of the participant's understanding of reproductive function, the participant's drawing, or body map, then becomes the focus for in-depth conversation with the interviewer.

A participatory action project in Zambia used body mapping to understand how Zambian youth conceptualize the reproductive system (Shah 1999). Small groups of adolescents divided by age and sex were asked to make simple sketches of the human body to show how the reproductive organs function. The researcher then asked each one to label the body parts and explain their functions, prompting them with questions such as "How does a woman get pregnant?" or "How can pregnancy be prevented?" Researchers were able to identify gaps and distortions that could be addressed through intervention. As the author of this report points out, body mapping can be combined with other qualitative methods or expanded into picture stories, or cartoons, as the basis for discussing sexual relationships. Although semi- and nonliterate people will not be able to write labels on their maps, research has shown that they can participate in a body mapping project, interpreting their drawings orally to the researcher (Shah 1999).

Social network analysis

Social network analysis is based on the premise that individuals seldom make decisions in isolation. Through network research, we are able to explore attitudes, beliefs, and actions of individuals in the context of group affiliations. Tracing a person's social network helps the researcher understand what people do and think in relation to group norms and expectations. It also reveals how people, as well as knowledge and information, circulate among different groups. Discovering the social network can be a first step in developing effective interventions to reduce behavior that puts people's health at risk.

Social network research has been used extensively to study risk behavior associated with sharing drug injection equipment and engaging in unprotected sex with HIV-infected partners. For example, network studies of heroin injectors have found that many were introduced to hard drugs, or regularly shared drugs and drug-using equipment, with relatives. Moreover, these studies show that cousins and other close relatives were heavily represented in the drug-using networks of people who had started injecting heroin as adolescents (Pino et al. 1999). These findings suggest that to be successful, interventions designed to prevent hard drug use among adolescents must address issues in family addiction as well.

Network analysis begins by identifying not only the network itself but also its members:

- What sets these people apart from nonmembers?
- What qualities do they share?
- What brings them together and how strong is the bond?

The task is to determine the criteria for inclusion or exclusion and establish network boundaries. This process may be as easy as obtaining a class roster or list of employees, or as difficult as patiently tracking down individuals through participant observation and key informant interviews. Clues to network boundaries can be discovered by asking people what makes a member. Once the network is defined and its members identified, the qualitative researcher proceeds by in-depth interviews and participant observation to explore the meaning of the relationships among network members.

In northern Thailand, where unwanted pregnancy and STI rates among young people are high, researchers turned to social network analysis to help develop new programs to reduce sexual risk (Bond et al. 1999). Snowball sampling was used to identify networks. Two young women selected randomly at each of three locales — public dormitories, workplaces, and entertainment venues — were each asked to name five friends they frequently went out with at night. These friends were contacted and asked to name five more friends. When no new names were mentioned, the process stopped, yielding three networks of affiliated youth at each site. In-depth interviews with individual network members explored cultural norms and behavior related to friends and romantic partners. Discovering sexual linkages led to identification of youth subcultures, communication channels, and patterns of risk behavior that varied among the networks. With this information as a base, program planners could then work with natural peer leaders to establish an outreach program that focused on healthier sexual decisions among different categories of youth at risk. Although the number of members in any one network may be small, the Thai example illustrates that knowing the characteristics of the network can help researchers and program planners understand the health risks of its members.

Social network studies often combine qualitative and quantitative techniques in the same research design. From a quantitative perspective, investigators use surveys and statistical analyses to measure relationships within, and linkages between, networks. Computer software for quantitative network analysis enables the researcher to create visual images of network relationships in which each member is connected to other members.

Qualitative analysis takes a more holistic approach in order to explore the meaning and context of the network relationships in a natural setting. Combining qualitative and quantitative methods is a powerful way not only to *measure* network characteristics, but also to *understand* the diffusion of ideas and behaviors within and among networks.

Participatory Methods

Participatory Research (PR) is not a specific method but rather the use of multiple methods to solve a problem through group action. Methodology depends on the research problem and the skills and resources of the group, but *the common denominator is local participation in decision-making and in implementing the study process* (Díaz and Simmons 1999). There are several ways to incorporate participatory action in a study, but all have in common the objective to help work groups or communities analyze their own situations and develop strategic interventions. Variations on participatory approaches are many and include Participatory Action Research, Rural Rapid Appraisal, Participatory Rapid Appraisal, and Participatory Learning and Action.

The concept of subject as participant in the research process is basic to qualitative design. However, PR takes the concept a step farther to cast participants as problem-solvers in their communities. The choice of topic therefore depends as much or more on a problem the participant group wants to solve as it does on the interests of the researcher. Participants typically are community groups that collaborate with the researcher to define a problem; identify information needed; collect, process, and interpret the information; and take action consistent with the results. Roles tend to blur as researchers and participants pool their knowledge to arrive at concrete solutions to problems.

Box 4.2

A Participatory Action Model: The PALS Program in Zambia

In 1996, CARE International in Zambia was planning to start a new project in adolescent sexual and reproductive health. Their goal was to reduce sexual and reproductive health morbidity and mortality by promoting behavior change and encouraging more adolescent-friendly health services.

Having had little experience with adolescents, the planners began by asking adolescents themselves to share their perspectives on reproductive health needs and concerns. Before any programmatic decisions were made, all CARE staff took part in a training workshop on the methodology of Participatory Learning and Action. Formal training was followed by a participatory appraisal with adolescents in one Lusaka community. The results led to establishment of the Partnership for Adolescent Sexual and Reproductive Health (PALS) Project and 12 more appraisals in Lusaka, Livingston, and Ndola, where the PALS Project was subsequently implemented.

Using results from the participatory appraisals, CARE submitted a proposal to donors and received funding for the PALS Project. The field methodology developed for PALS included an appraisal tool kit which adolescent participants could use in their own communities. The tool kit consisted of 17 participatory activities, including interviews, groups discussions, pictures and storytelling, role-play, mapping, and other techniques. With the support of clinicians and CARE staff, the teens used these techniques to identify problems and motivate peers to evaluate their own sexual decisions. Sharing and disseminating results from their appraisals also created an effective climate for helping young people work with health providers, teachers, and other community members on a peer education program that ultimately led to increased condom use and more effective use of family planning and antenatal and postnatal services.

(Shah 1999)

A PR project can use any qualitative method, usually multiple techniques and sometimes combined with quantitative methods. A common PR tool is geographic mapping. For example, a PR study to strengthen the link between an underutilized rural health center and the community might begin by mapping the community to identify geographic constraints such as the distances people have to walk to get to the center. Participants might then use their map to sample local residents for informal interviews in which they would gather information on experiences people had when they attended the health center and reasons they did or did not return. Their study would be likely to include direct observation of the health center itself aided

by a semi-structured guide. Based on their interpretation of these data, participants would arrive by consensus at a plan of action directed to specific policy-makers or providers willing to discuss and help implement the proposed intervention strategy.

Participatory research clearly has both rewards and challenges. On the one hand, PR builds knowledge from the ground up, involves stakeholders in defining problems and identifying solutions, links research directly to action, and increases local self-reliance through experience in systematic problem-solving. However, to make PR work, you must adopt attitudes and expectations that may be significantly different from standard professional norms of scientific research. You will have to make the transition from researcher to facilitator and trainer, stepping back from the dominant position, sharing ownership of the project, and encouraging participants to take an active role in project decisions. In fact, "the key difference between participatory and conventional methodologies lies in the location of power in the research process" (Cornwall and Jewkes 1995). Your skill as facilitator-trainer may be more important for the success of the project than your credentials as a research scientist. You may have to make compromises on the choice of methods, arbitrate differences among participants on interpretation of the data, or find alternative solutions to a problem when the group's recommendations are inconsistent with available resources. Finally, since any participatory study by definition has a specific activist agenda, it is important to understand that resulting grassroots social action may be as important as — or even more important than — the publication of findings in professional journals.

Topic Guides

Experienced qualitative data collectors often gather meaningful data with little more than a set of topics as a guide; the research questions are clear in their minds, and the techniques of qualitative data collection are their normal ways of working. In the course of designing the study, researchers may also have spent time getting to know the people and the setting through preliminary participant observation. By the time they are ready to conduct interviews or focus groups, topics flow easily from the research questions, aided by familiarity with the language of the study population. Interviewers may also have memorized the list of topics to be covered and can direct conversation spontaneously from one to another, stopping to clarify points or probe comments or perhaps return to earlier questions as needed to ensure that participants have gone as far as they can with each topic.

However, many who collect qualitative data are new to these techniques and will benefit from a more structured set of guidelines. Many researchers prefer a semi-structured topic guide with questions that reflect the initial themes and subthemes contained in the basic research problem. This kind of tool may be a set of standardized open-ended questions, but more often it shows examples of how questions can be worded, as well as being a reminder of the material to be covered (see Table 3.3, page 64). The topic guide can also suggest follow-up questions for various possible responses and examples of probes to elicit information at greater depth. If stories or other scenarios will be presented to stimulate ideas, they should be included in the guide.

Interviewers are encouraged to use their own words in the interview but to keep firmly in mind a statement of purpose for each question, referring to the guide as needed. For example, how well will this community accept emergency contraception or the use of condoms for dual protection against pregnancy and STIs? Interviews and group discussions can take many paths, moving toward and sometimes away from the key problem. Organizing the topic guide around a few central questions can help keep you oriented in the right direction, following possible new leads but always returning to the purpose of the study.

Although we urge all interviewers and focus group moderators to state questions in a natural way and not to read semi-structured guides as they would the questions on a structured survey instrument, many will feel more confident with some specific questions to help them manage the interview or discussion. Appendix 6 (see page 218) presents examples of several topic guides created for different purposes.

Box 4.3

Constructing a Topic Guide

Compose search questions. Reread the research protocol at least once, concentrating especially on the research objectives and associated problem statements. Turn the statements into a short list of broad questions that reflect what you want to learn in the study. Interviewers should commit this list to memory. Example: *I want to know how people in this community would react to a campaign to promote dual method use (DMU). Do they see themselves as needing protection from both pregnancy and STI? What factors would encourage or discourage DMU?*

Identify topic and subtopics. Subtopics are variations on the more general topics. There may be more than one topic in a single research objective, and each topic may have several subtopics. Topic: Acceptability of DMU. Subtopics: Understanding of DMU, experience with DMU, perception of partner's opinion.

Decide on a sequence. Arrange topic and subtopics in a logical sequence that suggests a natural flow for discussion. The pattern and sequence of themes do not have to follow the order of research objectives in the proposal.

Develop sample questions. Each topic or subtopic may have three kinds of questions: a main question, follow-up questions, and probe questions. The main question introduces the topic. Follow-up questions get more specific and take the discussion to a deeper level. Probe questions go even deeper, seeking clarification, asking for more detail.

Select projective techniques. Decide whether the addition of projective techniques will help participants identify with the issues. Examples are stories, photos, posters, and role-plays. Projective techniques are especially useful for encouraging expression on sensitive topics, such as sexual norms or illegal abortion, or on abstract issues, such as quality of life, self-esteem, or empowerment.

Prepare opening and closing statements. Compose sample statements that let participants know that the interview or discussion group is beginning or has ended. The opening statement includes an explanation of the project and information for informed consent. The closing statement thanks participants for sharing their insights and experiences, and reminds them again of the confidentiality of the data.

For examples of detailed topic guides on sexual risk, men's health and other issues, see Appendix 6 (see page 218).

Conclusion

Collecting qualitative data is a process of bringing what you want to learn together with what you observe and with what participants know and have experienced (Rubin and Rubin 1995). This chapter has emphasized the concept of partnership in participant observation, qualitative interviewing and focus group discussion. Although we advocate a semi-structured topic guide to help the interviewer or moderator keep the research problem in focus, flexibility is critical. Successful data collectors are prepared to adapt the tool and their personal styles to the natural flow of the discussion, wherever it takes them, as long as they are learning. Qualitative interviewing therefore demands versatility and sometimes quick change when the mood of the interview shifts or unexpected but important content interrupts the planned sequence. Similarly, participant observers return to the field each day open to new and possibly surprising discoveries.

Whether in observation, interview, or group discussion, researchers often feel bombarded with stimuli. Participants eager to share their experiences and ideas can quickly overwhelm an inexperienced data collector with valuable information. Information overload can be managed by careful planning and meticulous record-keeping. The conceptual framework, imprinted on the interviewer or observer, is a valuable compass, helping to keep a firm grasp on the purpose and main questions of the research and to locate what participants say or do in the emerging picture. And even the most experienced qualitative researcher does not expect to remember all the details of field experience. Clear transcriptions and detailed field notes are key to skillful management of large amounts of information which otherwise will be lost to science.

Each interview, each focus group discussion, each trip to the field can be an adventure. You will not know in advance exactly what will emerge, but with a clear sense of direction, flexibility, and enthusiasm for the unknown, your discoveries can become valuable contributions to qualitative understanding of sexual and reproductive health.

C H A P T E R 5

Logistics in the Field

*Reason and logic are needed to chart your
way through the woods … painstaking
planning, analysis, and execution, testing
the ground every step of the way. [But]
human compassion and understanding are
also necessary throughout the journey.*

(Fetterman 1992, 87)

Drawing on the experiences of many qualitative researchers, this chapter bridges the transition from study design to implementation in the field. In the following pages, we help you create a research-friendly environment by anticipating some of the pivotal decisions and tasks that will launch your study: from establishing contacts and involving key stakeholders to assembling a field team; training and monitoring interviewers; protecting confidentiality; developing and testing materials; organizing equipment and supplies; and recording, transcribing, translating, and storing data.

Logistics in the Field

Most qualitative research is interactive — composed of many face-to-face, often intimate, conversations with study participants. Ideally, we would spend long periods of time in the community or other setting, getting to know the people informally in their everyday lives. Researchers who are able to live in the research site during the study have found that participating in local events, observing both the routine and the exceptional, adds a great deal to their understanding of the social context (Hull 2001). Yet practical limits on time and resources may be constraints. In large studies, you may also be supervising the work of trained assistants who actually collect the data. In such circumstances, it is crucial to find ways to stay as close as possible to the field; for example, by frequent visits to the site, talking with local people, reviewing transcripts, and questioning data collectors about their observations and progress. If you are working across national, cultural, or language barriers, you may have a counterpart who will be your interpreter and guide. In any case, you or that colleague has to be there — listening, questioning, hearing, observing.

Although in this chapter we cover day-to-day issues in implementation, every field experience has its unique challenges, some predictable and some not. With careful planning, however, you will be able to identify and manage many of the risks and resources that will influence the outcomes of your study. And once you have become familiar with people at your study site and they with you, you will have no end of on-site expert advice to help you negotiate a successful field experience.

Contacts: Introductions and Approvals

Research textbooks that go from study design to data collection often fail to provide directions through the maze of introductions and permissions that stand between the researcher and the study participants. Yet how you approach these challenges may be key to the success of your whole project. In most situations, the researcher needs to be highly visible — an active participant, known and trusted in the community. In addition, a critical facet of interpretative understanding is knowing the study participants' world or the social context in which they live. You are more likely to be welcomed into that world if you have presented yourself and your study in a culturally appropriate manner. Pay attention to district medical officers, community officials, heads of organizations, and other local leaders, because they may have their own vested interests in your presence as well as your findings. Some may be protective of their constituents, others may fear possible negative consequences from your research. Still others may expect unrealistic support from you on some local issue. Take the time to explain the purpose and implementation of the study, turning potential adversaries into partners. Keep in mind that community leaders not only control access to the study site, but can also help you understand local culture, customs, and personalities.

Introductions to stakeholders

Most investigators start with introductions to district officers, medical and nursing directors, women's advocates, religious leaders, teachers, or others invested in the program or community. Is the political climate in this community or agency authoritarian, or do individuals generally make their own decisions on matters that would affect their participation in the study? Try to identify influential leaders whose views could potentially affect others' decisions on whether or not to participate. Do not overlook informal leaders, including influential women in the community and people who may not occupy positions of formal authority but tend to be consulted by others who know and respect them.

Visit these individuals, making appointments if possible, to introduce yourself and your study. In some communities, you may be expected to present yourself to a governing council who, along with the mayor or administrative head, will decide whether to approve the activity you propose. Similarly, a clinic director might ask you to explain your ideas to a board or to the clinic staff. Community leaders and local officials frequently take their cues from their constituents in deciding what stance to take on a proposal coming to them from the outside.

Remember that getting appointments and permissions can be time-consuming. The data-collection schedule you developed for your study probably has little relevance in the time frames of most community leaders and administrators. Take possible delays into account when you plan the study, and regard this introductory phase as a vital part of the research process. Approached this way, an otherwise frustrating delay can become an opportunity to become better acquainted with the research site.

Family influences

Individuals' decisions to participate in your study may also depend on the influence of family members. Many research problems in sexual and reproductive health contain culturally sensitive material;

women whose independence is limited by their subordination to more powerful family members may be fearful of consenting to participate in such a study. If they do consent, they may feel limited in how much of their lives they dare reveal without danger of recrimination. The same caveat applies to women in casual unions with sexual partners. In authoritarian relationships like these, the researcher may have to present the purpose of the study to a head of household, whether husband, father, mother-in-law, or unmarried partner. If so, the presentation should be honest but relatively general, with firm insistence on the privacy of the interview. Another approach to winning cooperation of powerful family leaders is to invite them to share their own views on the topic in separate, and equally confidential, interviews — whether or not such an exchange is part of your study design. Showing respect for the opinion of an otherwise resistant person not only involves him or her in a positive way, but may offer interesting insights that you might have missed.

On the other hand, in studies of particularly sensitive issues, full disclosure on the topic of the research may put the participant at risk in her family or community. In such a circumstance, your ethical priority is to protect the participant. In our study of clandestine users of contraception in Mali, researchers and providers alike were careful to help participants maintain secrecy from husbands who, the women felt, might punish them for attending a family planning clinic or even participating in the study (Castle et al. 1999).

Involving Policy-makers and Change Agents

Research can often influence policy or the way services are delivered. If your intent is to link your study results to local policies and programs, it is important to include policy-makers, service providers, and nongovernmental organizations (NGOs) early in the design and implementation.

For example, ask staff of the ministry of health to orient you to particular resources and needs of the study population; meet with a member of parliament who has a special interest in the problem you plan to study; introduce the study to the district commissioner or other local authority; or discuss the study with medical and nursing officers in charge of health services in the area. Invite suggestions for implementation and be open to possible new ways of articulating the research question for a better fit between the purpose of your study and policy-makers' goals for improving the well-being of the population.

Establishing reciprocity by including stakeholder questions not only facilitates access to the study population, but also may result in a stronger research design with findings more relevant to the problems and policy needs of the institution. As cited earlier, when one of the authors introduced a proposed study of contraceptive decision-making among women to the administrators of a family planning clinic in Bamako, Mali, they said they would like to know more about how women involve their husbands in the decision. Partner negotiation was therefore introduced as a major topic in the interviews and the results later shared with the entire staff. Similarly, NGOs often can use research findings to develop advocacy messages. Invite leaders of local women's or youth advocacy organizations to contribute to the research design by suggesting questions that would help them serve the needs of their constituents. You are not obligated to use stakeholders' questions, but if they are relevant to the basic research problem, you will win cooperation and respect by finding ways to obtain the information they need.

Project advisory committees

An effective vehicle for mobilizing the interest of policy-makers and community leaders is the project advisory committee. Depending on the nature of your study, you may want to establish an advisory group of influential people who will meet periodically to review progress on the study and advise on implementation issues. Such a group might include representatives from local and central government, schools, churches, women's advocacy organizations, youth groups, and other organizations. Since advisory committee membership may imply special privilege, it is best to include as broad a representation as possible so that selection of members does not seem to favor only one segment of the community.

Advisory committee members customarily do not participate directly in the design and conduct of the research. Their role is to advise. It should be clear from the outset that their purpose is to provide valuable consultation and review, not to make research decisions. Different members of the committee may take on different roles related to their interests and expertise, but typical activities might include reviewing protocols, suggesting culturally appropriate ways to ask questions, identifying key messages in the findings, linking results to recommendations, and participating in dissemination plans. You can help to ensure that these influential people will promote and use study findings if you begin by formulating clear research questions that address policy or programmatic issues; explaining or demystifying the research methods; and providing a role for stakeholders in the process.

Developing the Field Team

Never underestimate the value of local assistance. Including people from the study site in your field strategy not only helps in day-to-day management, but also enhances community rapport and increases the professional team's understanding of the site. Professional data collectors and local assistants will work well together if they appreciate the complementary roles that each can play.

Field assistants: the local team

When introducing the study to the community, identify a few local people who are especially interested in the project, who know the community, and who are willing to work with you. They will be your local field team. In Chapter 4, we discussed the role of key informants, people with special knowledge and insight into the phenomenon you are studying. The local assistants who help you implement the study should also be honest informants on the local scene and channels of information to their peers. But while a key informant is primarily a confidante and guide to the culture, local assistants are there mainly to help you with practical arrangements. They might be lay church leaders, community workers, or simply individuals who are well known and respected by their peers. As a general rule, it is advisable not to seek assistance from people who are controversial or in positions of authority in the group. Examples of people not to include on the field team might be the mayor or a member of his family, a prominent traditional healer or shaman, or the medical officer in charge of the health center. These individuals might provide valuable information but be perceived as intimidating or coercive by other participants. There may also be confidentiality issues involved.

The role of the local field team might include interpreting the study to people in the community, helping identify respondents who meet the sample selection criteria, welcoming participants (focus group members or interviewees), organizing refreshments, distracting curious visitors during interviews or focus group discussions, providing child care, or reminding individuals in the sample to come to the interview site. Local team members must not be present during interviews or focus group discussions and must not have access to data in any form. They should be strongly encouraged to respect the privacy of people in the study sample who have agreed to participate.

Using Qualitative Research Methods to Empower NGOs

Suzanne Smith Saulniers, Ph.D.

In Pakistan, nongovernmental organizations (NGOs) working in reproductive health service delivery have played a passive role as providers of information to donors. Donors, on the other hand, typically request, analyze, and use the information they get from NGOs, but generally do not reciprocate by communicating back new information. For the past 10 years, middle-sized family planning community service NGOs have received no written feedback from external monitoring teams or from the government agency that acts as the grant manager.

The role of local NGOs is confined mainly to collecting monthly and quarterly data on door-to-door family planning service delivery. They seldom analyze their own program evaluation results and are not taught how to use data they collect for program planning and assessment. Donor and government fund managers neither expect NGOs to assess service delivery problems nor encourage them to develop their own solutions to such problems. The result is that NGOs have become powerless to make fundamental changes and are discouraged from initiating reproductive health program improvements.

In 1998 the Asia Foundation, concerned about increasing decentralization of leadership and management capacity-building of NGOs, decided to adopt an innovative approach. The resulting research and intervention project, initially funded by the William and Flora Hewlett Foundation in 1996, aimed to promote the well-being of families and to advocate for smaller families by strengthening the role of men in family planning and women's reproductive health care. The project included a two-part formative research phase and a phase in which we tested an intervention model that used qualitative tools.

The remarkable empowerment of NGOs that took place during the research phase of this project convinced me that introducing qualitative techniques is an important capacity-building process in its own right. I believe this had as much to do with learning how to use the qualitative techniques — semi-structured interviewing, focus group discussions, and direct observation — as it did with the social responsibility that was promoted by the program.

Our research used the Trials of Improved Practices (TIPs) methodology, a social marketing approach in which trials are implemented by members of the affected groups. TIPS can be used to evaluate behaviors, motivations, instructional information, and approaches to overcoming barriers to a proposed change (Dickin et al. 1997). Five middle-sized NGOs were selected as participants, along with a four-member core research team of Pakistani health specialists.

Empowerment started from the beginning of the research. The key elements of empowerment were: a rigorous and closely supervised participatory training process, peer exchanges and collaborative support, and promotion of the message that the research teams were learning skills new to NGOs in Pakistan. I learned that when NGOs are directly involved in implementing research, they assume ownership and responsibility for the results of the data.

Three of the five NGO providers had been trained in TIPs research methods as part of a previous qualitative study. This project gave them an opportunity to reinforce their skills of focus group discussions, indepth interviews, direct observation, and NGO research management. The team worked collegially, benefiting from a non-hierarchical structure and mutual exchange during training sessions. When focus group discussions needed stronger researchers, not only would a core research team member step in, but also an experienced interviewer from another NGO might be invited to assist with discussions or refresher training of the interview team.

We found that peer-learning and reinforcement secured team members' skills in asking questions or knowing when to seek solutions to irregular use or non-use of modern family planning methods. They also learned how to engage in gender-appropriate needs assessments of female and male clients. This interactive peer approach and the qualitative results that emerged encouraged all the NGO participants to look critically at their current programs and to review their relationships with government.

Questioning the effectiveness of their current service delivery approach, the NGOs noted the absence of male involvement in their delivery design. They were surprised at how far removed they had been from their clients — delivering health messages without really understanding how people made reproductive decisions. They wondered why they had meticulously collected quantitative data without understanding their clients' attitudes, problems, and health care decision-making habits. In fact, NGOs were so optimistic about what they were learning that several approached the government minister to discuss service delivery policy.

They asked if they could receive funds to engage in self-monitoring, continue qualitative data collection, and collect quantitative data less frequently. They requested that greater attention be given to the role of men in family planning decision-making. And they asked that the government and donors also send them regular government monitoring reports on their activities and performance. Until this qualitative research experience, they had never considered raising questions to government or donors, nor had they considered themselves qualified to undertake program monitoring. Since then, this group has started a reproductive health network among middle-sized NGOs. Today, they are continuing their qualitative research training, applying for grants through the network and seeking funds to train others in qualitative methods.

Box 5.1

Characteristics of a Good Interviewer or Moderator

- Ability to feel at ease and to put others at ease
- Ability to project unconditional respect and acceptance of others
- Ability to convey warmth and empathy
- Good verbal and interpersonal skills
- Good listening skills
- Ability to project enthusiasm and genuine interest in others
- Awareness of own nonverbal reactions, using body language to project positive response
- Ability to interpret and explore what people say in light of the research problem, versus rote response.

(Adapted from Debus 1986, 36)

Local team members will know they play a vital role, especially if they are welcome to attend meetings of the whole team and if they receive a stipend consistent with the local pay scale. They may also appreciate a simple certificate or letter that documents their experience on your project. The certificate might be used to secure similar positions in the future.

The professional field team

Field supervisor. As researchers, we usually are outsiders, educated in research methodology but naive to the sociocultural matrix in which we conduct our studies. The gap may exist not only across countries but even within a country, where socioeconomic differences can create barriers between highly educated researchers and the populations they have chosen to study. When this situation occurs, a field supervisor can be an invaluable counterpart, a skilled assistant who understands the cultural context, is fluent in the local language, and has experience in qualitative techniques. Working closely with the researcher, this individual can help coordinate and supervise much of the data collection. Needless to say, the field supervisor must be a person who is liked and respected by interviewers and other members of the team as well as by participants and community leaders. A field supervisor who helps you gain access to information and serves as a cultural interpreter can also be a valuable key informant.

Interviewers. In the best of all worlds, interviewers are trained in a social science and experienced in qualitative data collection. Unfortunately, such individuals often are in short supply, because few universities provide training in qualitative research. However, we have found that less-experienced people with strong interpersonal skills and readiness to apply new interactive techniques can learn to collect excellent qualitative data. Since the task of a qualitative interviewer is to become a conversational partner with the participant (Rubin and Rubin 1995), personal attributes are important. A warm, empathic manner; sensitivity to different perspectives; and an ability to listen carefully and ask insightful questions are characteristics of a good interviewer, whether educated in the social sciences or not.

It is also important to know where potential interviewers would fit in the community structure. If interviewers or supervisors differ significantly from study participants with respect to distinctive characteristics such as education, economic status, or religious affiliation, they must be able to minimize the difference in status through an interpersonal style that is friendly and nonjudgmental. Would-be interviewers who, for whatever reason, are unable to put participants at ease, accept individual differences, or respond appropriately to the changing dynamics of the interview or group discussion, will not be effective.

Anticipating Strengths and Weaknesses When Training Data Collectors

Cynthia Woodsong, Ph.D.
Family Health International

The previous experience of field staff charged with data collection varies widely within and between projects, and this variability carries with it implications for training, monitoring, and supervision.

In providing training to field staff in an international multisite ethnographic study focused on HIV/AIDS behavior change, I have found it helpful to take into account the trainees' professional backgrounds, and how these might bias data collection. Field staff often come from the following backgrounds:

Health care workers (e.g., nurses, health educators, social services providers)

Strengths: (1) health care workers may be more comfortable talking about reproductive health issues, sexual behaviors, the body (especially genitalia) than most people; (2) participants may be more willing to discuss these things with someone they know is a health worker, a person whom they see as legitimately privy to such talk; and (3) health care workers know how to engage people, build trust, and offer reliable confidentiality.

Weaknesses: (1) health care workers may find it difficult to elicit data that are at odds with medical knowledge, feeling instead a need to correct misinformation; (2) they may be considered authoritarian, thus blocking free discussion of behaviors that the respondent knows are not considered correct within the health profession; and (3) participants may only endure the interview in order to receive treatment. This may bias responses as well as make participation potentially coercive.

Health care professionals enter the qualitative interview from the perspective of someone who is trained to provide for people, rather than learn from them. In training and supervising health care workers, I have found it helpful to remind the trainees that the respondent (patient) is the expert on the issue being discussed. Such trainees often need practice letting the respondent do most of the talking and remaining neutral to the content of what the respondent is saying. While it is a common practice to correct misinformation at the end of an interview, I learned that if a health worker interviewer says, "I can tell you more after we finish the interview," she may find it difficult to convince respondents that their opinions and beliefs are important. Additional skills training is often necessary to avoid a situation in which the respondent views the interviewer as the expert.

Survey researchers (usually trained or experienced in quantitative pencil-and-paper surveys)

Strengths : (1) appreciation for adherence to protocol and conscientiousness in covering all topics included; (2) awareness of the potential for biasing responses through additional explanations; and (3) efficiency and careful documentation.

Weaknesses: (1) rigidity and tendency to follow protocol in an almost robotic style; and (2) difficulty in grasping the concept of appropriate probing.

Survey researchers who have internalized the importance of staying closely within a structured protocol with strict question-by-question specifications are probably excellent interviewers and rightly proud of their expertise. However, they often find it challenging (if not unscientific) to switch to a conversational style of interviewing, with the extensive probing and disruption of question-flow order so common in qualitative research. When training survey interviewers, I rely heavily on role-play as a training tool, with trainees interviewing me as well as each other. Reviewing verbatim transcripts of practice and initial interviews is an essential training tool. Such review allows the trainer to more clearly point out missed opportunities to probe and to provide guidance on leading probes and questioning, while also reassuring the trainee of the things that they did correctly.

University-trained social scientists (anthropology, sociology, psychology)

Strengths: (1) strong theoretical background; (2) appreciation for and training in qualitative, in-depth interviewing; (3) awareness of cultural assumptions and worldviews of both respondent and interviewer; and skills in careful (sometimes excessive) documentation of the research process and data.

Weaknesses: (1) may spend too much time per data collection task; (2) lack of awareness of the nuances of applied research; and (3) devotion to favorite theories that may not be essential to the project.

Data collectors with university training in the underlying theoretical perspectives of social sciences and public health can be wonderful to work with. However, their solid training can be a hindrance if they are so vested in a particular theoretical perspective that they cannot adjust to the fast pace and practical requirements of applied research. In these situations, firm time limits, deadlines, and deliverable schedules help to keep the data collection on track.

With appropriate training and supervision, data collectors' different skill sets can be productively harnessed as an asset to qualitative data collection. Even novice field staff completely new to social science research may provide surprising abilities to connect their life experiences with data collection. If the research team leader and those involved in training field staff are aware of the trainees' potential strengths and weaknesses, they can move more quickly to spot and solve problems, and to organize the data collection efforts to make best use of appropriate skills.

Training

Unless you are collecting all the data yourself, you will need to conduct a training workshop for your interviewers, focus group moderators, observers, or other field staff. Most teams will benefit from at least one week of comprehensive training before they enter the field, but training and monitoring are a continuous process, even as data collection proceeds.

You may find that your study is the first time that otherwise experienced field staff have been exposed to qualitative principles and techniques. Survey interviewers are available in most countries, but we have often noticed that the more experience they have with structured protocols, the more difficult it is for them to be effective as in-depth interviewers and focus group moderators. When interviewers have been trained to phrase questions exactly as written and assign answers to preconceived response categories, as in a multiple-choice format, it is not easy for them to adapt and modify questions, probe answers with new questions, and control — but not dominate — a guided conversation or focused discussion. A tendency of experienced survey interviewers is to use a topic guide as if it were a questionnaire, asking questions verbatim, shifting topics too quickly, and forgetting to follow leads to deeper and richer sources of information. Similarly, field staff who have been reared and educated in relatively authoritarian families and societies may need considerable guidance in nondirective, nonjudgmental interviewing styles. This task is made all the more difficult by the same cultural constraints on participants who may have trouble being conversational in an interview. The interview may seem like a formal interaction, or even a duty.

In addition to orientation to the research objectives and materials, training must therefore include the elements of conversational style and instruction in nondirective interviewing, with ample demonstration and practice. A goal for successful data collection will be sufficient familiarity with the research questions that the interviewer can engage a participant in creative dialogue without having to read aloud from the guide but without losing sight of the central research problem. Experienced qualitative data collectors can also benefit from a refresher course on the use of qualitative techniques, including formulating questions, following leads, noting silences, and identifying field problems. Trainees will catch on to the conversational style more quickly if they can keep the main research topics in their heads.

We have found that the best training approach is practical and experiential, with liberal use of role-play and simulated data collection. A typical training program might take a week or longer if the field schedule allows, depending on the complexity of the research problem and skill level of the trainees (see Appendix 7, page 223). It usually begins with a thorough orientation to the research problem and purpose, and careful review of the interview guide or other protocol. Topics are likely to include the roles of the interviewer or moderator and note-taker, adapting what trainees have learned from survey research to qualitative data collection; different moderator or interviewer styles; the art of probing data; encouraging participation; observing nonverbal cues; managing problems that arise in the interview or group; and closing the interview or discussion. Interviewers should also be trained in the mechanics of taping and transcribing the sessions, including a backup plan for the occasional dysfunctional tape recorder or other mishap. Important elements of training are sensitivity to issues surrounding vulnerability and confidentiality, and the protocol for obtaining informed consent.

It is advisable to devote several days in the training program to practice of interviewing and observation skills, beginning with role-play and group feedback. As trainees become more proficient, consider bringing in outsiders to play participant roles in mock interviews or discussions. Actor-participants could be prompted ahead of time to simulate problems that commonly arise in interviews or groups, such as the argumentative participant, the silent participant, or the focus group member who dominates the discussion. Feedback from the group will help trainees gain confidence in handling these and other, often unanticipated, situations. If the team includes interviewers with qualitative experience, these individuals can assist with training, helping the less experienced at the same time they are reviewing qualitative techniques themselves. New interviewers might be paired with more experienced partners in role-play, switching roles as the less-experienced person becomes more comfortable with interview skills.

As you observe these practice sessions, take notes on the process to share with trainees. For example, note when an interviewer misses a cue to another question, or fails to probe a provocative comment. Trainees can also listen for gaps in the interview and prompt each other. If possible, tape and transcribe the practice interviews and distribute copies to the trainees to illustrate strengths and weaknesses of the interviews. Group critique of both novice and experienced interviewers' practice sessions is also helpful. Exercises like these can build confidence, at the same time underscoring the importance of attentive listening and flexibility in adapting the guide to the conversational flow of the interview.

It is also useful to include in the training sessions a brief overview of data analysis and in some settings, special training for staff who will help with the analysis. Understanding how the data will be analyzed reinforces for interviewers the importance of rapport in the interview partnership, as well as careful probing and flexible use of the interview or focus group guide. A simple explanation of coding and searching (see Chapter 6) will help interviewers understand that information will not be lost if it emerges out of the expected sequence of the interview.

A critical component of interviewer training in sexual and reproductive health is recognizing and responding to clues that a participant may be at significant risk. Survey interviewers typically are trained to be relatively passive on matters not related to the actual conduct of the interview, but in qualitative research, the interviewer as conversational partner cannot be impersonal and uninvolved. Confronted with disclosure of domestic violence, child abuse, or any threat to the well-being of participants, interviewers who collect sensitive data must learn how to give a caring and helpful response without jeopardizing the quality of the interview. They can also be prepared to offer referral for participants in need of counseling or other assistance. (See Chapter 4 for the interviewer's responsibility when a participant asks for help.)

Field Materials

Provide members of your field teams, both professional and local, with written instructions and summaries of the steps in the data collection phase. Such written communication might include:

- an overview of the project

- a summary of ethical standards for the study

- detailed task descriptions for the local field team and for each professional role (e.g., focus group moderator, note-taker, in-depth interviewer, field supervisor, or translator)

- a calendar with daily activities such as team meetings, training, pre-tests, and scheduled interviews or focus group discussions

- an activities schedule, including a time frame for collecting data and completing transcriptions or translations if done in the field

- a sample introduction to the project

- names and phone numbers of researchers who can answer questions and provide additional information about the project

Training Field Staff in Data Analysis

Cynthia Woodsong, Ph.D.
Family Health International

Analysis of qualitative data usually requires a minimum of three steps: coding the data, running the coded data, and analysing the data runs. In a truly iterative process, the final step usually leads to further coding, running, and analysis. The most common models for division of labor for data analysis are the following:

- staff who collect the data send it to other staff for analysis (most often based in the United States), and are not involved in the analytic process

- junior staff code the data (which they may or may not have collected) using a qualitative software package, and these data are then run and analyzed by more senior staff (again, often U.S.-based)

- the same staff who collect data are involved in coding and analyzing data

- the same staff who code the data are responsible for analysis

The realities of conducting applied reproductive health research often preclude participation by field staff in data analysis. Still, it is advisable to look for ways to involve those responsible for data collection in at least some aspects of the analysis.

Previous experience is probably the most important issue to take into account when making decisions about who should do which analysis task. Other factors include language and translation issues, the analysis approach, budgets, and timeliness. Whichever model you choose, your decision will have important implications for field staff training.

If staff are responsible for their own transcription and translation of data, it is reasonable to train them to do at least some basic high-level coding — i.e., organizing data into broad topic domains. Care must be taken to provide training and supervision for this high-level coding, and it is usually better to have data double-coded when in doubt. I have had good results training junior staff to use basic analysis software; their ability to quickly code pages and pages of transcripts is a real time-saver. When using junior staff, however, periodic inter- and intra-coder reliability checks after initial training are necessary. These quality control checks provide not only quality assurance for the research project, they also provide opportunities for further iteration and modification of the coding scheme.

Timeliness is, unfortunately, often the biggest driver in making decisions about whom to involve in analysis. Since fuller participation and inclusion in analysis takes more time, and more extensive training of field staff, inclusion usually falls by the wayside. For example, staff responsible for data collection in a Uganda HIV study recently told me that they would welcome the chance to be involved in computer analysis of the data. I was pleased to hear this until I learned that they did not have basic word-processing or typing skills. Due to time and budgetary constraints, as well as quality control issues, it would have been impractical to teach them the analysis software to be used in the study.

At a minimum, field-based researchers should be asked to review summaries of data once they are run. When those who have been involved in data collection are members of the culture from which the data were derived, they are in a unique position to make meaning of the data and advise on its application. Furthermore, by strengthening field staff capacity to serve more fully as partners in research, they can be better involved in seeing that the results are put to good use. An inclusive, learning approach is not only the correct thing to do, it also potentially increases research quality, especially for qualitative research.

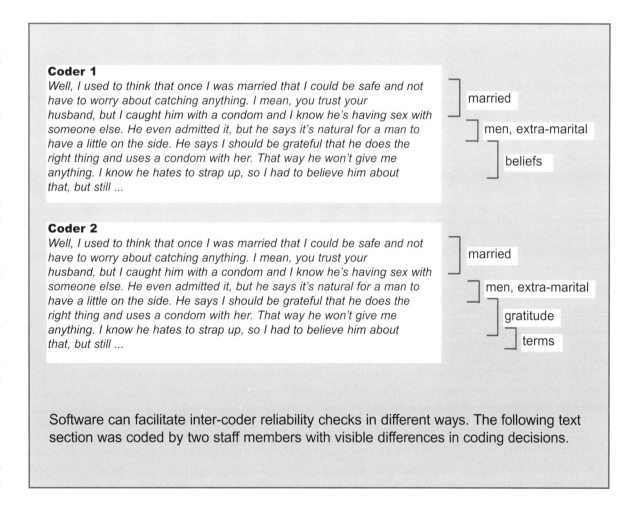

Coder 1
Well, I used to think that once I was married that I could be safe and not have to worry about catching anything. I mean, you trust your husband, but I caught him with a condom and I know he's having sex with someone else. He even admitted it, but he says it's natural for a man to have a little on the side. He says I should be grateful that he does the right thing and uses a condom with her. That way he won't give me anything. I know he hates to strap up, so I had to believe him about that, but still ...

married

men, extra-marital

beliefs

Coder 2
Well, I used to think that once I was married that I could be safe and not have to worry about catching anything. I mean, you trust your husband, but I caught him with a condom and I know he's having sex with someone else. He even admitted it, but he says it's natural for a man to have a little on the side. He says I should be grateful that he does the right thing and uses a condom with her. That way he won't give me anything. I know he hates to strap up, so I had to believe him about that, but still ...

married

men, extra-marital

gratitude

terms

Software can facilitate inter-coder reliability checks in different ways. The following text section was coded by two staff members with visible differences in coding decisions.

Copies of some of these materials might also be given to interested local leaders, especially if they are supervisors of individuals on your field team and have granted them time off for participation in the study.

Pre-testing

The pre-test is a dress rehearsal for all members of the field team, a mock venue with characteristics of the actual research setting. As in all social research, it is important to ensure that interview and focus group guides or topic lists, observation guides, photographs and stories, or other tools of data collection have been pre-tested in a group of trial participants similar to the participants in the actual study. If the study design includes subsamples of the population, each should be represented in the pre-test. Held at the end of interviewer training, a comprehensive pre-test gives data collectors additional hands-on experience and even more familiarity with the project. Interviewers who participate in this phase often add valuable suggestions for strengthening data collection materials and processes.

Pre-testing informed consent materials is as important as finding out whether participants will understand the interview questions. The pre-test should therefore include an introduction to the project and explanation of informed consent, worded as it will be presented to study participants. Is the language clear? Do participants understand the purpose of the research and the part they are expected to play? Are both women and men sufficiently assured of confidentiality to participate without reservation? If not, the statement must be revised until the researcher is confident that no one is taking part in the study without adequate knowledge of its purpose, expectations, and possible risk.

Ideally, pre-test interviews or focus group discussions should be recorded and transcribed exactly as they will be in the study. If possible, allow time to analyze the data using whatever computer software or other approach you have chosen. Analysis of pre-test data will point to the need for further revisions of the topic guides, instruments, or data collection process. It also enables the researchers to assess interviewing skills, retraining interviewers as needed.

As part of the pre-test, researchers should also conduct a trial run of administrative procedures for managing data and protecting the confidentiality of interview or focus group discussion tapes or other raw data in the field.

On the basis of the pre-test results, rethink your data collection techniques. Are you tapping the issues most relevant to the research problem? Are trial participants understanding and responding openly to these issues? Are interviewers tactfully probing responses, giving participants opportunities to think creatively about the questions? Review of pre-test data can be an excellent team-building exercise, involving all members of the professional team in reviewing and revising the data collection process.

Supervision and Monitoring

Have a plan for monitoring data collection and providing continued support to the field team. The researcher or a field supervisor should review all taped records or transcripts as soon after the interview as possible to pick up potential weaknesses that could jeopardize the quality of the data. If the researcher's or field supervisor's presence is not distracting to the participants, he or she should also sit in on some of the interviews, perhaps in the role of note-taker, in order to provide consultation later to the interviewer or moderator.

Even the most experienced qualitative data collectors will benefit from field supervision. Since the qualitative interview is not bound by a structured questionnaire, the interviewer is responsible for guiding the conversation, responding creatively to clues to new information, and helping each respondent to express him or herself openly. Unless you are doing your own interviewing, you will need to review tapes and, if feasible, observe interviews from time to time. If you are not fluent in the language of the interview, your field supervisor can be an invaluable aid in the monitoring process.

To ensure protection of study participants, review with the entire team, including local field assistants, the importance of respecting privacy and confidentiality. Pre-testing and discussion of the informed consent process is a natural way to remind data collectors of possible risks of participation. Moreover, interviewers and moderators who come from the same culture as participants may be able to heighten the researcher's awareness of sensitive areas where participants might be especially vulnerable. Discuss with data collectors how they will resolve situations that arise in the field; for example, family members who insist on being present in the interview, or individuals who seem not to respect the confidentiality of other participants in a focus discussion group. Although you cannot control what focus group participants tell others after they leave the site, most will welcome a basic rule for trusting and respecting each other's confidence, especially if they have helped to formulate the statement. Asking participants as well as staff to sign a confidentiality pledge will reinforce the message.

Researchers in the field must be always on the alert for ways to help data collectors improve or alter the process for more relevant information. Reviewing fieldwork as it happens helps you ensure quality and enables you to modify the process or address possible new questions or interesting ideas as they emerge. For most interviewers and moderators, probing beneath the surface is an especially difficult aspect of data collection. Valuable information can be lost if data collectors miss opportunities to probe significant comments. Appendix 8 (see page 225) summarizes some of the common errors that

occur in moderating focus groups and how they might have been avoided.

Generating Data Files

Take seriously the old adage, "Your research is only as good as your data." Since how you document your data will be a clue to their trustworthiness, we advise great care in creating and managing data files. You can record an interaction with handwritten notes while or soon after it happens, but audio recordings may provide a more complete account. Others will be able to review the tapes and decide whether they would draw the same conclusions from them. Using a computer to store and manage text facilitates the process of revising and updating your coding system as you review the data. You should also consider mechanisms for protecting the integrity of electronic data once it is cleaned and finalized for analysis.

Yet despite the value of recorded data, it is also important to collect it in as unobtrusive a way as possible. We try to use a small table microphone that can be placed slightly out of the line of vision between interviewer and respondent. As soon as you introduce yourself and the study, explain the purpose and anonymity of the microphone and ask permission to use it. We have found that participants usually forget the microphone quickly and may even be pleased that the researchers value what they have to say enough to record it. However, if at any point during the session a participant requests not to be recorded, you should turn off the tape recorder and resume taping only when the participant agrees. Good note-taking would obviously be an important alternative at this point.

While tape recorders are very useful, they should not be the only data record. The set of field notes that you generate from your observations or spontaneous conversations are also valuable data, complementing the records of interviews or focus group discussions that you transcribe from audiotapes.

Learning to Listen: How Qualitative Research Affected Novice Interviewers

Naveeda Khawaja, M.Sc., M.P.H.
Technical Alliance for Social Change

A seldom-acknowledged benefit of qualitative research is its impact on the people who collect the data. When interviewers are also health practitioners — for example, clinic staff or community-based family planning motivators — learning to listen and ask sensitive questions can open their eyes to the worlds of their clients and thus help them provide understanding and more sensitive care.

This is something we experienced when studying male involvement in reproductive health care in Pakistan.* The study's purpose was to learn more about the roles of men and women in family planning and reproductive health and how to help men understand women's reproductive health needs. Data collection was carried out in all four provinces by five NGOs.† A four-member core research team trained the interviewers in the field for in-depth interviewing and focus group discussion. Male interviewers collected data from male participants and female interviewers from female participants. At the conclusion of phase I of the study, interviewers provided oral feedback to all the researchers, the NGO managers, and the donor. Interviewers also completed an evaluation questionnaire to assess what they had learned from taking part in a qualitative research project.

Our careful examination of the questionnaire responses revealed that the interviewers had benefited professionally and personally from participation in what was for them a novel form of research. Their participation in qualitative research training and data collection had built self-confidence. The research process had enhanced their ability to think reflectively, which in turn had led them to question many of their own firmly held assumptions about how people live and manage their lives.

---

* The formative and qualitative study of men's role in family planning and reproductive health formed part of a larger program funded by the Hewlett Foundation and executed by The Asia Foundation Pakistan (TAF-PK).

† Mother-Child Welfare Association of Pakistan (Lahore, Punjab Province), Lyari Community Development (Karachi, Sindh Province), MEHAC Trust for Community Development and Welfare (Quetta, Balochistan), Anjumune Taraqiya Tanzeem Khawateen (Quetta, Balochistan), and Community Council Mardan (North West Frontier Province).

Learning the skills of interviewing also made them better listeners, able to maintain greater objectivity in interpersonal interactions, to build rapport, and to know when and how to probe. Some who had come recently to their respective agencies with little technical background gained specific knowledge about family planning and reproductive health.

Without exception, the interviewers reported that working together as a research team was satisfying and enjoyable. They described their participation in the project as a metamorphosis in their understanding of the relationships in marriage, between parents and their children, and between mothers-in-law (MIL) and daughters-in-law (DIL). Field experience had caused them to dismantle many of their own assumptions about sexual, reproductive, and family life and to give up stereotypes. One interviewer noted, "I liked doing focus group discussion with MIL. My assumption regarding them, that is MIL not cooperating and fighting with us, proved wrong. They talked so sweetly that I enjoyed talking to them."

Commenting on how field experience had increased their ability to listen reflectively to others' views, an interviewer said, "It was my opinion that I am correct in whatever I say or think. Now I give importance to conversation and thoughts of people and try to learn from them."

Another interviewer remarked, "Because of this research, I feel a change in myself. My skills of listening, understanding and making others understand through the process of a two-way communication has improved." And another described the research process as "similar to peeling of an onion. We peeled each layer till nothing was left inside."

Speaking about the training itself, researchers agreed that the experience of learning together had increased their motivation and their commitment to the whole research process. "The work and enjoyment went together," said one. "… the newness and novelty of the experience."

What they found novel seemed to be the access that qualitative interviewing gave them to people's private thoughts and personal lives. Within the comfortable exchanges of the interviews, they heard sensitive details that most people do not share even with their closest confidantes. The interviewers realized, too, that this information was available to them because they had indeed been successful in creating the trust and rapport that enabled the study participants to share their lives.

Another unanticipated benefit for some was the way that the research seemed to be working toward positive social change, especially around issues of gender. One interviewer said, "In this male-dominated society, this research was needed."

As rewarding as the interviewers found the research, there were also challenges to overcome. They had difficulty finding volunteers, and men in particular were often reluctant to be interviewed. Each team evolved a strategy to overcome this problem. In one case, women who agreed to participate were asked if they could persuade their husbands to be interviewed as well. Another team enlisted the help of a male colleague to recruit husbands of female participants.

Over the course of the research, the interviewers developed skills in crisis management, learning to be patient and persuasive, and to reduce heightened emotions. For example, "In one or two FGDs, hot words were exchanged and at times it came close to a fist fight. We just changed the topic to cool the matter," and "During research, we had the difficulty in asking questions because some women would hardly [ever] agree to give answers to questions. After a long wait, they would give an answer, but we would be patient and give them time to relax and answer."

Team work was one of the most valued aspects of the research design. Interviewers commented that working in teams prevented mistakes and contributed to completeness; reduced tension and anxieties; provided the opportunity for constructive feedback; and generally made the work better and easier. Because men and women worked together, they had the opportunity to question their own gender stereotypes.

As a result of their experience on our research team, clinic staff gained technical skill and personal confidence as interviewers in the field. But perhaps even more important, they acquired new interpersonal skills and understanding of common reproductive health and family problems in their communities. Their discovery of their own abilities as listeners and new respect for the people they serve in their health centers will add immeasurably to the quality of care they can provide.

Notes entered in brackets in the transcript are a good way to flag interesting observations or draw attention to contradictory responses. Analogous to the numbers generated in quantitative research, data from all these sources may be handwritten, typed, or entered in a computer file. But be cautious: *Observations that remain in the mind of the researcher will not be part of the research.*

Transcription and Translation

Audiotapes should be transcribed as soon as possible after the interview or discussion. When tapes accumulate on the shelf, only to be reviewed after fieldwork is over, you surely will miss subtle, nonverbal points as well as the opportunity to clarify ambiguities, investigate new leads, and follow up emerging hypotheses. Transcription services are available to take the drudgery out of this often lengthy and tedious process, but only the researcher can add nonverbal data, like a tone of voice or facial expression that could affect how you interpret the text.

Interviewer input is especially important in transcribing group discussions. In our experience, it works best for the moderator and the note-taker to transcribe each tape together, putting the spoken messages together with speaker identifications and nonverbal clues that the note-taker has recorded as the discussion develops. The note-taker's skill as observer and recorder of group process is obviously critical to the quality of the transcription.

When scheduling your fieldwork, allow two to three hours of transcription for each hour of focus group discussion, or plan to conduct your interviews or discussions in the mornings and work on transcription in the afternoons. Immediate recall is essential for capturing subtle nuances, verbal and nonverbal, in qualitative responses.

Good transcription is time-consuming, and inexperienced researchers are sometimes tempted to cut

corners by summarizing, rather than transcribing, the data. But language gives us important clues to meaning. How people say things is often as important as what they say. For insightful and powerful analysis, we advise taking the time to create verbatim transcriptions. A question often arises whether the transcription should faithfully replicate slang, jargon, obscenity, or incomplete or ungrammatical sentences exactly as spoken on the tape. For the purposes of most qualitative research, the transcript should be a faithful reproduction of the popular idiom, because that is how people express themselves. Even a pause in the conversation may be worth noting, because it may mean that the participant is tentative or unsure about what he is saying. And what about those grunts, sighs and barely audible murmurs that punctuate most conversations? Researchers vary on this issue and must decide whether such utterances are extraneous or might be further clues to the meaning of the data.

Notes and bracketed comments on the data collection process can be very useful. For example, the researcher might note in brackets that a particular question was loaded — phrased in such a way as to elicit a specific response. Methodological notes are red flags that alert the researcher later to points at which bias may be influencing the data and where questions might have to be modified.

Translation of vernacular expression is always challenging. Ideally, transcription and translation will be done at the same time, with input from the interviewer who collected the data for the transcript. Even if this degree of coordination is not feasible, the translator should work closely with the transcriber, trying to stay as close as possible to the original meaning. However, there are always words that simply have no translation. Many idioms and metaphors are culturally specific, and concepts that fit the conceptual framework of one culture may have no parallel in another. Describing symptoms and diseases is a case in point, since even when similar terms are used for an illness, they may have different meanings in different cultures. The best solution is to use the word or phrase that comes closest and include the original word in parentheses. If you have more than one translator, it helps to develop a vocabulary list so that there is agreement on terms to be left in the local idiom and to ensure that all staff fully understand the meaning of each term. Inclusion of particularly expressive terms from the original language enriches the transcript and may lead to discovery of new themes or ways of constructing familiar concepts. If meaning is not easy to understand in a long, discursive response, the translator might then paraphrase it and enter it in the transcript in brackets with a note. Chapter 7 provides more detail on transcribing and translating data.

Data Management and Storage

The researcher or field supervisor's job will be facilitated by a well-articulated plan for handling data as it is collected. Someone must be in charge of assigning identification codes to all individual records, including audiotapes, transcripts, demographic information sheets, and quantitative data if collected as part of the study. Documents are then stored in a secure location with access only by the researcher or field supervisor.

Preparation for efficient data management includes setting up a filing system with a place for each component of the study; for example:

- the original proposal
- protocols developed for data collection
- field notes
- maps of the study community
- topic guides
- informed consent forms
- socio-demographic data sheets
- codebooks
- instructions for data collectors and local field assistants
- interview or focus group transcripts
- other study materials

A good filing system will help ensure that important documents are not lost and that all materials will be at hand when you need them for analysis and writing results.

Timelines

Achieving an accurate estimation of time needed for data collection is never easy, but in qualitative research it is especially challenging. First, a qualitative interview or discussion is by definition flexible and open-ended. One to one and one-half hours is a comfortable time frame for most participants, but as experienced interviewers know, much depends on how the guided conversation develops. On the one hand, even with skillful encouragement, participants occasionally have little to contribute. More often, however, as trust builds so will the momentum and intensity of the interview or discussion. Participants will become more animated, and you will begin to hear the experience you are seeking and possibly the emergence of new themes in your inquiry. The interviewer must also be alert to participant fatigue, including distractions or loss of interest, and conclude the interview while it is still a positive experience. A thorough pre-test will help you gauge how long to stay on any one topic and how to move ahead without rushing participants. But however carefully you plan, expect to find many variations in the ways that different individuals and groups will respond to the study.

Other issues to consider when estimating your time in the field are the supervisory needs of data collectors, the time required to transcribe data tapes, and the importance of preliminary data analysis. The less experienced the interviewer in qualitative techniques, the more time that person will need with a supervisor. Additional assistance may be needed to ensure accurate and ethically derived information.

Inexperienced qualitative researchers sometimes pack each day in the field with more interviews or focus groups than they or their interviewers can comfortably manage. If transcription or translation will be done in the field, you may need to allow several hours for this task on the same day as the interview, depending on the length of interviews and the experience of the field team. A common time frame for a focus group study calls for one group discussion each morning: approximately one and one-half hours of discussion with time left for gathering and concluding activities. The afternoon is then devoted to transcription and translation, a process that typically takes three to four hours for each recorded session. On the other hand, if participants are employed outside the home or otherwise occupied during the day, it may be more convenient for them to meet in the late afternoon or evening. In that case, use the daytime hours for transcription, translation, and review of data. The important thing is flexibility to adapt the schedule to the needs of the men and women in the study. Remember also to include in your estimate an interviewer fatigue factor. Qualitative interviewing is intense and tiring; too tight a schedule may

exhaust interviewers or moderators, with a negative impact on team morale and the quality of the data.

Finally, as emphasized in Chapter 6, the researcher should try to plan time in the schedule to listen to tapes or read transcripts while still in the field. This preliminary analysis is an important element that distinguishes qualitative research from other, more structured investigations.

Conclusion

Most research methods texts offer their readers copious instructions on what to do and relatively little advice on how to do it. Their argument might be that since no two field experiences are the same, each investigator must negotiate the terrain individually, tailoring implementation to available resources. This is very true. However, the prudent investigator anticipates and detours as many potential roadblocks as possible. Knowing how to introduce oneself, use local resources, and build an effective team are fundamental to successful implementation. Success in the field demands diplomacy, respect for cultural differences, and an uncompromising code of ethics for the protection of participants and their families. A strength of qualitative research is that the researcher is continuously reviewing and evaluating the work in progress, clarifying questions, sharpening tools, and adapting techniques to new discoveries. We therefore urge researchers to keep ahead of the data collection, listening and observing, reviewing notes and transcripts as they are generated, being constantly on the alert to correct possible weaknesses, ask new questions, and strengthen the research process as it unfolds.

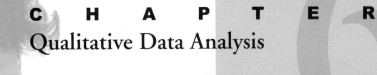

The core requisites for qualitative analysis [are] a little creativity, systematic doggedness, some good conceptual sensibilities, and cognitive flexibility.

(Miles and Huberman 1994, 17)

In all social research, whether qualitative or quantitative, the investigator systematically examines data to discover patterns and, in some cases, to identify cause and effect relationships. The process of investigation must be well documented so that others can follow it, understand the decisions that have been made along the way, and independently verify the results.

In other ways, qualitative and quantitative data analyses diverge. In quantitative studies, researchers carefully focus their questions, identifying key

Qualitative Data Analysis

explanatory variables and expected outcomes in advance. Contextual variables are either identified and controlled, or considered outside the scope of the study. Data collection and analysis remain distinctly separate phases of research. Analysis emphasizes prediction and testing of relationships between variables using statistical processes.

In contrast, qualitative studies are designed to understand the broader psychological, social, political, or economic contexts in which research questions are situated. As earlier chapters have emphasized, qualitative researchers typically begin with more general, open-ended questions, moving toward greater precision as detailed information emerges. Though previous research and theory may suggest that certain ideas are important to consider in a particular qualitative study, pre-defined variables are not usually identified beforehand. Instead, the meanings of certain ideas or concepts take shape as data are collected, making preliminary analysis an inherent part of data collection. Qualitative analysis begins with the first field activities and may lead to revisions or refinements in research questions as the study proceeds.

This chapter shows the reader how raw data — perhaps several hundred pages of transcripts, field notes, or other written materials — can be processed and interpreted to answer important research questions and address theoretical issues. It covers:

- principles of qualitative analysis

- terms used in describing the analysis process

- processes used to analyze qualitative data, including reading, coding, data display, and data reduction

- data management and logistical issues

- interpretation of data — moving from the minutia of study results to the main ideas

- integration of qualitative findings in mixed-method designs

Principles of Qualitative Analysis

Below are five principles that guide qualitative analysis.

1. People differ in their experiences and understandings of reality; how participants define a situation may not reflect assumptions made by the researcher. This principle is as central to qualitative analysis as it is to designing the study and collecting the data. Other chapters have highlighted the premises that social reality is complex, that participants often have different understandings of reality, and that their perspectives may differ substantially from assumptions of the researchers. In analysis, too, it is important for us as researchers to recognize and account for the cultural lens through which we inevitably view our research populations (Kelle 1997).

It is important to pay attention to the language used in our dialogue with study participants. Even when speaking the same dialect, we may in fact be speaking from different vantage points — attaching different meanings to the common words we are using.

Learn to recognize and become aware of your own perspectives during the data collection and analysis process. Account for them in field notes and bracket them in transcripts. Note what you think might be emerging explanations and check them against raw data. Be open to surprising findings but not too

quick to explain them. Always be ready to return to your study participants to understand better what you have learned. Actively seek out alternative explanations and see which ones stand over time. It takes patience and perseverance to understand the world that your study participants have presented to you.

As noted in Chapter 5, language can pose a serious challenge. If the researcher does not speak the formal language of the study participants, he or she will rely on others' translations of what was said. It is important to work closely during the analysis with key informants who are familiar with the languages and underlying perspectives of both researchers and participants.

2. A social phenomenon cannot be understood outside its own context. By context we mean not only the physical setting in which a behavior, attitude, disease, or process takes place, but also the historical, social, and political climates, and organizational or individual characteristics that influence the phenomenon. Qualitative researchers do not assume that such aspects of the context can be examined independently from one another. Rather, dependence and interdependence of phenomena are the working assumptions. We bring context into analysis by considering how informants' stories are shaped by their social position, economic opportunities, or religious convictions, and how narratives are situated in the broader physical, social, economic, and political environments in which informants live. For example, when investigating clandestine abortion practices, we might analyze context by seeking explanations in what we can learn about individuals, families, institutions, communities, or policies and events at regional and national levels. Documentation of past and present abortion legislation would provide insight into historical trends affecting access to abortion and ways in which the government might seek to shape popular opinion. Stories covered in the local media could provide important information about the key institutions involved in supporting or opposing abortion practices. Separate focus group discussions with clinicians, policy-makers, and religious leaders, and groups of men or women can provide a community perspective on abortion practice. Confidential interviews with abortion practitioners and recipients focus at the individual level on the economic, relational, and personal circumstances that influence abortion and how it is provided. Through analysis of information from many sources, you will identify the ways in which different groups' views converge or diverge and seek to explain what contextual factors lead them to do so.

3. Theory both guides qualitative research and is a result of it. As we introduced in Chapter 2, substantive theory offers a systematic explanation for some aspect of life, an explanation that has been tested and stands in multiple research settings. It does so by specifying a set of general or abstract concepts and their relationships to one another — the whole of which can be used to explain or predict the behavior, attitude, disease, or process under study (Glanz et al. 1997, 22).

Qualitative analysis can be informed by theory or it can generate theory. If the study is grounded in a theoretical framework, your plan for analysis should begin with the concepts and categories that have guided the research design. In other study designs, researchers avoid imposing a theoretical framework, letting theory emerge from the data analysis. (See the discussion of grounded theory in Chapter 2, page 19.) In either case, qualitative data lead to a rich, textured analysis and always the possibility of new theoretical understanding.

4. Exceptional cases may yield insight into a problem or new leads for further inquiry. Although analysis may seek common ground or consensus across different individuals or groups, it is equally important to understand how and why individuals or groups differ with respect to issues under study. Identifying and tracking exceptions may yield important insights and lead to a better understanding of the research problem.

In research involving sensitive topics, the individual who appears to be atypical or unique may in fact represent a much larger group of study participants who were unwilling to express themselves fully. Such might be the case if a physician is willing to relate circumstances and outcomes of clandestine abortions that are commonly conducted but rarely discussed. For some qualitative researchers, an important goal of such research is to make visible those whom society has overlooked. Hearing the voices of minorities and others whose voices are seldom heard in the scientific arena is an important contribution of qualitative research.

5. Understanding of human behavior emerges slowly and nonlinearly. As in design and implementation, qualitative analysis typically follows an iterative path. A flexible and integrated approach is therefore essential if the researcher is to understand complex issues from the perspectives of participants. It may, in fact, take numerous rounds of questioning, reflecting, rephrasing, analyzing, theorizing, and verifying. We emphasize again that qualitative analysis should begin in the field, continuing through (and beyond) the data collection period.

Sometimes analysis in the field can lead to unanticipated but consistent findings that the investigator will explore with related questions. In a study of new contraceptive users in Mali, participants often mentioned conversations they had with sisters-in-law about family planning. This clue led the

Table 6.1
Terms Used in Data Analysis

Theory. A set of interrelated concepts, definitions, and propositions that presents a systematic view of events or situations by specifying relations among variables.

Concepts or themes. Idea categories that emerge from groupings of lower-level data points.

Characteristic. A single item or event in a text, similar to an individual response to a variable or indicator in quantitative research. It is the smallest unit of analysis.

Coding. The process of attaching labels to lines of text so similar or related pieces of information can be grouped and compared.

Indexing. Process that generates a word list comprised of all the substantive words and their locations within the texts entered into the program.

Coding sorts. Compilation of similarly coded blocks of text from different sources into a single file or report.

What Are Qualitative Data?

Qualitative data may be generated from direct interactions with participants; from observation or secondary sources, including numeric or textual data from clinic records; or summaries or full texts from newspapers, popular literature, academic reviews, and other sources. In this chapter, we refer primarily to textual data in the form of expanded field notes or transcripts of recorded interviews. We do so with the understanding that even images or sounds must eventually be interpreted and their meanings noted on paper, to be systematically incorporated into analysis.

Text can be read at many different levels. As you become more experienced, you will begin to recognize and incorporate these different levels in your analysis. Among the characteristics to note when analyzing a segment of text are:

- the primary message content
- the evaluative attitudes of the speaker toward the message
- whether the content of the message is meant to represent individual or group-shared ideas
- the degree to which the speaker is representing actual versus hypothetical experience

Consider, for example, a text excerpt from a 34-year-old woman in Mali who works as a telephone operator and uses an injectable contraceptive.

I don't have a child on my back; I leave him playing with the other children. I leave him at home and I work until my lunch hour. Then I come back and work until the late afternoon and then go home. If I had a child on my back or if I were pregnant, do you think I would be able to do this job? Rather I would always be worrying about the state of the children and I'd be the laughingstock of everybody (Castle et al. 1999).

investigators to introduce questions about the influence of different family members in the decision-making process (Castle et al. 1999). Field analysis can also lead to inclusion of new participants. Looking at the data after every observation, interview, or focus group session keeps you alert to new discoveries and the potential for modifying the research process to strengthen the data.

Figure 6.1

Qualitative Data Analysis: Step-by-Step

Reading

Coding

I. In the field

Questioning

Intepreting

Verifying

II. At your desk

Reducing

Displaying

(Adapted from Huberman and Miles 1994, 429)

From the text we can assume that this woman has at least one child, but a child who is old enough to be left at home. Her main message is that contraceptive use has enabled her to work — something she feels would be difficult if she were pregnant or caring for an infant. We see the emotion in her words with her use of rhetorical questioning: "… do you think I would be able to do this job?" The phrase, to "have a child on my back" (referring to the West African tradition of carrying young children piggy-back supported by a large piece of cloth), evokes the constant attention, the burdensome quality of early child care. We sense a kind of relief from the speaker that she is not experiencing it now. The speaker also alludes to both psychological constraints and social expectations that could prevent her from working outside the home. Though she is expressing her opinion in this paragraph (rather than speaking for a larger group of working mothers), it is not clear whether she speaks from personal experience, from observations of others who have tried to work with young children on their backs, or from a more hypothetical

stance. The most we can say is that she believes she would have a hard time concentrating on her job if she were caring for a young child and would be ridiculed for trying to do both.

Basic Steps in Qualitative Data Analysis

Qualitative analysis emphasizes how data fit together as a whole, bringing together context and meaning. There are many approaches, but one way is simply to use the research questions to group your data and then look for similarities and differences. This approach may be particularly appropriate when you have limited time or resources for a more in-depth analysis or when your qualitative research is a smaller component of a larger quantitative study, conducted to provide further depth in predefined areas of interest.

A more in-depth and inductive approach to analysis is also appropriate. Figure 6.1, which outlines a

continued on page 143

Rapid Analysis of Qualitative Findings: A Case from South Africa

Theresa Hatzell, Ph.D.
Family Health International

Ministries of Health (MOH) battling public health crises often cannot wait for evidence from the published literature to make decisions. That reality became apparent when an STI/HIV unit director within the Department of Health (DOH) of South Africa requested immediate guidance from a public health research unit. The DOH was making decisions regarding resource allocations for condoms as part of the national HIV/AIDS prevention strategy. Working in collaboration with Family Health International, the public research unit had recently conducted a survey with women who had participated in a pilot launch of the female condom. The director of the STI/HIV unit asked our team for research findings indicating how well the national male condom promotion program was responding to women's needs to protect themselves, and whether there was any justification for spending money on the female condom as well. Pressed by budget-cycle deadlines, the director asked that we report preliminary conclusions from our survey results as soon as possible.*

We were able to provide the director with the information he needed. With analysis of a combined quantitative/qualitative structured survey instrument, our findings enabled him to justify allocating at least a small portion of the condom budget to female condom procurement. Here's how we did it.

We had collected data through face-to-face interviews during which we administered a structured survey instrument that included fixed-response questions, linked to more open-ended questions. For example, we followed the fixed-response question, "Have you ever tried using a male condom?" with several open-ended questions, including, "If not, why have you never used them before?" and "Is there anything in particular that has prevented you from trying them?" Therefore, the instrument yielded both quantitative and qualitative data which we were able to subject to an integrated statistical and content analysis. The design of our instrument proved crucial to understanding South African women's limited ability to control consistent male condom use, in spite of their own good intentions.

To respond to the priority concern of the STI/HIV unit director, we explored study participants' perception of their risk of STIs. All of these

---

* A limitation in conducting a rapid analysis based on combined qualitative and quantitative data is that the process tends to be purposeful and narrow in scope. Less opportunity is provided for iterative open-minded exploration of data than is normally advised in qualitative analysis.

people had been exposed to the nation's intensive male condom promotion initiative. We first used a statistical software package for quantitative analysis of the data derived from our survey's close-ended questions. This exercise provided us with results such as the percentage of women responding that they are worried about becoming infected with an STI; who say that protection from STI is completely within their control, somewhat within their control, or not at all within their control; and who say their risk of becoming infected with HIV is none, slight, moderate, or great.

We asked open-ended qualitative questions, such as, "Can you tell me why are you worried about becoming infected with an STI? What makes you feel that protection is completely within your control? Why would you say that you have no/slight/moderate/great chance of becoming infected with HIV?"

Verbatim written responses were entered into a single text document using a standard word-processing software package. The three questions served as headings, and each survey participant's response, marked by a unique identifier, was listed beneath the corresponding question.

Other team members read through all the responses to note both commonly repeated themes and rare points of view. Following this review of the data, we named and defined a set of codes that represented commonly cited ideas and unique but intriguing concepts that were relevant to the issue of risk perception. These included the following:

Code	Definition
NOTRUST	Cannot trust partners to remain faithful
FORCE	Partner uses threat of physical force to have unprotected sex
PLEASURE	Male condoms are associated with reduced sexual pleasure
YOUCHEAT	Asking for condom use implies suspicion of the partner's infidelity
MECHEAT	Asking for condom use implies an admission of infidelity on one's own part
MCBREAK	Male condoms are unreliable because they break
TAMPER	Male condoms cannot be trusted because partners can tamper with them
REFUSEMC	Partner refuses to use the male condom
ALWAYS	I use a condom for every sexual act
INCONSIST	Male condom use is irregular
PASTSTI	Had an STI in the past

Next, we copied the text into a file compatible with a computer software program for qualitative data analysis. We read through the data a second time and classified text by marking responses or segments of responses with the codes we had defined.

Once the text was coded, we used the program's computer-assisted search procedures to tally the frequency of selected concepts, as indicated by the codes. These simple frequencies helped us to identify major themes expressed by the participants; for example:

- feeling vulnerable to infection because women suspected their partner's infidelity but could do nothing about it

- doubts about the protection offered by male condoms because they are allegedly prone to breakage

- difficulty getting partners to use male condoms all the time

At that point we took another look at the quantitative data. We saw that 85 percent of the respondents said that protection from STIs was completely within their control. This finding really puzzled us, given that only 47 percent of the respondents said they were current male condom users. We ran a cross tabulation and found that the women who were completely in control were no more apt to report current condom use than those who admitted less than complete control.

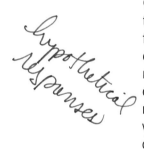

Once again we returned to the qualitative data. We used the capacity of the *Ethnograph* software to stratify searches and were able to tally code frequencies and retrieve coded text for a selected subset of respondents. In this case, we were especially interested in the qualitative responses of women who indicated that they were completely in control of protection from STIs. Once we took a closer look at the verbatim responses of those women, we surmised that many survey participants were probably responding hypothetically to the question about being in control.

Women were essentially saying, "*In theory* the ability to protect myself from STIs is completely within my control." They supported this assertion with normative statements such as:

> It is my responsibility to protect myself.
> It is my body. Only I can protect it.
> If I don't take care of my health, who will?

Meanwhile, this subset of in-control women commonly reported they are at risk of infection due to their partner's suspected infidelity or the alleged unreliability of male condoms. With the insight gained from our qualitative data, we were able to make an important clarification of the initial quantitative finding indicating most women felt they were in control of protection. We reported to the STI/HIV unit director that there was substantial evidence that many women continued to feel vulnerable to infection, despite their ready access to male condoms. This information, combined with evidence of women's ability to use the female condom in situations in which they could not manage to use the male condom, helped to convince the director that he was justified in using some funds for female condom purchase and distribution.

continued from page 139

qualitative data analysis process, identifies a sequence of interrelated steps in data analysis: reading, coding, displaying, reducing, and interpreting. The process begins with immersion — reading and rereading texts and reviewing notes. As you read, you listen for emerging themes and begin to attach labels or codes to the chunks of text that represent those themes. Once your texts have been coded, you explore each thematic area, first displaying in detail the information relevant to each category and then reducing this information to its essential points. At each step you search for the core meaning of the thoughts, feelings, and behaviors described in your texts — that is, you interpret the data. Finally, you provide an overall interpretation of the study findings, showing how thematic areas relate to one another, explaining how the network of concepts respond to your original study questions, and suggesting what these findings mean beyond the specific context of your study.

The five steps relate to one another in a way that is both structured and flexible. It is structured in the sense that each of these five steps builds upon previous ones. In general, you first carefully read your field notes and transcripts and then begin to code the data. Reading and coding should be initiated while the data are still being collected in the field. The data display and reduction processes are often conducted at your desk once all the data have been collected. However, even during these later steps in the qualitative analysis process, researchers may loop back through earlier steps to refine codes, reread texts, and revise certain aspects of the analysis.

Reading: Developing an Intimate Relationship with the Data

Most qualitative researchers would agree that qualitative analysis begins with data immersion. This means reading and rereading each set of notes or transcript until you are intimately familiar with the content. As we have emphasized, immersion does not wait for all the data returns, but starts gradually with progressive review as data are being collected. It is analogous to wading into a lake instead of diving head-first.

Reading for content

What do you look for as you read? First you should read for content. Are you obtaining the kinds of information that you intended to collect? Are the responses full and detailed or are they superficial? There are a number of reasons these first data may not be as rich or as topical as you would like. Perhaps the questions are not adequately framed or sequenced. Maybe the interviewers are not following up important leads with appropriate probes (see Appendix 8, page 225). Other aspects of the interview process may be inhibiting data collection — the venue, composition of groups, or style or characteristics of the interviewer. It is important to discuss these issues with data collectors or make note of them if you are the one gathering the data.

As you review the data, begin to identify emergent themes and develop tentative explanations. Make a note of any topics that have not been adequately addressed up to present, and ones that have emerged unexpectedly in the transcripts. You may find undeveloped or surprising new topics to explore in continued fieldwork. As recommended in Chapter 5, you might type these ideas directly into your transcripts, taking care to put them in brackets or italics so that you can distinguish them from original text. Or, record your ideas in a field journal or type them in separate memos. Some qualitative software programs allow you to link memos to specific text and then to print them together; this makes it easier to separate your interpretations from observations and other field data.

Noting quality

As you continue to read, begin to focus on the quality of the transcripts or notes. How were data obtained? If you are reviewing a set of field observations, how soon after the field activity were notes recorded? How vivid and detailed is the description? If they report an informal interaction in the field, how spontaneously was the conversation initiated and can you determine this from the notes? Were interview questions asked in a neutral way, or did the researcher suggest that some responses would be more valuable than others? These methodological problems will affect the credibility of your data — you must determine whether responses appear plausible, and whether there is sufficient contextual detail to add to your understanding. By including bracketed or italicized notes about such problems in your texts or in linked memos, you will give greater consideration to responses obtained through open-ended questions, and less to those obtained through leading questions. You will also begin to develop a system, or audit trail, by which others can review your analytical work. Ultimately, the researcher's skill will enhance or reduce the trustworthiness of study findings.

Identifying patterns

Once you have field notes or transcripts from several different sources (i.e., different kinds of participants or different methods of data collection), review them as a set to identify important themes. Then start to examine how these themes are patterned. Patterns may include those that occur in all or some of your data, possible relationships between themes, contradictory responses, or gaps in understanding. Gaps suggest new questions for more exploration. As you collect additional data, this process is repeated and formalized as discussed later in this chapter. It may lead you to adapt your study design, to seek different sources or types of information, or to modify your interview or discussion guides to explore new topics.

Coding: Identifying the Emerging Themes

After you have read and become familiar with your first texts, you can begin to code the themes. Codes are like street signs, inserted into the margins of your handwritten notes or typed after segments of text to remind you where you are and what you see. In qualitative analysis, using words or parts of words to flag ideas you discover in the transcript can make analysis of a large data file easier and more accurate. With key themes coded in this way, you can later search and retrieve interesting segments and look at them as a separate file. Having all the pieces of the text that relate to a common theme together in one place also enables you to discover new subthemes and explore them in greater depth. Though most qualitative researchers use some process of coding, there are no standard rules about how to do it. Researchers differ on how to derive codes, when to start and stop coding, and the level of detail they want. When more than one person is involved in coding, develop a process to negotiate or reconcile coding decisions. Be guided by what is most useful to you as you organize and make sense of the text, and remember to document coding decisions as you make them.

What aspects of the text do you label?

Some researchers develop codes that closely match the ideas or language found in the textual data. They want to avoid imposing words or concepts that might prevent them from seeing their data in a new way. Others borrow terms from the social science literature that represent more abstract concepts important to their field. These have the advantage of being understood by a wider audience. Whether borrowed or emergent, labels allow you to assemble under one concept many seemingly disparate pieces of text and to search for connections among them.

Consider the following text, excerpted from an interview with a 27-year-old Egyptian woman who had used the intrauterine device (IUD) several different times, having had one inserted shortly after the births of each of her three children. She participated in a study to examine how changes in menstrual patterns affect the use of certain contraceptive methods.

Analysis

ID#RX234
27-year-old single woman
12/11/99
Interviewer: QRM

The IUD is good and everything, but during the first year I used it, my period used to come every three months, every two months, so I felt worried. <Worry about Delayed Cycle> I thought that I had become pregnant while using it. So, I went to the doctor and she told me that I'm not used to the IUD yet. As you get used to it, your period will come every month. <Device-Body Relationship> [Comment: This explanation seems to suggest that the woman's body rather than the contraceptive method determines suitability of a method and that there is a natural period of adjustment. Do providers or women have similar ideas about other types of contraceptives?]

Then, I used to forget about it, because I came and asked the doctor <Treatment-seeking> and she told me that it was going to regulate itself <Reassurance by Physician> and, sometimes she used to give me injections and tell me that they were injections for pregnancy. If the period had stopped, it would come. [Comment: What kind of injections is she giving? DMPA?] Sometimes she used to do that. [Comment: How common is this practice? What are the repercussions of bringing down the menses in this way?] And when I take it (the injection) the period comes <Treatment for Delayed Cycle>.

The last time, when it stopped for five months I got frightened, thinking that I might be pregnant, <Worry about Delayed Cycle> though I didn't feel that I was. [Comment: When her physical symptoms did not point to pregnancy, did she worry about other illness or problem?] There was no appetite for anything special or dizziness or anything. <Pregnancy Signs> So, the doctor told me: "By Allah, there is nothing wrong." <Reassurance by Physician> And I said: "No, I feel worried." Then she said: "Ok, I will prescribe injections for you to take. If it is just that the period has stopped, it will come. If there is a pregnancy, then we will know." <Treatment for Delayed Cycle> I thought about taking a pregnancy test, [Comment: Did she actually request a pregnancy test, or did the provider offer one? If so, why didn't she take one?] but she told me: "By Allah, there is no pregnancy," but I still didn't feel comfortable. <Worry about Delayed Cycle>

Several important themes emerge from this excerpt and help us understand the relationship between menstrual bleeding and contraceptive use. They include:

- a description of certain changes in the menstrual cycle from the woman's perspective
- the woman's attitudes towards delays in the menstrual cycle
- the provider's explanation of their cause
- attempts to treat those changes

These categories might be sufficient initially to label the texts. However, if you have more than a few interviews you will find that such broad headings give you little sense of the main ideas emerging from your data. You will need to develop new codes that divide these themes into smaller components, or subthemes.

To illustrate, we start with concrete terms from the above excerpt of text. You might insert the code <Worry about Delayed Cycle> into the first and third paragraph. But, suppose that additional data from the field suggest that a delayed cycle was just one of many different changes related to contraceptive use that affect the menstrual cycle. And suppose that while some women worried about these changes, others did not — in fact, that delayed or reduced cycles were actually welcomed by many women. Your task now becomes one of grouping these different messages so that they make the most sense. You might choose to focus on individual side effects, comparing <Increased Bleeding> with <Delayed Cycle>, noting within each coding category which contraceptive methods are most often associated with menstrual change and how different women react to it. Or, you might choose instead to focus on different kinds of reactions to cycle changes, grouping negative attitudes toward increased bleeding and delayed cycles together, separate from women who were not concerned about, or even welcomed, certain changes.

A more abstract set of codes could also be developed for this example. The provider gives the woman an explanation for her delayed cycle, <Explanation for Cycle Change>, suggesting that a period of time was needed for her to adapt physiologically to the IUD. Furthermore, this delay was not unusual, but to be expected in adjusting to an IUD. Other texts from this same study suggest that some women's bodies accept IUDs while others reject the device. It might be useful to capture more detail in the connection between the device itself and women's physical reactions to it, using <Device-Body Relationship>.

During the coding process, you may want to insert notes into the text. For example, the physician's explanation for the woman's delayed cycle is surprising in some ways. Each time this woman began using an IUD, it was inserted within 40 days after childbirth while she was breastfeeding. One might in fact expect her not to have a menstrual cycle for a number of months, depending on how frequently she was breastfeeding and her own pattern of postpartum menstruation. But why does she or her physician not relate the delayed cycle to her breastfeeding status? It is a good idea to capture such questions by inserting memos in the text when data are ambiguous, contradictory, or missing, so that you can attempt to clarify information in continued fieldwork, or account for it during the analysis.

Finally, give some consideration to the words that you choose as labels. The provider's explanation for the delayed menstrual onset and her attempts to reassure the IUD user could be coded <Counseling>. On the other hand, in the field of family planning, the term counseling is already laden with meaning. Sometimes terms from knowledge, attitudes, and practices (KAP) studies or Demographic and

Health Surveys reduce the tendency to overuse labels or stereotype data.

In addition to inserting codes, the researcher in the example on page 145 has included comments and questions in brackets. The bracketed notes will remind her to probe these aspects more deeply in future interviews.

The evolving coding scheme

As additional texts are coded, the researcher will notice that certain labels begin to cluster while others separate out. For example, one might discover that many different kinds of people (husbands, neighbors, or friends) provide reassurance to contraceptive users about menstrual delays, and that they provide similar kinds of explanations for temporary cycle changes. On the other hand, the researcher might find that the physician in this particular interview is the only one who subscribes to the idea of physical adjustment to a new method. In that case, the code <Device-Body Relationship>, which seemed relevant initially, might be less important in the analysis. A qualitative investigator should be always be alert to new and surprising ideas and be ready to code them accordingly. For this reason, a coding scheme is never rigid, but evolves over time. (See Buston 1999 for more examples of the evolution of coding.)

It is a good idea to track changes in your coding scheme. One way is to keep a notebook or computer file in which you list each code, its definition and an example of how it is used, and record any revisions of codes and the dates on which these revisions were made. When multiple coders are involved in a study, it is important to involve them as a group in coding decisions so they understand

Common pitfalls include: (1) coding too finely (too many distinctions) so that important unifying concepts are missed; and (2) forcing new findings into existing codes instead of adding codes that could extend analysis in new directions.

how codes are to be applied to text. Be sure that everyone is clear on who has authority to alter the master file with the most updated version of the coding scheme. (See page 124 for more on training staff for data analysis.)

A Word about Software

It is possible to conduct qualitative analysis without the use of a computer. For many decades, qualitative researchers have used handwritten notes or transcribed verbatim interviews by hand. They have underlined text, written codes into the margins or pages, or otherwise highlighted segments of print to distinguish ideas and messages. They have cut and pasted, sorted, and piled — organizing data around central themes. In fact, some researchers still worry that relying too much on computer shortcuts will impede the process of analysis by distancing them from the text.

However, modern computer software programs can greatly enhance qualitative analysis by performing a number of basic data manipulation procedures. These procedures include creation and insertion of codes into text files; indexing; construction of hyperlinks; and selective retrieval of text segments (Kelle 1997).

Some software packages make the coding process quicker and more consistent. For example, instead of typing every code into computer-stored text files, *NUD*IST* keeps a record of codes that you create and allows you to select already created codes from drop-down menus. This feature protects you from inadvertently altering your coding scheme

continued on page 153

What to Look For in Software for Qualitative Data Analysis

Kate MacQueen, Ph.D.
Family Health International

The software options available for qualitative data analysis (QDA) have been steadily increasing in recent years. This is both good news and bad news. Good, because it means it is getting easier to match the best tool to the task. Bad, because it means there are more opportunities to choose a tool that works poorly, or not at all, for the task at hand. How to make the best choice?

Concerns in choosing QDA software include:

- How complex are the data?
- How complex is the analysis?
- What resources — staff, time, and technology — are available?

As these questions suggest, QDA software decisions are an important part of the research design process. When those decisions are put aside until after the data is collected, researchers often find that they have collected more data than they can manage or analyze in a systematic way.

How complex are the data?

Qualitative data present organization and management challenges that are different from those presented by quantitative data. Data such as field notes, recorded and transcribed interviews, video recordings, written responses to questions, and photographs can contain many layers of information that will need to be carefully peeled apart during analysis. The greater the amount of data, the greater will be the complexity of organizing and managing it.

Choose software that helps you organize the computer files containing your data. Look for software that lets you decide where to store your data files and that doesn't require you to place data files in a particular directory on your computer.

How complex is the analysis?

The more complex the analysis goal, the more important it is to choose software that is up to the task. Analytic goals can range from simple summaries of responses to complex theoretical modeling or hypothesis testing.

- At the simpler end, the goal of summarizing responses about individual topics may be fully met using a word processor to insert topical codes in the text, conduct word searches on those codes, and copy text excerpts to summary tables. Depending on the volume of text, this goal could also be achieved using paper, highlighters, scissors, and tape.

■ A somewhat more complex goal would be a description of the way different topics are related to each other. For example, you might want to code issues from discussions on multiple topics. Software that produces reports on the co-occurrence of codes would be helpful. If the data are rich with layers of information, the software should also let you organize your codes into hierarchical trees and networks so that you can easily go from a broad overview to a detailed view of content. Look for software that will generate summary tables that show which codes occur together and how often, as well as text sorted by the codes assigned to it.

■ If complex modeling or hypothesis testing is the goal, then you may need several software programs so that you can go beyond text analysis to decisional analysis, cluster analysis, and multidimensional scaling. A key issue here is the ability to import and export data. Of course, such complex approaches also require equally sophisticated research design and data collection strategies. Unless you already have at least some formal training in or experience with most of these methods, you probably should not choose this as your goal.

■ Another issue is the amount of socio-demographic data that will be used as part of the qualitative analysis. For example, for a single analysis you may want to contrast responses for men and women, for different age groups, for different ethnic groups, and for different research locations. The more kinds of groupings you want in the analysis, the more important it will be to choose software that lets you link this type of information to the qualitative data so that it will automatically sort the data in different ways.

What staff, time, and computer resources are available?

The number of staff who will be working on an analysis will impact your choice of software. As staff increases, so does the need for organization. This includes tracking who is doing what, ensuring that everyone is using the same standards, and merging the results of each team member's analysis task. If there is a lot of data, or the analysis goal is fairly complex, you should choose software that helps with these tasks.

Many QDA packages require a significant amount of time to learn, and the packages may cost hundreds of dollars. Therefore, if you are familiar with a particular software package, it may be worthwhile to continue using that package if it meets most of the needs for a new project. But if you are attempting a project that is more complicated than your previous work, you should make a detailed outline of the data management and analysis steps that will be required. Then test them out using the software you intend to use to make certain it will work and what will be required in terms of time and effort. Also, you will want to make certain that your computer(s) have enough memory to store the data and run the program without crashing (or straining your patience).

Software needs based on study complexity

Simple qualitative study. Such a study would have most of the following characteristics:

- A limited descriptive goal, e.g., to summarize the range of responses on five or fewer major topics
- Limited data needed to achieve that goal, e.g., less than 250 pages of text, no more than 20 in-depth interviews, or no more than 10 focus group discussions
- Analysis will be done by one or two people
- Little or no socio-demographic data to be used during the analysis, e.g., only sex and ethnicity differences will be noted

Example: In preparation for a larger community-based intervention trial to enhance access to prenatal care, a qualitative researcher conducts 12 in-depth interviews with women who gave birth at the local hospital without previously receiving care. The goal is to describe some of the experiences of women in this situation to enhance the training of the staff who will implement the intervention. The interviews elicit information on each woman's home environment, her access to transportation, the extent to which she relies upon traditional healers, her perceptions of the value of prenatal care, and her experience with the hospital during her recent birth. Two focus groups are also held with hospital staff to determine what they perceive as the major barriers for women seeking prenatal care. The interviews are audiotaped and transcribed. A research assistant helps with data analysis.

Software requirements: Minimal; the objectives can be met by using a word processor with search, copy, and paste tools.

Moderately complex. This type of study would have two or more of the following characteristics:

- An explanatory goal, e.g., why a particular outcome is observed
- A moderate amount of data, e.g., 250 to 1,000 pages of text, 20 to 50 in-depth interviews, or 10 to 20 focus groups
- Analysis team to have two to four people
- More than five major topics to be covered by the study, with overlapping issues within at least some of the topics
- Limited socio-demographic information to be used during the analysis, e.g., no more than 20 variables

Example: Once the intervention trial described above is underway, it becomes clear that first-time mothers are not being effectively targeted. The researchers implement a sub-study to find out why. They begin by conducting five focus groups with a variety of women to find out how to locate and enroll women who are pregnant for the first time or are likely to become pregnant for the first time. They initially use the interview guide developed for the simple study, but after conducting eight such interviews, they identify a new set of issues that have not been previously addressed. They modify the interview guide accordingly. In addition, they note that income, education, employment, and housing appear to influence access, so they develop a set of standardized questions on these factors. Another 20 interviews are conducted. All focus groups and interviews are audiotaped and transcribed. Another research assistant joins the analysis team.

Software requirements: This type of study is best done with the help of software specifically designed for qualitative data analysis. Almost any QDA software package can be used for this type of study.

Complex study. This study would have two or more of the following characteristics:

- A major scientific goal, e.g., theoretical modeling or hypothesis testing
- Data collection on a large set of topics that are organized into hierarchies or networks of information
- Very large volumes of text, e.g., more than 1,000 pages or more than 100 text files
- Detailed quantitative measures or descriptors that will be linked to the qualitative results
- Coordination of one large analysis team (five or more people) or multiple small teams with discrete analytic tasks

Example: The community intervention trial to enhance access to prenatal care is successful but a follow-up study two years later shows a subsequent decline in access, especially for first-time mothers. The researchers hypothesize that this is related to a combination of local cultural values that tend to isolate childless women, in combination with economic factors that increase the dependency of young women. They suspect that long-term, sustainable improvements in first-time mothers accessing prenatal care will require greater involvement of their spouses or partners. They design an ethnographic study that will collect information on all of these issues (gender roles, age roles, family roles, socioeconomic status, pregnancy, motherhood) through a series of interviews with men and women aged 15 to 45. Data collection strategies include structured interviews that are audiotaped and transcribed, informal interviews for which notes are taken and then compiled, and field notes describing observed interactions in a variety of settings. Data analysis is conducted in stages by two senior researchers and four research assistants. Several structured interview guides are developed, based on interim data analysis.

Software requirements: A project of this magnitude requires systematic file and data management, the ability to link text and quantitative data, the ability to export summary data for use in other software programs, and the ability to track and replicate analysis decisions. Most QDA software packages will support some of these tasks, but not all of them. In this situation, it is important to carefully evaluate the options included in a software program to determine whether it will meet your needs.

Information on QDA software

The Centers for Disease Control and Prevention has developed two QDA software programs with a special emphasis on facilitating team-based analysis projects and the integration of qualitative and quantitative data. They are free and available online. *CDC EZ Text* is designed primarily for use with open-ended responses to structured questionnaires. It is available at *http://www.cdc.gov/hiv/software/ez-text.htm*. *AnSWR* is designed for more complex qualitative projects and is available at *http://www.cdc.gov/hiv/software/answr.htm*.

A number of popular QDA software programs are available commercially through Scolari Software, including *ATLAS.ti, Ethnograph, HyperRESEARCH, QSR Nvivo, QSR N5, winMAX, and C-I-SAID*. Free demos are available for some. Online information may be found at *http://12.22.103.11/*.

The following web sites provide a variety of resources as well:

(1) *Content Analysis Resources for Quantitative Analyses of Texts, Transcripts, and Images* at *http://www.gsu.edu/~wwwcom/content.html*

(2) *Computer Assisted Qualitative Data Analysis Software (CAQDAS) Networking Project* at *http://caqdas.soc.surrey.ac.uk/*

continued from page 147

and helps you later to assemble related text segments for further analysis. It also enables you to revise automatically a particular coding label across all previously coded text. One change in the master list changes all occurrences of the code. Other programs with this capability include *AnSWR, CDC EZ Text, ATLAS.ti, and QSR Nvivo.*

Another function that most software packages provide is the construction of *indexes*. An electronic index is a word list comprised of all substantive words in the text and their locations in terms of specific text, line number, or word position in a line. Once texts have been indexed, you can more easily search and find a specific word or combinations of words, or move to the next occurrence of the word or phrase.

Most word-processing software enables you to conduct simple word searches. Packages like *DT Search* extend the word-search function by allowing you to:

- find all words with similar root: (menses, menstrual) (mens*)
- specify a range of synonyms: (cycle delay *or* amenorrhea)
- join two concepts together: (cycle delay or amenorrhea) *and* worry
- restrict the search of one word or phrase to another located within a specified number of words: (cycle delay or amenorrhea) *w/5* worry
- exclude words or phrases: (IUD, not Levonorgestrol)

Hyperlinks enable you to cross-reference or link a piece of text in one file with another in the same or a different file. For example, you can write memos about a text segment or identify text from another source that relates to your original segment and then link them. If, for example, a husband and wife both talk about contraceptive side effects in separate interviews, you can link text segments from the two interviews for comparison. Hyperlinks also are used to relate codes and their related text segments to one another. A number of software programs permit hierarchical ordering of codes. That is, you can identify a general code <Reaction to Cycle Change> and link subcategories of codes <Wait, Seek Treatment, Stop Method> under the main heading. Depending on what your data say, you may find that each of these three reactions is an equally viable option; no visible pattern exists in the different actions. Or you may find that women in the study tended to follow a consistent path — first waiting to adapt to the method, next seeking treatment if side effects do not subside, and finally discontinuing the method. Some packages allow text segments to be linked to each other without using codes, or enable you to build non-hierarchical networks of codes or text segments (Kelle 1997).

Advantages of continuous coding

Continuous coding as data collection proceeds has many advantages. First, it imposes a systematic approach, assisting the analyst to identify gaps or questions while it is still possible to return to the field for more data. Continuously reviewing the coding structure in light of new texts may also reveal early biases and help you move beyond them, allowing you to redefine concepts without imposing unnecessary structure. As noted in the Field Perspective on software (see page 148), some software packages make it easier to code texts and revise coding schemes as you go.

For practical reasons, researchers sometimes wait until all the data have been collected before starting to code. When using a transcription service, it may be necessary to submit all transcripts at one time rather than sequentially. However, coding cannot begin until you have text, whether handwritten or

Figure 6.2
Coding Sort to Label Text by Theme

Segment 1. *Country 1: Male FGD #1 (8 participants)* — FGD identifier

Let us imagine the study is completed, and one day your wife secretly inserts this gel. Will you be able to tell that she has applied the gel when you have sex with her? — Moderator's question

  E *There will be no difference. The pleasure will be the same.* — Participant ID

  J *I will not be able to notice the difference.*

  ? *We cannot know, since women are usually wet during sex. We can't tell if it is because of the gel or not.*

  H *I think it is possible to notice, because there is a difference in the sexual feeling when the gel is applied and without the gel. I will feel some changes because of the gel.*

Segment 2. *Country 1: Female FGD #1 (7 participants)*

In the future, this product may be available for use without [having to use] condoms. So, we would like to know whether you would be able to use this product without your partner's knowledge.

  S *It would not be good for me to use the product without my partner knowing, because we are one body. And, I would be in trouble if he discovers that I am using a product that he doesn't know about. But if I tell him, everything will be fine and he will be aware of whatever is happening.*

  V *If this product was on the market and I used it without my partner wearing a condom, can't he develop sores on his penis?*

Segment 3. *Country 2: Male FGD #1 (7 participants)*

Do you think that it is possible for a woman to use the product without her husband's or partner's knowledge?

No. 5 It is not possible, because if you find out later on … you might start suspecting that there is something wrong in her body. So, she should tell you, "We are doing this." And, then you agree. If she has a disease, she should tell me that she has a disease. Then we go together and seek treatment.

No .6 For a woman to use [it] without your knowledge, aah, I don't think that is fair. As a couple, we are one when we are in this house. If there is something you have to do, don't do it without telling your partner … I don't want to find out about it accidentally. That is not good.

There are some who are not married, but have girlfriends. Do you think that such a girl can use it without her partner's knowledge?

No. 5 Aaah, it depends on the girlfriend — whether she is a genuine girlfriend or she just does what girls do nowadays. Because, if she is your real girlfriend, a man and woman who love each other, she should tell her partner about what she wants to do. But, if she is like these prostitutes …

Let's say your wife just uses it, but you have sex. You, as a man, would you be able to tell that something has been used?

No. 6 You can feel it. Because, with someone you have known for a while, you know what she is like.

No. 2 I would add that the sexual pleasure changes, and the wetness.

Who has the power to decide whether the product should be used or not?

No. 3 The man has the power. He has the power because the woman cannot say that she wants to use it. What does she want to prevent? Because it is for preventing the virus.

typed into a computer. Waiting too long to type your notes could cost you the opportunity to revise and refine your questions and thereby gain richer information on your research topic. In this situation, good field notes and regular reviews of those notes as a team are critically important.

Coding sorts: building theme-related files

As you read, reread, and code text, begin to formulate ideas about what the data are telling you. You are then ready to start a more formal analysis, examining separately and fully each important theme as it emerges from the data. The first step is to conduct a *coding sort*, which is a collection of similarly coded blocks of text entered into new data files. Coding sorts can be done manually, using highlighting or cut and paste techniques; with simple word-processing software; or with qualitative data analysis software.

Figure 6.2 shows an example of a coding sort for a theme developed to label text concerning whether a woman can use a vaginal gel to protect herself from HIV without the knowledge of her partner. We name this theme <Secret Use>. The transcribed and translated conversation is adapted from a multi-country focus group study that examined the acceptability of this new microbicide product to married couples in two African countries (Bentley et al. 2000).

We constructed this coding sort by blocking and copying computer text segments from original transcript files into a new computer file. If you do this work manually, you will need to enter identifiers that indicate the original source files for each block of text in the new, sorted file. However, many qualitative analysis software programs track this information for you. In Figure 6.2, note that each block of text is identified by country, gender of group, and a group identification number. Letters or numbers typed into the original transcripts identify participants while ensuring confidentiality. When the speaker's identity is unknown, a question mark is used.

In most qualitative studies, coding sorts consist of numerous text segments for each theme. The three segments in our example have been selected to illustrate how comments on one theme, clandestine microbicide use, can be identified in different transcripts and clustered in a single file.

Displaying Data: Distinguishing Nuances of a Topic

Having extracted and combined all the information on a theme in a coding sort, you are ready to examine the theme more closely. Displaying data means laying out or taking an inventory of what you know related to a theme. Now you can turn your attention to capturing the variation, or richness, of each theme, separating qualitative and quantitative aspects and noting differences between individuals or among subgroups. The first step is to identify the principal themes and subthemes that emerge from the data. In our illustration of the coding sort above, participants are expressing opinions on whether it is possible, or feasible, for a woman to use the microbicidal gel in secret. Since most participants have taken a clear stand on this issue, their responses could initially be classified as supporting or rejecting clandestine use. As analysis continues, you will identify subthemes that reflect finer distinctions; for example, reasons for support or rejection.

Once you have identified the principal organizing themes, return to the data and examine the evidence that supports each theme or subtheme, both quantitatively and qualitatively. Quantitative aspects of a theme might include information about frequency or duration, size or quantity of a phenomenon. A qualitative examination of each would include attention to specific vocabulary participants use to discuss the topic. Consider differences in

intensity or emphasis. Notice whether an attitude or experience is related first- or secondhand. Examine the text for nuance, identifying different contexts in which the phenomenon occurs and considering what was not said. Below is one example of how a researcher might flesh out details on the theme of *secret use*.

Quantitative examination of secret use

While a full-scale quantitative treatment of data is beyond the scope of this book, it might include a variety of analysis techniques including frequency distributions of important codes, cluster analysis of themes, and multidimensional scaling. Whether or not more sophisticated approaches are used, it is important to determine how commonly themes occur in the data and whether they tend to emerge in specific subgroups or through particular data collection methods, or more generally across groups and methods.

Secret use might be possible. At first glance, it appears that most participants believed that the product could not be used without a partner's knowledge. Only three participants from one group, the men's group from Country 1, directly stated that "we cannot know" when a woman uses the microbicide.

Secret use not possible. At least some participants in all the groups believed that the product could not be used secretly. Though the majority remained silent on the subject, about one-third said they were fairly certain that a partner would discover secret use.

Qualitative analysis of secret use

Secret use not possible. Two reasons emerged to explain why most participants believed clandestine use would not be possible. One concerned physical signs of microbicide use, namely that the male partner would feel "something different" — particularly if he were not wearing a condom. (Most participants in this conversation were somewhat vague about what exactly the man would feel.) One woman was worried that he might develop sores from direct contact with the gel. The same woman felt that some of the gel might leak out, while a man suggested that the amount of wetness would change. All discussions of this idea were short, emotionally detached — even rather clinical.

The second reason that secret use of the product was considered impossible related to betrayal of the emotional bond between a man and woman and expectations about that relationship. In fact, such concerns were offered more as an objection to secret use than belief that secret use is impossible. They relate to the subtheme of partner bonding, raised by both men and women with comments such as:

> It is better for us to know as a family.
>
> Our partners are part of our body.
>
> As a couple, we are one when we are in this house.
>
> ... if she is your real girlfriend.
>
> If you have known (her) for a while, you know what she is like.

Included in the concept of partner bonding is the idea of obligation and an element of fear if that obligation is breached. For example, women remarked that, "I would be in trouble if he discovers," and "he should not be disappointed." Men also implied that such a breach could have negative consequences for a woman. They commented, "You might start suspecting," and "I don't want to find out about it accidentally. That is not good." Such comments also hinted at the importance to men of control in the relationship, another subtheme that invites further exploration.

Secret use might be possible. Several men indicated that they might not be able to detect microbicide use ("The pleasure will be the same," "Women are usually wet during sex."). There was also some suggestion that secret use of microbicides might be acceptable in certain relationships but not without risk. One man suggested that a woman who doesn't love you — a prostitute — might not inform you that she is using it. Without explicitly stating it, he seemed to suggest that a man might be unable to detect microbicide use by a prostitute.

Others implied that a wife who does not consult her husband about such matters might succeed in hiding it for a while but not in the long-term, and that the consequences of detection could be serious. It would break the bond between husband and wife. "If you find she uses the gel without my knowledge, she is not my real wife. Your real wife would not fail to tell you what she is doing." For a woman, it would risk her security. "He will catch you using [it] and he will divorce you." "It is dangerous to do something without your partner's knowledge."

Alternative responses. Some women and men redefined the question. Instead of focusing on secret use, several women talked about women's need for protection when their partners are unfaithful. A woman in one group and a man in another both suggested that behaving or changing risky behavior is better than using a microbicide, clandestine or not. Other participants said that a partner's unfaithful behavior is reason enough for a woman to use a microbicide. (Whether it can be used secretly is unclear). For some men, a woman's infidelity is reason to deny her use of the gel, because it would only reinforce her assumed promiscuity.

Developing Hypotheses, Questioning and Verification

We have shown how, by clustering segments around a theme, <Secret Use>, you can extract meaning from data. As you continue organizing information associated with each theme, you will start to form hypotheses — hunches about the data that you want to investigate further. In fact, throughout the entire process of collecting, reading, coding, and displaying data, the qualitative researcher is formulating questions, interpreting responses, developing theoretical explanations, and trying to validate or reject emerging conclusions.

- Do the categories that I have developed make sense?

- What pieces of information contradict my emerging ideas?

- What pieces of information are missing or underdeveloped?

- What other opinions should be taken into account?

- How do my own biases influence the data collection and analysis process?

Attention to data credibility

How do you determine whether a research participant is giving you a credible response to a question? How do you make sense from the jumble of responses from different groups or individuals? Not all responses should be treated equally. It is important to examine how information was elicited and how it was delivered. Information is likely to be more credible when:

- the participant is responding to open-ended questions rather than highly suggestive ones

- he is talking about his own beliefs, motivations, or experiences rather than someone else's

[handwritten note: more credible when talking about him/herself]

- she does not contradict herself in subsequent dialogue

- he speaks in detail rather than generalities

In the microbicide study there were contradictions in the data regarding whether physical signs of product use would be visible to a partner. A minority indicated that they would not, but some said that condom use (advised to all participants in this clinical trial for ethical reasons) would mask the wetness of the gel. Data collectors could have probed more fully, comparing the perceptions of couples who failed to use condoms consistently with those who said they always used condoms. Another potential biasing factor could have been the selection requirement that in order to be in the trial a woman had to obtain her partner's cooperation. It is not surprising, therefore, that many women in this sample rejected the possibility of secret microbicide use. Would women outside the clinical trial see more potential in secret use? Would women in the trial answer differently if they were interviewed individually or if their partners were not also participating in the trial?

It is important to weigh the credibility of your data as you interpret what you "hear" and attempt to confirm early conclusions. From a tactical perspective, it is helpful to question your data at every stage of the analysis. Some researchers enter questions, uncertainties, and misgivings directly into their transcripts, distinguishing commentary from raw data with brackets or parentheses, italicizing them or bolding them. Others link interpretive information as separate memos. As you review transcripts, if you are still collecting data, you can integrate new or revised questions into the interview or discussion process. On the other hand, if data collection is complete and you are now working from the coding sorts, you may want to enter separate memos about emerging conclusions, reminding yourself to return to your raw data for evidence to validate or reject your ideas.

Table 6.2

Example of a Matrix Summarizing Data on Secret Use

Country 2	Not Possible	Possibility Not Ruled Out
Women Group 1	He will feel it.	Consensus unclear. (1/23/99, p24)
Group 2	Dangerous to do w/o your partner's knowledge. He may ask you to leave the house! He will catch you using [it]; he will divorce you [b/c assuming female promiscuity]. Better to be honest with him. (4/24/99 p39-40)	If he feels that, it may cause problems. (p27) If a small amount, he may not notice.
Men Group 1	It cannot be done. I will feel something ... why did it get wet so quickly?	If she uses gel without my knowledge she is not my real wife. (4/25/99 p23)
Group 2	You can feel the difference. Sexual pleasure changes.	It is not possible b/c if you find out later on, you might suspect something wrong with her body ... I don't think that is fair.

Data Reduction: Getting the Big Picture

Data reduction means distilling the information to make visible the most essential concepts and relationships. Along the way you have read through transcripts, identified important themes and developed a coding system to mark these themes. You have sorted data from your original transcripts into new files organized by theme. You have explored the rich variation of each thematic file, identifying key concepts and discovering the perspectives of different subgroups in your study.

It is time to step back from the data. The reduction process usually happens once all the data are in and you have become familiar with their content. The goal now is to get an overall sense of the data and to distinguish central and secondary themes. It is

also a process of separating the essential from the nonessential. To get this wider perspective on the data, it is often helpful to use visual devices (Ryan and Bernard 2000).

One such visual approach to data reduction is to develop matrices, diagrams, or taxonomies for each thematic file that has remained central to the study. We return to the microbicide example. Table 6.2 is an illustration of one approach to data reduction: a matrix constructed for the code <Secret Use>. For one country (Country 2), it identifies key phrases that relate to the theme's two main components: 1) secret use not possible or feasible under certain conditions; and 2) possibility of secret use not ruled out. Page references identify the source of the comment in the text file. If more than one focus group participant has expressed essentially the same idea, it is noted after the phrase (e.g., 2x). By including other countries or population segments in this matrix, the researcher is able to visualize and compare responses across different groups and subgroups.

A matrix enables the researcher to assemble a lot of related fragments of text in one place, abbreviating comments from the coding sorts to reduce a complicated data set to a manageable size. Other matrices that were developed for this study included: acceptability of the gel and intentions about using it if available; experiences with actual use; effect of product use on sexual experience; and one-word descriptors that participants used to describe the product. Some software makes it easy to develop such matrices, although they can also be developed by hand. While the process can be time-consuming, doing so helps the researcher establish the boundaries of important themes. In fact, when multiple researchers are involved in the analysis process, each can pursue different themes and present findings to the group. Lively discussion may ensue as the group explores how themes connect, overlap, or contradict each other.

While it makes sense to develop matrices to capture the essence of some themes, different mechanisms may be more appropriate for other themes. For example, the theme <Treatment for Menstrual Change> emerged out of the study cited earlier on menstrual changes from contraceptive use. The cultural model, shown in Figure 6.3, might help clarify why some women acted while others did not after experiencing changes in their menstrual cycles, and what kinds of actions women took who did act.

Data reduction may not be necessary for all the codes you develop. Some codes may be discrete enough that further refinement is not needed. The code <One-Word Descriptors> used in the microbicide study would be one such example. Other codes may contain multiple ideas and necessitate

Figure 6.3
Cultural Model for Menstrual Change from Contraceptive Use

development of several different matrices, diagrams or taxonomies in order to reduce complex constructs to main themes and subthemes.

Interpretation

In this last section, interpretation, we focus on three questions: how to arrive at the essential meanings of qualitative data; how to ensure that the interpretation you offer is trustworthy; and how to approach interpretation when your study includes both qualitative and quantitative data collection methods.

Interpretation is the act of identifying and explaining the core meaning of the data. It involves communicating the essential ideas of your study to a wider audience, remaining faithful to the perspectives of your participants. The purpose of interpretation is not simply to list a handful (or pages full) of interesting themes and their examples, leaving readers to draw their own conclusions. Rather, it is to identify ways that the many different pieces of your research puzzle (emerging themes and subthemes, connections, and contradictions) fit and what it all means. Although the meaning that you extract from your analysis should reflect the intent of your study participants' responses, it must also have relevance to a larger population and provide answers to questions of social and theoretical significance.

Developing credible or trustworthy interpretations of qualitative research includes arriving at understandings that would make sense to the men and women who have agreed to be observed, to answer questions, or to participate in other ways in the study. Of course, there may be times when comments reveal that some or all study participants do not want certain information acknowledged and will publicly deny or suppress it. This might be the case, for example, if release of findings could undermine the relatively more powerful or privileged positions that certain individuals hold over others. Or, conversely, participants might deny or want to suppress information if they fear it will put less-advantaged individuals or groups at greater physical or social risk. In such situations, checking the trustworthiness of your interpretations against community understandings may be difficult to achieve. In addition, credibility of qualitative results does not necessarily mean that the findings are reproducible. Other researchers might examine the same data and interpret them differently. This is not dissimilar to arriving at different conclusions about the relationship between quantitative data when different statistical analysis techniques are used. In both qualitative and quantitative scenarios, the

researcher must re-evaluate the first analysis, looking for factors that contribute to the different results, use his best judgment in deciding which procedure to favor, and present his process for external scrutiny. This convention is part of the scientific process and the accumulation of knowledge.

When both qualitative and quantitative data have been collected and analyzed, the interpretive process must include integration of the two types of data. Qualitative and quantitative researchers working together identify where different approaches produce similar or complementary findings, and where they are contradictory. When findings are contradictory, the researchers must decide how or whether to reconcile or prioritize them to arrive at an overall interpretation of study findings.

Synthesizing findings: gaps and connections

Following the steps recommended in this chapter, you have read and reread your texts and developed and refined codes, noting the detail of each coded theme and extracting the central ideas. Novice researchers are often tempted to conclude their qualitative analysis at this stage, presenting a list of themes and examples with little thought to how different elements of the analysis fit. But as experienced qualitative researchers know, the main task now is to determine how the themes or concepts identified in the study relate to each other and to their context. Doing so can be difficult because of the large number of themes and subthemes that often emerge in qualitative research. One way to accomplish this step is to develop diagrams or other visual representations that map out relationships in the data.

Tip: Concentrate on one "coding sort" at a time — selecting the most central themes to begin with and then working your way out to related themes as they appear important. If you work in this fashion, you will to begin to see how certain themes are connected.

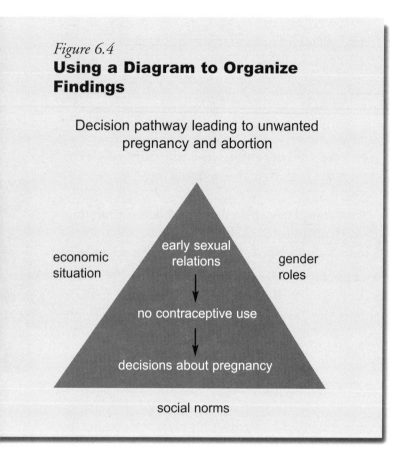

Figure 6.4

Using a Diagram to Organize Findings

Decision pathway leading to unwanted pregnancy and abortion

economic situation

early sexual relations

↓

no contraceptive use

↓

decisions about pregnancy

gender roles

social norms

In a qualitative study on adolescent abortion, teams from two West African countries conducted a study to identify social, economic, and cultural factors that lead to unwanted pregnancy and result in illegal abortion for some unmarried adolescents (Tolley et al. 1998). A number of themes emerged, including:

- adult and adolescent perceptions of current sexual mores

- boys' and girls' expectations about relationships with the opposite sex

- the role of economic pressures and how they influence decisions about sexual partnerships, contraception, and pregnancy outcomes

- communication patterns between adolescents, teachers, and parents about sexual and other issues

- adolescent and adult knowledge about reproduction and contraception, as well as abortion techniques

- reported contraceptive behavior

- providers' attitudes and behaviors related to reproductive health services for adolescents

- adolescents' experiences of clandestine abortions

The researchers struggled to make sense of so many different themes, wondering how to present them in a way that could be understood and useful to a larger audience. Through the process of coding and sorting data and developing thematic matrices and diagrams, they found that three contextual factors seemed to explain differences in adolescent sexual behavior and reproductive decision-making: the different ways in which boys and girls are socialized, economic differences, and the influence of adults and peers. Teachers, parents, and youth offered different perspectives on why or under what circumstances adolescent couples had sexual relations, how they made (or avoided making) decisions that might lead to pregnancy, and how they eventually made the choice to keep or abort the pregnancy. However, their different perspectives could be explained by examining sexual relations, contraceptive use, and pregnancy-related decisions through the lens of three broad areas: economic roles, gender roles, and social norms.

After several attempts to represent visually the different themes, the research teams developed the diagram in Figure 6.4. The centrality of contraceptive use (or its lack of use) as a pathway to pregnancy enabled the researchers to focus on the policy implications of their findings. This diagram enabled them to present all their data in an organized way. The final report presented in greater detail how each of the three sets of factors influenced sexual and contraceptive behavior and decisions related to pregnancy outcome.

Interpretation of qualitative data in a mixed-method design

Before you can link the findings from qualitative and quantitative data analysis in a mixed-method study, you must first analyze each data set according to procedures associated with its paradigm (see Chapter 2). How you then integrate these findings is guided by the purpose of each component in the study design. Their respective purposes influence whether qualitative and quantitative components are given equal weight in the study design, whether one is primary and the other secondary, and whether qualitative and quantitative components are conducted sequentially or at the same time (Tashakkori and Teddlie 1998).

Often the two components of a mixed-method design are conducted sequentially, but one is considered the main study. If, for example, qualitative data were first collected to inform development of structured data collection instruments for a quantitative survey on dual protection, analysis would focus on identifying those issues that lead individuals or couples to consider, request, or reject use of methods to protect against pregnancy and sexually transmitted diseases (STIs). It would also investigate the language people use to talk about such issues. Qualitative analysis would then be completed first, resulting in a list of topics, perhaps even specific questions with a range of structured responses — words or phrases, examples, or metaphors that could easily be understood by the intended audience. On the other hand, if qualitative data were collected post-survey to help explain differences in reported contraceptive use and pregnancy rates, qualitative data collection and analysis might focus on understanding why people consistently use contraceptive methods, why some switch methods, and how they explain their decisions.

When qualitative and quantitative analyses are conducted sequentially, or when one set of analyses clearly dominates the study design, linking the findings from the two research approaches can be fairly straightforward. However, linking qualitative and quantitative findings may prove more challenging when both methods in the study design have equal status (Tashakkori and Teddlie 1998) or when they are conducted in parallel. In these more truly integrated studies, a combination of methods may be used to confirm research findings or to increase their explanatory power.

Difficulty arises when qualitative and quantitative methods uncover dissimilar, or even contradictory, conclusions. What should a researcher do when the data do not agree? A first step is to look for explanations that reconcile initially contradictory explanations. Reconciling the findings may require additional analyses of either or both types of data. In the Field Perspective on rapid analysis in South Africa (see page 140), qualitative findings on women's feelings of vulnerability and the difficulty of negotiating condom use conflicted with the quantitative finding that, for most respondents, protection from STIs was within their control. After returning to the qualitative data and examining the language that women used to express their understanding of control, the researcher concluded that most women were giving hypothetical answers to the structured (quantitative) questions on control of STI prevention methods. They also appeared to have answered these questions from the standpoint of desired, rather than actual, decision-making responsibility. Another way to resolve contradictions is to stratify or regroup quantitative data for further analysis on the basis of the qualitative results. Or, you can stratify the qualitative results by significant predictive variables in the quantitative analysis.

But despite all attempts to reconcile contradiction, different findings are sometimes irreconcilable. In such cases, the researcher is advised to present the divergent interpretations and allow readers to draw their own conclusions. It is especially important in this situation to provide sufficient information on the data collection and analysis strategies to allow readers to evaluate for themselves the credibility of your interpretations and perhaps to arrive at different conclusions. Following are ways to maximize the credibility of your qualitative findings.

Establishing trustworthiness

Qualitative data analysis is intense. Having immersed oneself in a process of reading and rereading, labeling, dissecting, questioning, and synthesizing, it is sometimes difficult to step far enough back from your emerging interpretations to determine their ultimate trustworthiness.

In Chapter 2 we introduced four criteria — credibility, dependability, confirmability and transferability — by which to assess the truth value of qualitative findings. Below, we discuss these four criteria and how they may be incorporated into your analysis process.

Credibility. Credible interpretations of qualitative data offer explanations that are consistent with the data collected and are understandable to people in the study population. Such interpretations are contextually rich. They are sensitive to differing perspectives in the study sample, perspectives that sometimes diverge or even clash. Credible interpretations develop explanations that somehow reconcile or show how divergent findings relate to the context under study.

There are several techniques for ensuring that interpretation is credible: (1) looking for negative cases for emerging hypotheses; (2) testing rival explanations; and (3) seeking explanations for inconsistencies arising from triangulation of respondents, methods, theories, or researchers (Patton 1999; Kidder 1981; Kreuger 1998).

In a study to assess the quality of Norplant* services in Senegal, for example, one issue we examined was access to Norplant removal after fewer than five years of use. The study included a group of women who were currently using the method, a second group who had discontinued Norplant after five years, and a third group who had used the method less than three years before stopping. It also included providers.

All providers recognized — in principle — that a woman had the right to have her implants removed whenever she wanted. However, on further probing, fewer than a third of providers said they told their clients that removals could be requested at any time for any reason. Interviews with current and past Norplant users confirmed that few providers gave them information on Norplant removal. In addition, reports from some past users that they had trouble convincing providers to remove their implants early led us to speculate that women were actively discouraged from using Norplant fewer than five years. However, our data showed that some early discontinuers had little or no problem getting their implants removed.

We delved further into the stories of early discontinuers who did and did not have problems. Most women who had problems said they requested removal because of increased bleeding. In contrast, most women who obtained removal easily did so for other reasons, either health-related or to get pregnant. Furthermore, almost all women who gave health-related reasons had stopped using the method on the physician's advice, not at their own request. Were there any exceptions? We returned to the transcripts to find that one women had, in fact, requested removal of Norplant on her own volition

---

* Norplant is a system of five capsules containing progesterone that are implanted just under the skin of the upper arm and provide contraceptive protection for five years.

because she could not tolerate changes to her menstrual cycle. Her situation seemed different from other women in the study. She herself was in the medical profession, and it was her colleague who had removed the implants.

By looking for cases of women who got their implants removed early without objections from providers, we arrived at three interwoven notions related to Norplant removal. One was that providers often held different views from users about acceptable and unacceptable reasons to discontinue the method. The second was that women differed in their ability to negotiate removal for reasons that might not be viewed as important by providers. The third was that users often resorted to strategic explanations for their desire to have it removed. Thus closer analysis revealed that these seemingly contradictory results did, in fact, reflect real issues for users.

Showing that you have moved beyond your initial understanding of a research question to gain a more in-depth perspective also builds credibility. One way to show this progression is to consciously compare your final interpretation with what you first expected to find. By identifying and documenting your motivations, interests, and perspectives initially and throughout the research process, you will be better able to navigate around those biases to represent the study respondents more fully and credibly. Some researchers write down what they expect to find before implementing the study. If there are no surprises in the data, no contradictions or revisions to theories, then you may not have dug deeply enough, but instead, discovered only what you originally set out to discover (Lincoln and Guba 1999).

Dependability. In quantitative research, an important test of reliability is the extent to which findings can be replicated. The goal is not only to replicate the results of a study (which, given intervening time and change may not be perfectly possible), but to be able to replicate the processes used to obtain these results (King et al. 1994).

To increase the dependability of qualitative findings, on the other hand, you might incorporate a team approach or use multiple independent coders or analysts. This tactic will help to offset the subjective bias of one researcher. The process of resolving differences in interpretation can be a check against individual bias to some degree — but differences in individual power or status might still influence process. Or you may have a second independent investigator analyze data. In this way, the potential for individual influence over interpretation is reduced, but there is no way to rectify differences in independent interpretations. If two significantly different interpretations of the data emerge, you might need to resort to a third independent investigator, or present both interpretations of the results, allowing the reader to draw conclusions from both perspectives.

Qualitative researchers should also address issues of process dependability — the ability of other scientists to replicate the study procedures. Because qualitative data collection is often more fluid and researcher-dependent than quantitative interviewing, such documentation should include information about the researcher's background, and professional and project-specific training. Other important information includes field decisions to change methods, revise questions, and so forth. For example, in the Norplant study cited earlier, we originally intended to use the same technique (focus group discussion) to gather information from current method users — those who had completed four or five years of use — as well as from early discontinuers. During pre-testing, however, we discovered that women who had stopped using the method early were not showing up for group discussions. In follow-up visits to these women, we discovered that many were anxious about sharing personal opinions and experiences in a larger group. Most, however, were willing to talk to us privately in their homes.

Confirmability. By definition, qualitative research recognizes the central role of the researcher in defining issues for study, interpreting information and guiding the research process. Qualitative researchers do not claim to be detached and neutral scientists, unencumbered by their own experiences and values. They do believe, however, that by being conscious of their own subjectivity, they can better understand its effects on their efforts, thereby allowing participants to express their experiences, values, and expectations. Qualitative researchers can check whether they have sufficiently maintained the distinction between their own and their subjects' ideas by opening the study process to outside inspection and verification.

One such approach is the audit trail (Lincoln and Guba 1985). This technique entails collecting and storing six categories of information:

- Raw data — uncoded transcripts, tape recordings, field observation notes

- Data reduction and analysis products — list of codes, theoretical notes about working hypotheses, matrices

- Data reconstruction and synthesis products — diagrams and notes showing how different themes relate, a final report

- Process notes — methodological notes, notes about trustworthiness, audit notes

- Materials relating to intentions and dispositions — study protocol, personal notes about motives and expectations of the study

- Instrument development information — interview guides, data collection protocols

By creating an audit trail, you enable other researchers to review the analysis decisions you have made along the way and verify that your interpretations are well grounded in the data.

Transferability. Because qualitative analyses are so firmly rooted in specific contexts, some researchers believe it is not possible to make inferences to other populations. Others appear to draw general conclusions from their research too casually. While the first limits the usefulness of qualitative research, the second limits its potency or effectiveness. There is a middle ground, however. It is to apply lessons learned in one context to similar contexts. But how can we do this?

First, as qualitative researchers, we should draw our conclusions carefully, ensuring that they are supported by data. Second, we can provide enough description of the research context, the characteristics of the study participants, the nature of their interactions with the researcher, and the physical environment that others can decide how transferable the findings are to other contexts. Finally, the results are more likely to be transferable if the original research design had a model-testing or theory-building objective. Such designs will explicitly identify theoretical constructs or components of a conceptual model to be tested within, or adapted to, the new study population. Results from the proposed study are then used to: (1) support the model or theory; (2) refine the model or theory; (3) limit the generalizability of the model or theory; or (4) postulate an alternative model or theory.

CHAPTER 7

Putting It into Words: Reporting Qualitative Research Results

Writing up qualitative research "convert[s] private problems into public issues, thereby making collective identity and collective solutions possible."

(Richardson 1990, 28)

Applied reproductive health research frequently has as its goal to influence policy, strengthen programs, or change health provider practices. The main product of qualitative research, however, is text — papers, reports, articles, books, and data archives.

As researchers, what can we do to make our writing matter, have an impact? What influence do we have over how people will interpret or use the text we have generated? How can we present results convincingly, especially to people who may be more accustomed to understanding issues in quantitative terms?

Putting It into Words

Writing up qualitative data is a process that includes determining whom to address, and why; revealing one's point of view in relation to the data; and dealing with special issues of trustworthiness. This chapter discusses presenting qualitative data in reports and scientific publications, including how to organize methods and results sections; the importance of distinguishing between presentation and interpretation of findings; treatment of quotes; appropriate length; and techniques for combining quantitative and qualitative findings.

Ethical Norms in Writing

The very nature of qualitative research — the active generation of insights and meaning by study participants sharing their stories — has important practical and ethical implications for how researchers report study findings. Be aware of qualitative reporting conventions even before you begin your study, and use them to guide your work.

In general, the ethical norms that govern how we write about people's lives include "the four non-negotiable journalistic norms of accuracy, nonmaleficence, the right to know, and making one's moral position public" (Denzin 2000, 902-903). When you write up sensitive information on human sexuality, contraceptive decision-making, and client-provider interaction, keep four basic principles in mind:

Aim for balance and accuracy, not neutrality.
Qualitative writing aims for balance and accuracy of reporting of findings, not neutrality. It presents multiple sides of the particular reproductive health issue being studied. It aims to elicit the knowledge, understandings, and insights of the research participants and to present their insights in context.

Assure that no harm comes to participants. You must not only assure that no harm comes to those interviewed as a result of their participation in a study, but also to assure that no harm comes to them as a result of the publication, presentation, or dissemination of their views or experiences. Even when names are not given, there may be information that could reveal the identity of some participants.

Give public voice to findings by sharing participants' own words. The aim of most social scientific inquiry is to generate knowledge and insights for the scientific community and ultimately to benefit society. The tradition in qualitative research of presenting insights of study participants in their own words is both a philosophical commitment and a qualitative writing norm. Try to include quotes or even brief phrases (if possible, in the participants' original language, along with translation). By presenting participants' perspectives in their own words, you both empower them and convey important contextual information to readers, such as depth, detail, emotionality, and nuance (Denzin 2000).

Describe the context of your interactions and disclose your role. Generally, qualitative researchers learn about other people through interaction in specific roles such as interviewer/interviewee or participant observer/persons observed (Richardson 1990). For readers to be able to judge the quality of the research, they must have adequate information on when and how you gathered information, the nature of your relationship with those studied —

your conversational partners — and knowledge of your standpoint and motivation in carrying out the study. At some point in your report, clearly state all sources of funding for your work.

The concepts of voice and reflexivity are of central importance in qualitative writing. Reflexivity in writing means letting our readers see our individual insights as historically, culturally, and personally situated. Because qualitative research always explores the context in which phenomena occur, qualitative writing involves presenting relevant aspects of the larger historical, political, cultural, or scientific context of the issues we study and the findings we generate.

Getting Ready to Write

Many investigators new to qualitative methods ask when they should begin writing up research for publication. Because qualitative research generates rich information, determining where to focus one's attention, getting organized, and deciding on the level of detail to be shared is often difficult. How do you know when research is ready for writing? Do you have other considerations — time, money, donor interest, etc. — that may necessitate ending the study and beginning to write?

Recognizing when to write. When you have come as close as possible to the point of saturation in your analysis, where additional data are not yielding new insights, you are ready to write. At this point, if you have followed a systematic research process, you should have a full set of files that document your reflections on what you learned. You will also have:

- a final list of codes
- tables, matrices, or other summary devices that identify aspects of the reproductive health concepts you have studied
- a clear understanding of the thematic structure: how your themes fit together and how they relate to your conceptual framework

In conducting your study, you have generated information in the form of text, photos or images, and sometimes numbers. As you interpreted and analyzed the information you gathered, you also began to write up your thinking. You may have made notes on the margins of your transcripts (e.g., "most married women are reluctant to ask husbands to use condoms") or determined text headings to depict sort categories (e.g., "fear of pregnancy" or "fear of sterility"). Now your task is to put what you have learned from the study into a narrative: to produce text that weaves everything together and will make sense to your intended readers, text that would also be considered accurate and complete by members of the group you have studied.

Chronicle what you have learned. There is an intermediate step between data analysis and compiling a report, writing for scientific publication, or preparing a presentation: writing a chronicle of your personal discovery. Some people call this the "writing it out of your head" (and onto paper) phase. In this intermediate step, you take the insights you have gathered and start writing the story of what you have learned. Your task is to take

all you know and make it concrete for yourself in a relatively concise summary — typically about three to four pages.

To do this, begin by clustering the fragments of thematic ideas, and integrating them into a meaningful account of what is going on. Talk about linkages and interrelationships you see among ideas or themes. You may take different vantage points on the findings — a gender or economic perspective, for instance — but focusing on a clearly defined aspect of the material will help you organize your account. Often, there is more than one analysis for a study, and you will need to focus on a particular set of findings.

As you write, keep asking yourself, "What is this (really) a study of?" Having a clear understanding of how your concepts are linked is the most important signal that your analysis is finished. If you are getting ready to write and do not yet have a clear understanding of how key themes fit together, go back to your data before proceeding. As described in Chapter 6 (see pages 160, 162), some qualitative researchers develop a visual or graphic diagram of how their key themes or concepts fit together, making sure this relates back to their conceptual framework. In writing, they then touch on each aspect of the diagram, describing how the concepts are related. Another approach to sorting out the links between study themes is to convene a meeting of key informants and the research team, break into small groups to discuss how the themes fit, then reconvene as a larger group to work towards consensus on the meaning of the data and relationships among key ideas.

One of the greatest challenges that qualitative researchers have in writing up findings is to remain focused on the research questions and objectives, while linking the questions to the findings. In qualitative research, the study findings — which are the product of analysis — are the researcher's insights from sorting the data, identifying a small handful of key themes, describing how they fit together, and understanding how they fit in the larger socio-cultural context. Quotes from participants, the raw data, should not be considered or presented as results, but rather as illustrations of insights arrived at through your analysis. Just as a quantitative researcher would not provide raw line listings in the results section of a paper, a qualitative researcher must do more than present strings of quotes. The results, or findings, represent a synthesis. The quotes provide richness and detail.

Choosing a Format, Audience, and Voice

Qualitative research is primarily about text, although in some research, images, body maps, and photos are considered and analyzed as forms of visual language. Like modern scientific writing, which reflects conventions first developed in the late nineteenth century, qualitative research writing has its own traditions and conventions regarding presentation of data and the visibility or invisibility of the author-researcher in the writing itself. However, these conventions are still evolving as qualitative research expands in its use and application.

An array of stylistic conventions can be used for presentation of qualitative data on reproductive health. Not all qualitative researchers choose conventional scientific formats for presenting findings; many experiment with form, format, voice, shape, and style. Reporting people's insights can be accomplished through genres such as fiction, poetry, performance, graphic arts, photographs, videotapes, and multimedia presentations (Gergen and Gergen 2000). Other approaches range from testimonials, such as first-person accounts by hospital obstetric patients regarding the quality of labor and delivery services, to scientific papers, which might include selected quotes from study respondents on contraceptive acceptability. The range includes such familiar formats as research reports, scientific journal articles, reports for donors, field reports, evaluation reports, operations research reports, oral presentations, fact sheets, and slide presentations. Even when using familiar formats, however, certain conventions differ from quantitative research reporting and writing, including use of quotes and the sequencing of certain information.

Determining how to write — which presentation style to choose — requires first determining your purpose. Are you writing to influence community opinion leaders, to inform policy-makers, or to promote changes in health provider practices? Is your purpose to further academic discussion with scientific colleagues, to satisfy your faculty tenure committee, or to fulfill an obligation to share findings with study participants? Being clear about your purpose — and identifying secondary objectives — will help you determine what audiences to write for. At the same time, balance your aims with available resources by undertaking a frank assessment of your time and resource constraints.

In general, those writing for academic audiences commonly write papers for presentation at conferences or for publication in social science, health, or medical journals. Such papers typically articulate conceptual frameworks or theories, describe methodologies used, and present and interpret data. Qualitative research journals usually allow longer length for articles than quantitatively-oriented journals, while scientific monographs provide space for the fullest exposition of results.

Like the choreographer, the researcher must find the most effective way to tell the story and to convince the audience of the meaning of the study. Staying close to the data is the most powerful means of telling the story, just as in dance the story is told through the body itself.

(Janesick 2000, 389)

Papers published in journals for less academic audiences, including some health practitioners, may also provide theoretical frameworks for better understanding an issue, such as the gender dimensions of risk behavior and sexually transmitted infection (STI). Writing that targets an audience of health providers often includes concrete suggestions for better practices, as well as broad policy recommendations. It is important to include appropriate scientific references or citations in materials written for health professionals.

Tip: For examples of scientific journals, university presses, and commercial publishers that accept articles that report on qualitative studies, see Appendix 10.

Writing intended for lay readers or the public typically presents the human face of a persistent reproductive health problem; for example, abortion-related morbidity and mortality. Such writing should either suggest reform of current practices or policies, or outline guidelines for how to alleviate a problem or improve practices (Denzin 2000).

Determine the basic story you are going to tell, who is to do the telling, and what type of narrative format you plan to use to weave your data. Your choice of presentation style will depend on your audience, purpose, and obligation to the study participants. The format you select may also depend on the characteristics of your study. For example, a narrowly focused ethnographic study of commercial sex workers in one establishment may lend itself to a narrative style, but a more widely focused study may not. Your selection of a format may be influenced by various other factors as well, including availability of staff time or financial resources for writing, upcoming opportunities for presentation at conferences, or a tradition in your organization to write reports instead of to publish in journals. Once you have ascertained which primary and secondary audiences you intend to reach with your report, you will be able to assess which writing practices would be appropriate for a presentation of methods and findings.

One way to get an audience of health professionals to pay attention to your findings is to *imitate conventional scientific writing styles, but modify them to suit the presentation of qualitative findings* (Miller and Crabtree 2000). If you are writing for clinicians, for example, you might use certain biomedical writing conventions in your report — such as visual presentation of findings through tables, charts, diagrams, and data matrices — or present case reports, a narrative approach familiar to clinicians. A case study approach typically includes the presentation of a detailed description of the cultural context, assumes the researcher will *seek* rather than *test* hypotheses, and relies on the author to integrate and interpret the findings in a historical, cultural, organizational, and political context (Cernada 1982). Selected use of such scientific writing conventions may increase the likelihood that readers more familiar with quantitative science will pay attention to what you report.

Variations in the standard report format

Depending on your study, purposes, and audience, you may need to modify the standard scientific report outline to fit your material. Your outline should reflect your audience's information needs and other factors, such as the importance you assign to discussion of theory. Other widely used approaches to organizing qualitative writing include much of the same material as presented in a standard scientific report but with certain variations in the ordering of contents:

Problem-solving approach: a) State the problem and describe the importance of the research topic and its implications for health policies or practices, or its impact on theory. b) Briefly describe your methods. c) State what you have learned about individual reproductive health themes or concepts. d) Offer your conclusions.

Narrative approach: a) Tell your story by way of a chronological narrative, illustrating a problem or process — such as barriers to contraceptive services — step-by-step or from multiple perspectives.* b) In your conclusion, explain why and how the process occurs. For example, if your study examines community perspectives on female genital cutting, and adherence to the practice varies from village to village, you might organize your findings site by site.

Policy approach: a) Present a conclusion as to why a process or behavior occurs or fails. b) Walk through the evidence to show how you reached this conclusion. Journalistic and policy-oriented reports typically follow this pattern, for busy readers who have little time for reading a lengthy article until they have grasped the relevance of the material.†

Analytic approach: a) Organize your findings in terms of the theoretical or conceptual framework you used to develop your study. b) Describe what you have learned and how it fits in the larger framework.‡ If you use a locus of control model to

continued on page 176

---

* A narrative approach can be very dramatic. See an example in Ronai 1995.

† See an example in Appendix 11, page 237.

‡ For an example, see Kaler 2001.

Box 7.1

How to Organize a Standard Scientific Report

If you want to publish in a prominent academic journal or prepare a report for ministry of health officials, you may choose to follow a fairly standard scientific format. Most journals limit articles to 12 typed pages (2,500 words) plus references and two to three tables, following a general outline:

I. Introduction
  A. Literature review
    1. Relevant facts from previous studies
    2. Questions unanswered by previous studies
  B. Purpose of the study
    1. Main question and summary of basic approach used to answer it
    2. Anticipated contribution of study results
  C. Brief description of the study
    1. Who did the study, where, and when
    2. Brief description of the methods and participants
    3. Description of relevant cultural or contextual information (e.g., religion or religiosity, socio-economic context)

II. Methods
  A. Study design
  B. Sampling methods
  C. Data collection methods
  D. Data analysis methods

III. Results
  A. Presentation of the results
  B. Interpretation of the findings
  C. How the results relate to earlier studies and your conceptual framework
  D. How methodological difficulties could have affected results

IV. Conclusion
  A. Importance of the results to others thinking about the problem
  B. Logical next steps for research
  C. Implications of findings for the specific purpose of the study

V. Recommendations
  A. Policy or service delivery recommendations
  B. Community action recommendations (if applicable)

VI. Acknowledgments

VII. Bibliographic references and citations

What One Editor Looks For in Qualitative Research Papers

Marge Berer, M.A.
Reproductive Health Matters

Reproductive Health Matters (RHM) is an interdisciplinary journal in the sexual and reproductive health field with a diverse international audience. It commonly publishes papers that report on qualitative research, e.g., social science research or users' perspectives in conjunction with clinical trials in the field. What follows is what I, as an editor, look for in a qualitative research paper and what it needs to include in order to be publishable.

RHM's editorial policy states that it is looking for papers that identify and help us to understand women's reproductive and sexual health needs, and to evaluate and improve upon existing policy and practice for women's benefit. Qualitative papers can raise fundamental concerns and dilemmas and expose the multifaceted nature of problems and their solution. *RHM* looks mostly for papers that have a women-centered perspective and that foster new thinking and action in the field, whether at the local, national, or international level. Findings need to be relevant cross-culturally and able to be put to good use by others, no matter where they happen to live.

Good qualitative research requires as rigorous a process of research implementation and reporting, within accepted and broad guidelines, as does quantitative research. It is at least as difficult to do and to write about well. Much has been written about how to do this sort of research. For those who have no training, it is worth reading about how to do it before starting out. A paper is only as good as the research upon which it is based, with good writing skills added in. If the research itself is flawed, there is nothing an editor can do to help, except to point this out.

Describing the Research

A paper needs to start off by stating what problem or situation led to the research, followed by the aim of the research, where, when and how it was carried out, and by whom. If the study was an integral part of a larger research project to collect quantitative clinical or other data, then the larger research study must be described as well, in order to place the findings in the context in which they were gathered. If these wider aspects of the study are described in detail in one or more other papers or reports, whether published or unpublished, these should be summarized briefly and referenced.

Study Participants and Methodology

Qualitative research by its very nature takes time and cannot easily include large numbers of participants because it involves in-depth, field-based methods. Even so, to be relevant to others, especially at the international level, the findings must have sufficient value to be worth knowing about and publishing. For example, they must be important enough to affect future work on a new contraceptive method, or to alter some aspect of health education, counseling, service delivery, or policy. This means that the research methodology must be as carefully thought out and implemented, as with quantitative research, and reported in enough detail so that the process is clear. For example, the participants must in some way be representative* of the group from whom they are drawn, such as young, unmarried women attending family planning clinics in a particular city. The way in which participants are chosen must be described. If they do not make up a random sample, how were they found? Why them and not others? If key informants were consulted, how and why they were chosen and not someone else? What participants were asked to provide should also be described. Procedures for obtaining consent to participate in the study should be detailed in the paper.

The methodology for obtaining the information also needs to be described, i.e., the questions participants were asked, who interviewed them, how the data were recorded and analyzed, etc. Qualitative research may be on a sensitive subject, e.g., sexual relationships and behavior, illegal abortion. It isn't always easy for participants to tell the whole truth, especially in one possibly short interview with a stranger. Hence, in order to judge the quality of the information being reported, the reader needs to know the means that were used to elicit the information. For example, sometimes researchers go back to talk to all the participants two or three times, or have tested and found successful sensitive ways of probing for details. If efforts were made to get in-depth responses and not superficial or normative responses, such as holding focus groups to find out social norms and then in-depth interviews to find out actual behavior or practice, this should be explained.

Findings

The paper needs to be about who the participants are, what was learned from them and why it is important, but not about the process of finding the information out. Hence, the presentation of the findings does not need to follow the order in which the questions were originally asked. It makes a difference whether all the participants, half of them, or only a few of them have experienced a problem or believe something that is described.

Possibly the most common mistake authors can make is to think that because their research is not quantitative, it need not contain any quantitative data or follow any accepted process of reporting. While too many

---

* This does not mean representative in a statistical sense. See the discussion of sampling in qualitative research in Chapter 3.

numbers can clutter up a paper of this kind, no sense of numbers in participants' responses means it is difficult to know the significance of what is reported. Nuances and distinctions are worth teasing out as well.

Quotes from participants should illustrate points being made better than the text — but they should not repeat what is in the text or vice versa. It isn't necessary to include more than one quote to illustrate a point, but rather to make it clear that a certain number of participants said something similar. Sometimes, when a striking comment, a point of view, or an experience is uncommon but important and relevant, it is worth quoting as an exception.

Translation of quotes into English, where required, does not need to make people sound stupid or foreign. It should be in correct English (current usage) appropriate to the participants' style (colloquial, formal) in their own language.

Discussion and Recommendations

The discussion should not summarize or repeat the findings but interpret them and discuss their significance. What potential effect they will they have? The author(s) should make recommendations about any changes that should be made as a consequence of the findings. If the study had limitations in this regard, these also should be discussed. Further research would provide work for the researchers, but recommendations of further research should be restricted to taking knowledge or practice forward more broadly.

If the research team disseminated their findings to others, this process should be described. If they went back to the study site and consulted the participants for their input into the report or provided information to them about the findings or on the subject of the research for their own benefit, this also should be reported.

RHM's editorial policy is to appreciate research that is linked to action, i.e., in which the results of the study are used to benefit the participants and others in similar circumstances and not done only for its own sake or to benefit mainly the researchers. A research team may not be in a position itself to carry out an action component, but they can work with others who can.

If I were permitted to make only one recommendation to authors about how to proceed, I would recommend that they read the papers of researchers and authors in the field whose work is valued and study those papers well before designing a study, going out to do fieldwork, and writing their papers. Worthy goals in the pursuit of knowledge, the ability to hear and understand the significance of women's and men's experiences, creativity and sensitivity in the research process, using proven research methodology — together these will result in excellent research reports which are well worth publishing. Good writing and editing skills help too!

continued from page 172

examine domestic violence, for example, explain how your findings support or differ from the model and related thinking.

No matter what format you choose, be sure to follow the basic principles that hold for all scientific writing: demonstrate a knowledge of available scientific literature, and get your facts right (Rubin and Rubin 1995).

Once you have determined your audience and the basic format you will follow, find and read samples of excellent writing that address similar audiences. Analyzing styles and formats by other researchers in your field can help you organize your data and insights effectively.

For example, if you are writing about a series of focus group discussions on sexual decision-making, try to find articles that describe research that uses comparable methodologies:

- How is the material organized?
- Does your material lend itself to this kind of format?
- How does the author describe his or her methods and analysis strategy?
- Where is the author in the text? How has the author dealt with reflexivity — i.e., how has the author revealed his or her standpoint vis-à-vis the subject of sexual decision-making? (Richardson 1990)

You will need to anticipate the approximate length of your manuscript, so that you can balance detail with space considerations. Aim to provide enough description to convey meaning, but do not overwhelm the reader with length. The level of detail you will provide about your study and the length

of your writing will depend to a large extent on the audience you choose to address. Choosing a specific journal for submission or determining a specific format to emulate will also help you identify an appropriate length for your material. (See Appendix 10, page 233 for information on where to publish qualitative studies on reproductive health.)

Finally, if you are writing as a research team, it is helpful to determine from the outset who will be an author, and to agree on roles before you begin (see Appendix 12, page 239).

How to Begin Writing

Write a statement of purpose. This helps you find and maintain a focus (Wolcott 1990). Here are some examples:

This paper examines the dynamics of condom use among female commercial sex workers (CSWs) in Durban, a large coastal city in KwaZulu-Natal province. Our objectives were to explore the socio-behavioral determinants of condom use between CSWs and their partners, both in professional sexual relations with clients and in personal relationships with domestic partners. We also sought to examine the extent to which HIV/AIDS influences CSWs' condom use in these situations (Varga 1997, 75).

In this article, we describe our methodology for exploring conjugal physical and sexual violence. In addition, we present some of our initial findings concerning informants' perceptions regarding the nature of this violence, its antecedent causes, its consequences, and the strategies employed to deal with it. It is our hope that this research will not only contribute to academic knowledge but will help to resolve people's problems by means of the application of the results in education, health, political and other fields (Glantz 1998, 377-378).

Do not continue writing until you are satisfied that your brief statement of purpose captures the essential components of your study: what you looked at and where, how, and why you studied it.

Next, put together a detailed written outline, a sequence, or an expanded table of contents (Wolcott 1990). In addition, decide first how you are going to present your authorial voice (Wolcott 1990). To use a dramaturgical metaphor, will you be offstage but clearly directing the performance, or will you be the narrator interpreting meaning between scenes? Your stance or voice should reflect the basic processes of data collection used in your study. Rubin and Rubin recommend that "if the interviews were deeply interactional, with the parties exploring ideas together and coming up with a joint conclusion, then the researcher's voice and role should be apparent in the report" (Rubin and Rubin 1995, 268).

Once you have written a clear statement of purpose, identified your audience, chosen a presentation format, and written an outline, you should be ready to begin your report or article. What is typically included in the main report sections — introduction, methods, results, and conclusion — and where that differs from scientific writing on quantitative studies, is described below.

Introduction

Begin by describing how your topic and design fit within the existing body of literature. If you studied maternal mortality by interviewing husbands of women who died in childbirth, be sure to cite both epidemiologic and ethnographic literature on maternal mortality, as well as literature that would cast light on the use of family members as key respondents for reporting reproductive health events. Some investigators find it useful to write both their statement of purpose and this section on the study's relationship to existing literature even before they begin the study.

Methods section

Describe how you went about your study in as much detail as space allows, presenting those aspects that most affected collection and analysis of data. Explain how you identified whom to interview, how you gained access to the interviewees, and why they were willing to talk to you (Rubin and Rubin 1995). When did you conduct the fieldwork? How extensive was your involvement? How long did you stay, and what was your role? Present a straightforward description of the setting and events and invite the reader to see through your eyes. Make sure to describe your sample, including socio-demographic characteristics such as age, marital status, religion, sex, education, and other descriptive information related to the research problem. Presenting this information in a table format is often reassuring to audiences more familiar with quantitative methods.

Also, describe important aspects of the local context or culture. For example, if abortion is among the topics investigated in the research, provide background on the legal status of abortion in the country, and describe prevailing cultural or religious beliefs and whether the study population's beliefs differ from these. Studies in sexual and reproductive health often include reproductive history as well as; for example, number of pregnancies, age at first birth, and contraceptive use.

Content Checklist: What to Include in Study Write-ups

Whether you write up your data as an oral history, final report, or a social science journal article, your manuscript will need to answer the following questions:

- What was the research question, and in what context does the problem exist?
- How was the research designed?
- What techniques or methodologies did you use for data collection and analysis? What types of data were collected?
- Why were the research design, sampling strategies, data collection approaches, and analysis techniques appropriate to the question you posed, in the particular context of your research?
- Was the research process iterative?
- Is the interpretive process used in the analysis clearly described?
- What did you find out, and what do you think it means?
- What was your relationship with informants, and how did you and they influence each other during the research process?
- Have you demonstrated an understanding of the world portrayed in your text in a way that readers will feel accurately represents the local perspective?
- Have you conveyed adequate levels of detail about the people and context you studied, including specialized or commonly used language regarding the aspect of reproductive health you examined?
- Have you grounded your findings by systematically integrating negative cases and contrasting them with cases that are very different? (Flick 1998, 244)
- Have you explicitly shared with readers your own personal biases, perspectives, and motivations, and how these might affect your research?
- What were the limitations in your study?

(Adapted from Miller and Crabtree 2000; Golden-Biddle and Locke 1999)

As you write, be sure to detail how you "navigated" while in the field, including how closely you interacted with the interviewees (Golden-Biddle and Locke 1999), how you involved others at the research site, and how you created a friendly and trusting climate for the research. You will need to discuss the ways in which you collected and analyzed the field data. How did you modify your design? Did you use more than one data collection technique? Under what circumstances was information cross-checked? What were the limitations of the study? What aspects of your decision-making had the greatest impact on your research? Answers to these questions will help your readers understand how to evaluate the merits of your findings.

Results section

Make a clear distinction between presentation and interpretation in writing up your results. Virtually every stage of your work will reflect simultaneous analysis and interpretation: your study findings are interpreted data. When you present findings, define them as such. When you discuss what you believe the findings mean in relation to other data or concepts, let the reader know you are interpreting those findings.

A typical way to write qualitative research is to move through themes sequentially as you follow the evolution of some issue. With this approach, you first present study findings, then share your insights on what they mean. How you order your presentation of themes is like constructing an argument. "Qualitative theory is developed by elaborating and interpreting the unexpected and the apparently contradictory. If you have evidence for both sides of an argument, then present it and explain it" (Rubin and Rubin 1995, 263).

Box 7.3
How to Organize and Report Findings from Mixed-Method Studies

A structure that works particularly well for studies using more than one methodological approach is to organize the presentation of all findings by key themes. You will need to be selective in your choice of themes — with so much data it will be essential to leave some material out. As you write, guide the reader through findings from one methodological approach, then present the findings from a different approach, and then tell the reader what you think the combined findings mean regarding that theme. After treating all your key themes sequentially in this way, write a conclusion that explains the linkages between themes, explains the findings in light of your theoretical framework, discusses how applicable the findings would be in other contexts or with other groups, and discusses whether the findings are consistent with other studies.

Sometimes a study that uses both quantitative and qualitative methods gives different results when examining the same phenomenon. It is not your responsibility to reach a unifying conclusion regarding discrepant findings, but you should present these contradictions and offer supporting data for the reader to assess.

In his combined methods study of sexual cultures and sexual health among young people in Lima, Peru, one author (Cáceres 1999) begins by presenting his study objectives and discussing the social theories or philosophies he employs. Second, he outlines the qualitative and quantitative phases of his study, describing the tools and processes used in data collection and analysis, stating ethical considerations, and providing socio-demographic information on the study population. Next, he leads the reader through each thematic topic, alternately presenting qualitative and quantitative findings, as available. The findings are organized by thematic areas — gender images and norms; factors in sexual socialization; sexual experience; the process of sexual initiation; the structure of sexual risks; and special contexts for sexual experience (paid sex, coercive sex, and concomitant use of alcohol or drugs).

Like Cáceres, you can successfully alternate between presentation of qualitative and quantitative data on specific points — even where themes break into sub-themes — and still retain your focus. In writing on sexual risk, Cáceres presents quantitative data on the proportion of young women who report having experienced undesired pregnancy [*embarazos no deseados*] and on cofactors for undesired pregnancy. Without interrupting the narrative flow of his elaboration on this phenomenon, he shifts into qualitative findings regarding young people's thoughts on factors that lead to undesired pregnancy, factors such as the relative stability of the couple or the use of tricks by one partner to achieve pregnancy as a way of trapping the other in the relationship. In his analysis, he provides selected quotes by adolescent study participants to illustrate key insights. Finally, once all relevant findings are presented on a given theme, he provides a unifying conclusion: his interpretation of what the findings mean, how variations in the findings can be understood, and what is important about what he learned.

In a qualitative study in Haiti of women's roles in sexual decision-making, the authors lead the reader through five themes to illustrate how Haitian women's capacity to negotiate safe sexual behavior, including the use of condoms, may be related less to their knowledge of the disease than to their customary role in sexual relationships (Ulin et al. 1995). Expanding on key thematic ideas, they present a range of study participant perceptions, descriptive information about participants who offer comments and quotes that illustrate both themes (e.g., beliefs about vulnerability and consequences of AIDS) and subthemes (e.g., social rejection, destruction of family, uncertainty about a spouse's fidelity) that they determine to be important. Following this presentation of results, which includes some explanatory interpretation, the authors offer a conclusion, which is comprised of their analysis of the findings with regard to the eight specific study objectives posed at the outset of their investigation. They present the conclusion section much like a series of distinct discussion sections for a scientific journal article, each about a page long. Finally, the authors end with a recommendations section, presenting their viewpoint on the study's implications for intervention.

The approach you take to organize your presentation and discussion of findings can be chosen to reflect aspects of your research design, whether you have conducted in-depth interviews, focus group discussions, or participant observation. Instead of separating the presentation of data from interpretation, some authors choose to weave the presentation of results into their analysis in a way that parallels their conversations with study participants over time. This kind of writing is similar to storytelling, with the researcher-author serving as narrator.

For example, in a study of adolescents in Detroit, Michigan, who intentionally infect themselves with HIV (Tourigny 1998), the author presents key themes in a series of case studies. Interview transcripts from a larger study had revealed that a subgroup of teenagers infected themselves with HIV in order to feel visible and important; others to access care and social services; and still others to elicit community or family support. The author decided to focus on this phenomenon through case studies of six self-infected young people she knew well, and to present her interpretations by way of personal commentary woven throughout the six case studies.

If your presentation of findings is logical and coherent, you increase the probability that your work will be accepted by the audiences for whom you are writing. This principle is valid even when dealing with multiple sources of data and presenting highly complex issues. Having a consistent structure for presentation of results helps you organize the material more efficiently and helps those who read your report make sense of the information.

However you structure the presentation of your findings, offer your interpretation and use your field notes to provide concrete illustrations and examples. Sharing the process allows readers to arrive at their own conclusions as to the meaning of the data.

Make use of numerical tables and other quantification where you can. It can help your readers, for example, to learn that "Individuals in all but one of the six focus groups believed in some form that young women cannot get pregnant the first time they have sex." Using numbers gives readers an indication of the relative importance of an idea and allows them to weigh the evidence you present. But be careful: One of the most common mistakes in reporting qualitative research is to treat data from qualitative samples as if they were quantitative data. For example, since the sampling for qualitative studies is not representative, *overemphasizing numbers and distributions is erroneous and misleading*. This is why it would be helpful to provide appropriate examples.

As you write, get your facts and references right the first time, and if you make generalizations, use specific instances to support your conclusions (Wolcott 1990). Write about whether you feel the findings from your study would make sense to a study participant and why. Tell the reader what steps you took in the study to ensure that the study question and the results were consistent with participants' views of their world.

Conclusion section

In the conclusion section of your paper or report, tell the reader whether the research has generated information that you didn't expect. Relate your themes to your statement of purpose and original question(s), and describe how your data support your explanation of the question, or your conceptual framework, if you used one. If you have created a visual diagram showing how your themes fit together, reflect on your original framework and whether it was borne out or not. What do your findings, the cluster of ideas, mean in a broader context? How might these findings apply beyond the original study population? Be careful not to suggest that your findings can be generalized, but rather state or show why you believe they are extensible (meaningful to a wider public health community) or not.

Your report will be more credible if it is organized around a conceptual framework, if the framework is elaborated throughout the report, and if it is supported with adequate qualitative evidence (Lofland 1974).

Describe findings that indicate controversy or polarization. If these relate to gender, say so. For example, if you conducted a series of focus group discussions on the influence of religious beliefs on family planning, note where women say one thing and men say another. Likewise, if you find that contraceptive discontinuation is associated with changes in menstrual bleeding patterns, be sure to discuss whether the results fit with findings from similar studies conducted elsewhere. If not, can you explain why they do not? Make clear the multiple and sometimes contradictory perspectives reflected in your data.

State the policy or programmatic implications of your findings, if applicable. Some writers place these in a separate "Recommendations" section that follows the "Conclusion" section.

How to Use Transcript Quotes in Narrative

Your use of quotes in your writing depends on what you are trying to accomplish. Also, as you select and present quotes, take care to represent participants' viewpoints fairly and respectfully.

It is important that you choose quotes that illustrate significant findings, that you manage the marking of quotes in transcripts efficiently, and that you present them in ways that preserve the contextual information necessary to understanding them accurately.

How to select appropriate quotes

Use representative quotes to illustrate norms or shared perceptions. These quotes should succinctly represent concepts that many who were interviewed would recognize as their ideas. For example, in one West African study of service delivery for the contraceptive implant Norplant, the majority of respondents independently mentioned the phrase *va-et-vient* ("coming and going" or "being given the runaround"). Hearing so many women say that to get Norplant removed, they must endure being given the runaround by service delivery personnel alerted the researcher that this service delivery phenomenon was entrenched. The women's shared phrase pointed to this phenomenon as a key theme to be explored in future research.

Use provocative quotes to highlight insights not generally held but perhaps innovative or pioneering. For example, if a focus group participant mentions that women like the female condom "because they can insert it before they leave work," you might explore whether potential users in that area perceive themselves to be at high risk of rape when commuting, and whether they feel the female condom would offer disease protection. Be careful not to give undue importance to quotes that may reflect atypical positions.

Draw on different people's voices, not just the most articulate. Be sure to check whether the range of people you quote reflects the range of people interviewed. One way to illustrate a range of perspectives and variations in language is to list short phrases related to your theme:

> *My wife and I decide together how many children we'll have.*

> *It's up to the man to decide how many children he can afford, because he's the one who earns the money.*

Use quotes to show that it is important not only what people say, but how. Language use, or tone, can indicate decision-making, discord, ambivalence, underlying emotion, or social expectations. Things said with great emotion, or powerful word choices, may indicate provocative issues below the surface.

How to prepare transcripts and manage foreign language translations

Mark key quotes to use in writing as you read through your transcripts. Have a good system for flagging possibly useful quotes as you read through the text; for example, participant or group ID code and line numbers on the transcript. As you write or make notes on your interpretation of the data, you can use the code as a temporary shortcut for the illustrative segment; for example, FG2-UM, 75-120, where the reference is to lines 75-120 in the transcript from your second focus group of urban males. Otherwise, trying to relocate a memorable quote when you need it can be a frustrating search. If you are using software to do your analysis, you can designate a code to retrieve salient quotes (see Chapter 6, page 153).

As a general rule, use verbatim quotes. However, minor changes may be needed to make a quote clearer — especially if it is a translation. Do not let clarification change some subtle meaning. If you need to shorten a quote or change some words, the convention is to put your substituted words in brackets [ ] and replace omitted words with a space and then three dots, called ellipses. For example: "My boyfriend and I want to protect ourselves from these [sexually transmitted] diseases, but … we don't always have condoms when we need them."

Many words or expressions in other languages have no literal translation or if translated, lose the subtlety of the original statement. The best way to handle these is to use the word that, in the translator's opinion, comes closest to the original but also to include the original word or phrase in italics within parentheses. For example: "An [informally] married (placé) woman agreed that 'life on the streets is hard … a woman without employment can't stand up to her partner.'"

Include key foreign words or phrases to enable readers who do know the language to judge the validity of the translated data. For example:

> Moderator: *What kind of people can contract the AIDS disease?*
>
> 1st Haitian respondent: *People who are fooling around (viv deyo), living promiscuously (nan epav), but if both people are not living like that, you will not get it.*
>
> 2nd Haitian respondent: *What she says is right, [but] some women who live with men are not involved with other men (li pa nan anyen), while their men may be involved in everything (nan tout afel).*

Weave explanatory quotes into your interpretation. The usual approach is to make the point in your narrative and follow it with an illustrative statement from a participant. You can wrap the quote into the narrative:

> *Most women seemed to believe that men expect to make the decisions about family size. As this 32-year-old woman lamented, "I really wanted only two kids, but my husband — you know how men are — insisted on a big family."*

Or for longer quotes, you can set them off as indented paragraphs, usually with a slightly smaller font. Note that quotation marks are used when the quote is embodied in the narrative but not when it is set off in its own indented paragraph:

A 42-year-old nonliterate mother of six volunteered the following illustration to explain how friends help each other:

> *When two women meet, they talk about the disease. I will say, "My dear, the AIDS disease is out there. Are you being careful?" And my friend might say, "I have this man I've been sleeping with, but I don't know if he has other women. Do you think I should break off this relationship?" And I say, "You can use a condom."*

Note that quotes become more alive if they are labeled with descriptive information; for example, a 16-year-old woman pregnant for the first time, or a 40-year-old unemployed factory worker. Remember never to put the name of the respondent in your report or quotation. You may have descriptive information in background data sheets (see Chapter 5). Your choice of descriptors will depend on the information you consider most relevant to the point you are making in your narrative. These descriptors can also follow the quote, for example:

> *I hide the pill packet in my clothes when my husband is home. I don't want him to find it, because he does not know I'm going to the family planning clinic.*
> Market woman, primary schooling, 27-year-old

You can also link several short, related quotes, indicating clearly that they are different speakers; for example:

> *I hide the pills in my clothes when my husband is home.*
> 27-year-old market woman
>
> *I take my pills before he comes to bed — I go to bed before he does.*
> 33-year-old teacher

When my husband asks, I just say I'm not using them.

30-year-old farmer

Keep quotes down to short segments of text — enough to suggest the context and not so long the reader loses the thread. Ask yourself whether the segment is a good reflection of the point you want to make. Since very long quotes tend to distract the reader from the flow of the narrative, they should be just long enough to give some life to the text. The narrative should speak for itself, i.e., make the point or show how the quote illustrates something you have written. You can also provide interpretation after the quoted remarks; for example, pointing out that the clandestine users above have different strategies for keeping their contraceptive use secret.

When using quotes in oral presentations of your research, keep them short. Just as presentations of quantitative studies are usually accompanied by slides or transparencies that summarize the data in statistical tables, qualitative researchers use words, or brief excerpts from transcripts, to illustrate the points they are making. These displays can be prepared exactly as they would for a written report, except that you should avoid presenting long passages on the screen. Short quotes, using some of the conventions discussed above for abbreviating verbatim statements, can help an audience visualize the data, or hear the participants speaking through you, the researcher. Presenting verbatim expression of your study participants enables the listener to share in the excitement of discovering life from the perspectives of the people living it.

Box 7.4
Does Your Study Matter?

■ Have you identified gaps in the literature and suggested ways your work offers new thinking in an area of importance?

■ Are the results consistent with other studies? How applicable are the findings in other contexts or with other groups?

■ Does your study rebut accepted thinking on the reproductive health topic you addressed, at least to some extent?

■ Does your writing provoke readers to reexamine their assumptions underlying prevailing theories or lines of thought?

(Adapted from Golden-Biddle and Locke 1999; Lincoln and Guba 1999, 398)

Establishing Credibility through Effective Communication

Despite potential skeptics — possibly including audiences more familiar with the logic and methods of quantitative inquiry — your obligation is "to gather the most highly credible information possible within the constraints of your situation and to present your conclusions in a form that makes them ... understandable and useful" (Morris et al. 1987, 8). Whether or not you communicate effectively with specific audiences will influence whether your study will be considered credible by those groups. Policy-makers, fellow researchers and community members will determine their confidence in your reproductive health study by examining both what you say and the manner in which you say it.

Three basic strategies can be used to enhance the credibility and communicability of your study report:

- Make sure the study question and results matter to your intended readers (relevance)

- Understand your audience's needs (length, level of complexity, conventions regarding credibility)

- Attend to the basics of good writing (clarity, accuracy, logical development of ideas)

No matter whom you communicate with, your readers will consider your text in light of their own needs and interests — both personal and professional. For example, if you report on in-depth interviews with married women who discontinue use of an intrauterine device (IUD), your intended readers will interpret and act on the text by relating what you present to their own views on the subject. These may relate to client-provider interaction, spousal decision-making, or even the value they assign to qualitative, as opposed to quantitative, approaches to studying contraceptive use. In order to convince readers that your findings hold merit, you will need to achieve a balance between challenging their assumptions and reiterating the familiar — in terms of the format, style, and content of your report.

Take care that what you say and the evidence you marshal to support your insights will seem realistic to your intended audiences, as well as to those you interviewed or observed in your study. Does your writing convey to readers "a sense of familiarity and relevance as well as a sense of distinction and innovation" (Golden-Biddle and Locke 1999)? Most readers will judge your written presentation as a direct reflection of the quality of your research. To convince the reader that you have accurately recorded and understood the meaning of what study participants said, present detailed descriptions and key quotations, and back up your argument with evidence (Rubin and Rubin 1995).

Then check your work by reviewing the content checklist on page 178. If you follow these steps, you will go a long way toward convincing your readers of the credibility of your report.

An important related issue is effective communication — writing that engages your readers intellectually and emotionally. The goal of qualitative writing is "to represent the world of your interviewees accurately, vividly and convincingly" (Rubin and Rubin 1995, 261). Your results will be important "if your report is read and its vividness influences decision-makers" (Rubin and Rubin 1995, 53). Writing has the potential to motivate readers to change practices, to explore new avenues of research, to inform health advocacy efforts, or to spur communities into action. Your responsibility is to make your study report as accessible, credible, and engaging as possible. Vivid stories can provide convincing descriptions of health conditions or issues, touching your readers more profoundly than abstract discussions alone. Hearing reproductive experiences in people's own words is gripping and powerful. Individual stories convey excitement, fear, drama, and realism. Do not be afraid to share emotion in bringing the interviewees' insights to life for the readers of your report (Rubin and Rubin 1995).

The ultimate interpreter of the quality and usefulness of your work is the reader, who interacts with what you have communicated and decides whether to integrate it into his or her work and worldview or to dismiss it. The credibility and communicability of your report will determine to a large extent whether readers will use your findings and whether the findings will have an impact on health policies, practices, and behaviors.

CHAPTER 8
Disseminating Qualitative Research

The ultimate goal of qualitative research is to transform data into information that can be used.

(Rossman and Rallis 1998, 11)

W hen we write about men's notions of HIV risk or dissemi-
nate women's perceptions about quality of care, we are fulfilling a practical
and social mandate common to applied research on reproductive health: the
creation of information for use by programs to improve services or by decision-makers to inform policies. The end-product of applied qualitative
research on reproductive and sexual health should be to give public

Disseminating Qualitative Research

voice or visibility to private or hidden issues; to cast new light on puzzling
questions; to make invisible problems clear (allowing solutions); and to
make reproductive health problems more understandable (allowing better
solutions) (Rubin and Rubin 1995, 51-52).

Because applied research aims to generate information that can be used, the
dissemination of study findings — what, why, by whom, to whom, and
how — needs to be considered from the beginning. If you want your results
to be used, start planning for dissemination even when you are designing
the study and developing a budget. Your specific purposes for dissemination
can vary, and may include the following processes or products:

- Strengthening and increasing the frequency of communication between
  the researcher and study participants
- Providing tools or materials for researchers and health advocates to communicate in support of policy change
- Helping other researchers, scientists, or decision-makers understand the
  social, cultural, political, or economic factors that influence reproductive
  health
- Empowering marginalized, silenced groups (such as victims of sexual
  violence)
- Providing practical information to solve programmatic problems
- Keeping reproductive health issues alive in the media, donor, and public
  health communities

Dissemination activities may include individual or group discussions before, during, or after study completion; meetings; publication in peer-reviewed journals; distribution of fact sheets; use of traditional media (e.g., songs, posters, puppet theater); coverage by news media; audiovisual presentations; or training workshops.

Contrary to the popular notion that dissemination implies only end-of-study activities, such as a seminar to brief senior health administrators, *research dissemination is a process, not a one-time event.* You do not have to wait until you have analytic saturation to disseminate. From the first day you introduce your study to ministry of health officials or community leaders, you are actively disseminating information on the purpose, scope, and potential impact of the study. When you return to key informants to say "This is what I'm hearing; does it make sense to you; why or why not?" you are sharing preliminary findings and opening a collaborative dialogue on their meaning.

In short, dissemination is an ongoing part of the dialogue with stakeholders that characterizes applied qualitative research. The methods used in qualitative research bring you into repeated contact with opinion leaders, community members, and other stakeholders; these interactions serve both to gather and to share information. Having unearthed in-depth, often deeply personal, information on what people say about reproductive health issues, it is then your responsibility to share study insights as widely as possible — whether such dissemination is formal or informal, direct or indirect.

As you develop a research dissemination strategy appropriate to your study, you will likely encounter obstacles. These can range from resource constraints, or skepticism about the validity of findings on the part of policy-makers and scientists unfamiliar with qualitative methods, to personal reservations regarding your interpretive role, or resistance on the part of health bureaucracies to information suggesting new practices. Many researchers believe either that research dissemination is outside their professional capacity or that it is not their responsibility. Others think they are responsible for dissemination only to the research community. It is important to consider from the outset where your research responsibilities will end, and whom to involve in order to promote effective utilization of results.

While many of the strategies and activities used to disseminate qualitative research are identical to those used to disseminate other types of studies, there are a few issues specific to qualitative work. For example, a frequent complaint among both scientists and policy-makers who have previous experience with qualitative studies that were poorly designed and implemented is "Why should we believe that these results mean anything? This information is anecdotal!"

To accomplish the ultimate purpose of applied research, to produce new and useful information, you will need a strategy for presenting your results effectively and persuading audiences that your findings are credible. We recommend at the very least disseminating your findings to study participants, health advocates, and the local or international research community. Incorporating participatory dissemination from the beginning, a process to which qualitative methods lend themselves, will generate better data and give your research results a better chance of being used.

Research Ethics Require Dissemination

The obligation to disseminate information back to study participants has been considered part of the professional code of applied sociologists, anthropologists, and other social scientists for decades, as has the public disclosure of findings. The Association of Social Anthropologists of the Commonwealth, for example, states that a researcher's "obligations to the participants or the host community may not end (indeed should not end, many would argue) with the completion of their fieldwork or research project … [Researchers should] communicate their findings, for the benefit of the widest possible community" (Association of Social Anthropologists of the Commonwealth 1999).

Qualitative researchers are ethically bound to disseminate findings for several reasons. First, we share the fruits of research — namely, information on study findings — to ensure that community members will continue to cooperate in future studies. Second, the use of qualitative research methods — whether focus group discussions with commercial sex workers or structured interviews with health educators — is based on creation of trust. We reciprocate that trust by sharing information, returning the benefits of research to the individuals and communities that have contributed their insights. This ethical commitment to reciprocity has become more formalized in guidelines on the informed consent process for international research involving human subjects, including qualitative research. In large part because community members in countries where AIDS research is being conducted have demanded that the benefits of research accrue to them more directly, international guidance documents are increasingly recommending that communities as well as study participants be informed of study findings after research is finished (Heise et al. 1998, 37; UNAIDS 2000b, 19).

There are other reasons to take seriously your role in dissemination. For example, effective dissemination of findings is a cornerstone of the research partnership and a proxy indicator of research impact (Harris and Tanner 2000, 818).

An Inclusive Dissemination Process Promotes Utilization

Ideally, qualitative study designs include a component in which study participants are contacted and asked whether the preliminary findings appear valid to them. For logistical and financial reasons, this phase is not always possible. Nevertheless, do what you can to check that your findings would make sense to your conversational partners. You might, for example, conduct exit interviews with stakeholders before leaving the study site. Every time you ask your conversational partners how they understand the meaning of the data you are generating, you are inviting them to contribute to shaping the messages that will emerge from the research, while at the same time disseminating information on the study. Such interactive dissemination leads to more grounded and therefore credible study findings.

Communication and participation are actually two words sharing the same concept. Etymologically the Latin communio *relates to participation and sharing.*
(Dagron 2001, 33)

Experts in diffusion of information agree that an inclusive and ongoing approach to research dissemination also leads to a greater likelihood that findings will be utilized (Rogers and Storey 1987; Havelock 1969; Cernada 1982). To foster a climate in which research is seen as relevant, involve stakeholders in as many research dissemination activities as possible. Stakeholder participation can mean very straightforward, simple activities. Maintaining frequent communication with key groups through visits, telephone calls, e-mail correspondence, or technical support is a powerful way to promote interest in and use of study findings. A recent study on the dissemination of research-based HIV prevention models to community service providers in the United States found that dissemination efforts are more successful when they "occur in the context of ongoing relationships between researchers and service providers, and when staff-training technical assistance is followed by opportunities to plan and problem-solve how to implement the research-based intervention" (Kelly et al. 2000, 1087). The authors of this randomized control trial concluded that the frequency of outside contact reinforcing and supporting initial dissemination messages to health administrators and providers had a significant impact on adoption of research-based HIV service delivery approaches.

How to Develop and Implement Dissemination

To develop a strategy for disseminating study findings and promoting their use, you will need to make decisions on what to say, to whom and through which means — and make sure you have the staff and financial resources to conduct your plan. In practical terms, a modest but effective package of dissemination activities might include facilitating the development of an information resource center in the study community (e.g., a mini-library containing the study report and relevant materials), publishing a newsletter with research results, collaborating on research reports, publishing journal articles, defining messages of importance to stakeholders, determining appropriate dissemination vehicles, or translating results for policy audiences.

At a minimum, aim to:

- write a report and discuss it one-on-one with key decision-makers

- plan a half- to one-day presentation meeting for health professionals and advocacy organizations

Box 8.1
Ways to Foster Two-way Communication in Research

Research stakeholders are more likely to utilize study findings if they feel they have participated in creating the results and are consulted and kept informed throughout the research process (Rothman, 1980, 68-69). To promote utilization of study findings, plan to include two-way communication steps such as:

- Collaborative development of subprojects

- Regular two-way communication and consultation with stakeholders

- Regular written feedback to stakeholders on study purposes, progress, findings

- Substantial face-to-face dialogue about progress, preliminary study results, implications of results for programs or policies

- Field trips with managers and stakeholders to view activities in order to create understanding, enthusiasm, ownership of study results

- Collaborative seminars to interpret findings

- Joint development of a family of related print materials written at appropriate levels for different audiences

- Follow-up visits to ministry of health officials or other key parties to personally deliver and review the study report

- One-on-one discussions with stakeholders for informal discussion of results, with written communication regarding next steps

(Adapted from Population Council, 1994)

- return information to the community through community discussions, a brochure on findings,* or other means

- distribute copies of your report to local universities, libraries, and key local and international organizations

To increase the likelihood that your study results will be used, keep in mind that the information must be communicated to the appropriate potential users (primary and secondary users). Study findings must address issues that users perceive to be important, and reports presented in a form that is understood and considered credible by the potential users. Information must be delivered to each audience in time to be useful, such as during revision of national guidelines on family planning service delivery practices (Morris et al. 1987). Special events such as World AIDS Day or International Women's Day may offer an opportunity to focus attention on your study. Also, try to make your communications as pleasant as possible — consider serving lunch at your dissemination seminar, or combining tea and an informal talk with government officials to whom you hand the report.

No matter how modest or ambitious your dissemination goals are, develop a written strategy based on audience needs, your needs and resources, current and emerging opportunities, timing, and the power of your study findings (Rogers and Storey 1987).

Box 8.2

Dissemination Factors that Promote Utilization

- the information needs of specific audiences are considered when designing the study

- the credibility and reliability of the research findings are accepted by users of study findings

- findings are disseminated to multiple audiences using a variety of channels and formats

- presentation of findings emphasizes the important lessons learned, especially from the point of view of the intended audience, rather than the need for more research

(Adapted from Sharma 1996, 20)

If you intend to influence an audience, know its motivations and its idiosyncrasies.
(Morris et al. 1987, 15)

---

* See Appendix 13, page 240 for an example of a brochure designed to share study findings with the communities that participated in the research.

Involving Librarians, Researchers, and the Media in Dissemination Planning

Edmond Bagdé Dingamhoudou
Population Council, Senegal

In 1997-98, the Centre d'Études et de Recherche sur la Population pour le Développement (CERPOD) and Family Health International (FHI) conducted a qualitative study in Mali of women's experience with contraception — what they expect from it, why many are reluctant to try it, and why some start but do not continue (Castle et al. 1999). Researchers followed 56 new contraceptive users in Bamako, the capital, over an 18-month period to see how family pressures encourage or discourage contraceptive use, focusing on communication, support, and strategies women use to control their fertility. Women were recruited during their initial visit to the Association Malienne pour la Protection et la Promotion de la Famille (AMPPF) clinic and interviewed three times at eight- to nine-month intervals. Eleven focus group discussions were held with approximately 100 experienced users, married men, and older women with daughters-in-law. Thirty-two women who had never used contraception also were interviewed.

The study yielded a number of findings that the research team thought were useful for family planning program staff and others. What good are findings that are shared only among the people who have conducted the study, without further dissemination? This question is becoming increasingly relevant to research endeavors on the African continent. It follows that no dissemination process can achieve its desired results as long as the messages that it seeks to convey do not address issues of public concern.

While CERPOD was finalizing a written report on the study (CERPOD 1999), our documentation center was also organizing a regional workshop on disseminating population and reproductive health research findings. We hoped to set up a regional reproductive health network of librarians and documentation specialists who could work with both journalists and researchers. The program included a training session on dissemination concepts in which participants developed practical ways of disseminating research findings using drafts of unpublished brochures.

The workshop participants were split into four groups. Each group was asked to list the elements of a dissemination campaign and to present their ideas on how to distribute the family planning study brochure. All possible means of dissemination were recorded. An introductory session on the Internet was even offered to the many participants who were not yet familiar with this tool. During the plenary session, all the ideas were synthesized and discussed to see which ones converged. At the end of the workshop, each participant went home with a written dissemination plan for the CERPOD materials.

Direct contact with journalists, documentation specialists, librarians, and researchers made it possible to examine closely the barriers to an effective dissemination process. The researchers, documentation specialists, and librarians were very open about their fear of working with journalists. They considered them to be too hurried and motivated by sensationalism. Importantly, they believed that journalists tend not to credit the source of the information (the researcher) or the contribution of the documentation specialist or librarian. In turn, the journalists criticized the others for being suspicious and overly cautious about distributing information.

Eventually, participants discovered the complementary roles of the different groups involved in the dissemination process. The journalists showed the researchers, documentation specialists, and librarians how to write a press release for the media, announcing the availability of the new publication. The journalists then learned from the others how to conduct documentation searches.

Any dissemination process must pay special attention to the support materials; the message itself; and areas of technical, professional, and even artistic design. My advice to qualitative researchers planning study dissemination is to use any opportunity to reach those who could use the information in their work or lives. Also, I recommend involving other relevant groups, such as librarians and journalists, as we did in the CERPOD workshop.

A strategy should include the following 10 general steps and considerations:

Conduct a needs assessment to help shape the dissemination of findings. One of the most important elements in dissemination to promote utilization of research findings is adequate understanding of what users need (Havelock 1969). Determine the degree of interest among researchers, health professionals, stakeholders, women's groups, and others who work to improve reproductive health.

Make a list of what people want to know and why they want to know it (Morris et al. 1987). Consider the decision-making process and the most influential people working on this issue in the setting you are studying. Your stakeholders can also help create this list. Do not assume you know all the groups that could benefit from the information. Also, be aware that sometimes stakeholders may not want to disseminate information to certain groups; try to ascertain whom they do not want you to talk to and why. Remember that different groups of people need different kinds of information in different forms and at different times (Morris et al. 1987). Ask who might be influential in action to improve reproductive health conditions, attitudes, programs, or policies suggested by research findings or recommendations and whether such individuals or groups have an explicit advocacy agenda.

Audiences that may be appropriate to involve in dissemination, either as creators or recipients of information related to your study findings, may include other researchers, reproductive health program directors, planning ministries, donor agencies,

All information is subject to misuse; and no information is devoid of possible harm to one interest or another. Researchers are usually not in a position to prevent action based on their findings; but they should, however, attempt to pre-empt any likely misinterpretations and to counteract them when they occur.

(Association of Social Anthropologists of the Commonwealth 1999)

news media, or nongovernmental organizations (NGOs) that focus on women's health, human rights, adolescent health, or civil society.

Ask yourself if your findings will or should matter to your audiences. Be realistic. Ask if the information in your report is:

- *relevant* to the user's real and compelling problems

- *practical* from the user's perspective

- *useful* and applicable to their situation

- *understandable* to potential users

- *timely* (Morris et al. 1987)

Ask if the findings will have a negative impact or be controversial. When you originally designed your study, you should have considered the potentially disadvantageous uses of the data you planned to collect. In planning your dissemination strategy, be sure to revisit these issues. Anticipate whether your study results might be embarrassing to program administrators, parliamentarians, or other community leaders accountable for decisions and oversight of health programs and policies (Hess 1989). Consider whether the news media or citizen groups may take the findings out of context. Be aware that "the study will be used, one way or another, and sometimes those uses are different from the ones [the researcher] intends" (Rossman and Rallis 1998, 11).

Sometimes study findings lend themselves to misinterpretation and therefore need special consideration in dissemination planning. For example, in a combined qualitative and quantitative study of the social and economic consequences of family planning use in the southern Philippines, researchers

Box 8.3

Working with the Media

The media play a key role in conveying health information to researchers, clinicians, and the general public (Grimes 1999).

Mass communication using news media, advertising, and marketing channels works particularly well to publicize new information and influence social norms. Media coverage of reproductive health issues can demonstrate the benefits of particular policies, articulate obstacles to health services, or model behaviors such as responsible parenthood (Smith WA 1995). If your study purpose involves communicating results to a wide group of people, and you have sufficient resources to do so, seek out a media professional or health advocate who can help you plan effective activities, keeping these guidelines in mind:

■ Establish your message.

■ Consider your audiences and direct your messages to them. Your audiences are mostly interested in how they are affected by what you say.

■ Know your facts.

■ Use human language. Everyone relates best to human experiences, so use stories drawn from your research to make your key points easier to absorb. Try to avoid technical terms. Use quotes from research participants to illustrate your message.

■ State your conclusions clearly, from the beginning. For example, you might say "This study showed that prophylactic provision of emergency contraception prevents abortion, and let me tell you why" (Seidel 1993).

■ When interviewed, stick to a couple of key points; practice articulating a very brief message that broadcast journalists can use as a sound bite.

found that one-fourth of all women, rural and urban, reported ever having been physically harmed by a spouse (Cabaraban and Morales 1998). The study found that among the significant correlates of violence were the wife working for pay and the husband sharing household chores. When initially presenting these results in the community, some audiences mistakenly concluded that male involvement in cleaning and washing leads to violence. One man griped, "Therefore, in order to avoid violence, we must not do household chores." To correct further misinterpretation of the results, the research team met with stakeholders to develop a dissemination strategy (Cabaraban 2001). Jointly, they developed an approach to serve the community interest while avoiding potential distortion of the data. They recommended that churches use the research results in developing guidelines for marriage counseling, that local institutions be encouraged to provide safe haven and legal services for battered women, and that health providers — including midwives and traditional healers — be trained to provide assistance and referrals for women experiencing violence.

How your study results will be used may be outside your control, but you are responsible for anticipating the potential negative uses of the information. By planning ahead, you can assist stakeholders and members of your research team to prepare for findings that may be controversial or lend themselves to distortion.

Find out what criteria the audience uses to consider information credible and useful for decision-making. To promote effective communication, determine which sources of information the group considers to be credible, useful, or timely (Goldstein et al 1998). Assess which style of dissemination best meets this group's needs. Some may prefer brief, or graphically interesting materials, while others require either comprehensive or academically oriented materials. Sometimes written dissemination is not culturally appropriate, but a

Transforming Research Findings into a Telenovela

Patricia Bailey, Dr.P.H.
Family Health International

Toward the end of Family Health International's (FHI) five-year multinational Women's Studies Project (WSP), those of us who had worked on WSP studies and dissemination planning in Bolivia discussed how to share project findings with groups outside traditional academic and public health circles. As the research projects in Bolivia were ending, we planned a final dissemination conference for ministry officials, non-governmental organizations (NGOs), and women's health advocates. The conference format, which included panels on specific themes that emerged across the studies and activities, allowed participants to synthesize findings and articulate practical recommendations. We also contracted with a local video producer, Fundación Solón, to take these themes, write a script, and produce a video, which was transformed into a four-chapter mini-series produced for television. This short *telenovela* fictionalized the lives and voices that were revealed to us and became an instrument of entertainment, education, reflection, and controversy. As a coinvestigator on several of the Bolivia studies, I found the popularization of scientific findings to be a unique and exciting experience.

The five studies used a range of qualitative and quantitative methodologies, including a case study of women-centered health care services; a cross-sectional survey of couples; in-depth interviews with men and women; a longitudinal survey of women; and a situational analysis of services that included interviews with clinic staff, clinic users and non-users. In different ways, each generated rich insights into our research question: how the use and non-use of family planning services affected women's lives.

We met several times with the video producer, who was convinced that the qualitative nature of the findings translated well into a drama with great human interest. The producer intertwined several subplots to reflect the complexities of urban life in El Alto, a fast-growing city filled with immigrants who arrive from rural areas with their cultural traditions and customs intact. The producer chose to depict the tensions of everyday life through: a character who loses his job and, humiliated, must turn to his wife for financial support; discrimination between social classes and ethnic subgroups; a young woman seeking to ensure a better life and her partner who is threatened by her independent behavior and desire to delay childbearing; an adolescent who is faced with an unwanted pregnancy and in desperation seeks an abortion; and an unhappy physician who finds neither his personal nor his professional life satisfying. All these themes came directly from the findings of the five studies. In the *telenovela*, these difficulties and challenges are mediated by images of the rising sun in the altiplano, the poignant hilarity of a tuba-playing drunk, a coy flirtation between two elderly clinic workers, and the compassion that individuals express when faced with the suffering of others.

Subplots in the *telenovela* illustrated perceptions and conditions that study participants shared with us:

■ An adolescent discovers her unwanted pregnancy and resorts to an unsafe abortion with severe complications. She almost loses her life, but the young physician intervenes and saves her, restoring his faith in himself and his professional calling to help others.

■ A middle-aged man loses his job and drinks excessively; his wife becomes the sole support for the family. In order to cope with this new responsibility, she wants to use a contraceptive method to avoid future pregnancies. Together they attend the physician's clinic, are counseled, and leave with condoms.

■ A young woman, a university student, seeks an intrauterine device (IUD) without telling her partner. She wants to delay childbearing in order to finish her degree, but when her partner finds out, he attacks her and goes to the clinic and assaults the physician.

■ An elderly cleaning woman at the clinic and the clinic gardener begin a relationship, but she has misgivings about sex after menopause. The physician assures her that sex at her age is fine.

■ The physician suffers a personal and a professional crisis. His wife throws him out when she discovers he has visited a prostitute, his car is stolen, and he decides to quit his work to take a job as a car salesman, like his friend.

Reflecting tensions revealed in the research, the physician character stands for the superiority of western medicine while the older indigenous clinic cleaning woman, a traditional herbalist, represents traditional medicine. When the irate young husband beats up the physician, the cleaning woman successfully treats the physician, who gains new respect for traditional medicine. Class/social/ethnic tension is exhibited between the indigenous older woman at the clinic and the young doctor who treats her poorly — e.g., he won't give her a ride in his car because she might be dirty.

Besides being shown on television, the video will be used in pre-service training for medical and nursing students in Bolivia and elsewhere in the region. It is to be used also among health care professionals at NGOs and in the public sector to promote discussion of the many factors that influence sexual and reproductive health. Differences in gender, ethnicity, culture, and social class all translate into an imbalance of power and lack of recognition of human rights within civil society as well as among health care professionals. Meanwhile, we await the public's reaction to this human, powerful, and accessible teaching medium.

series of community discussions would be. Different groups need different information, in different languages, using different terminology, delivered in formats that respect cultural or other norms. Timing and opportunities will also differ by group.

Identify people to work with. If you have determined that you have time only to disseminate your findings through written reports, consider working with local groups that could plan and implement broader dissemination of the findings. These might include professional associations, librarians, broadcast journalists, NGOs, or folk media committed to disseminating health messages.

Find as many ways as possible to report results back to key groups interested in the findings. Ask yourself who could best deliver the information. The knowledge dissemination and utilization literature shows that information produced internally — in contrast to information imported from the outside — is often more acceptable and credible. Consider various options, including co-presenting the information with a health program manager who intends to use the findings. Find out if there are existing consortia, such as a national reproductive health task force, that can either integrate their dissemination efforts with yours or reinforce your efforts with supporting messages. Offer a local health Web site the opportunity to post the executive summary of your study report.

Identify opportunities as well as potential problems. Identify other relevant activities going on in the setting (conferences, events, or ongoing media coverage of a related issue), and consider whether information can be an element for empowerment of study stakeholders. Research summaries or fact sheets can sometimes be used by community organizations as supporting information in their proposals to donors for service delivery project funding.

In short, plan specific ways to reach out to each important audience through channels that have appropriate "reach, frequency, and cultural impact" (Seidel 1993, 2). If time and financial resources allow you to collaborate with a communications consultant or a local NGO skilled in dissemination, ask them to develop and pre-test materials and messages for various intended audiences.

Identify dissemination priorities using a collaborative process as you develop your strategy. Perhaps you work at a major university and have conducted in-depth interviews on the use of emergency contraceptive pills in collaboration with research partners in several locations. You might decide — and your study participants might tell you — that health professionals, women's advocates and policy-makers all could benefit from the findings. In this case, your strategic priorities, developed with appropriate input, might be to:

- widely disseminate technical data on emergency contraception and the specific study results (locally, nationally, internationally)

- help local experts or other partners understand that how they translate findings and technical information into political or programmatic terms is key to gaining support for policy or program changes

- build local capacity for ongoing dissemination and policy reform related to provision of emergency contraceptive services (Porter and Hicks 1995, 32)

You likely will not implement a comprehensive dissemination strategy without assistance — you may be too busy, may not consider it appropriate, or may not have the needed resources or skills — but your role in identifying dissemination priorities is crucial: You have sifted through the data and articulated what they mean.

Begin disseminating from the outset. From the first day of your contact with stakeholders, inform them of the purpose of your study, its limitations, and its potential outcomes. Help your study participants play an active role in informing others. Simple dissemination activities, such as handing out a short letter describing the goals of your study, may help to create a climate conducive to research and empower research stakeholders to support your work. Be cautious to present such material in a way that avoids the appearance of being a public announcement, being clear that it is an internal communication to the research team or participants. Consider also that once you have provided written materials to individuals or groups, your materials may be inappropriately used or be printed in the local newspaper.

Help your readers identify the most important information. If developing printed materials, use headings, write topic sentences, and pay attention to spacing, margins, and graphic design. In short, do what you can to improve the readability of your material (Morris et al. 1987).

How to Reach Policy Audiences

Health policy reform is a process comprised of three dynamic, interactive activities: problem definition, the generation of solutions, and political consensus-building (Porter and Hicks 1995). If shared effectively, your research findings can influence policy in defining reproductive health problems and shedding light on possible solutions. Translating research findings into terms that address the interests and concerns of decision-makers and other groups active in public policy is not easy, but it is vital (Porter and Prysor-Jones 1997). As Rist notes, "Qualitative research can be highly influential ... with respect to problem definition, understanding of prior initiatives, community and organizational receptivity to particular programmatic approaches, and the kinds of impacts (both anticipated and unanticipated) that might emerge

Dissemination

What We Learned from Conducting Qualitative Research on Reproductive Health in China

Baochang Gu, Ph.D.
China Population Information and Research Center

A study on the impact of family planning on women's lives in China (Xie et al. 2000), conducted as part of the Women's Studies Project of Family Health International (FHI),* was the first study conducted through international collaboration in China that had the explicit goal of investigating directly how family planning has affected women, both positively and negatively. The study employed both focus group discussion (FGD) and a questionnaire survey. The FGDs, which allowed hearing the voices from both women and men whose lives are immediately affected by family planning, turned out to be a novel study methodology that provided valuable information for program implementation.

A number of studies have been conducted since the mid-1980s using quantitative data to assess the abnormal sex ratio at birth in China. However, the FGD approach used in this study revealed how people rationalize sex preference in children and why people in rural China so desperately want to have a son. Some women in North Anhui said:

> To have high status in the community you need a son. Otherwise you are looked down upon in the family and community.

> Without sons, your husband will dislike you; you will be very much discriminated against by the mother-in-law and the family.

> These women live miserable lives, especially if they are sterilized. Then there is no more hope. You terminated your family line.

In fact, our fieldwork suggests that the methodology greatly altered the relationship between the researcher and the researched. With a questionnaire survey, people tend to act as information providers, seeing the study as unrelated to their own interests and well-being. Sometimes, respondents are unmotivated, or even become bored and uncooperative in responding to a long list of questions. But in FGDs, participants tend to use it as an opportunity for their voices to be heard. They feel respected and heard.

At the beginning of the project, the research staff were worried about whether women would be willing to talk openly, especially on sensitive topics related to their personal reproductive lives. During the sessions, once the purpose and subject of the session were explained, there was an initial silence, and then women would start to speak one after another. Sometimes, several women were vying for the chance to speak out; they did not

---

* The Women's Studies Project was funded primarily by the U.S. Agency for International Development. This study in China was funded by the Rockefeller Foundation and the Ford Foundation.

want to miss the chance to talk. In all of the study areas, participants often had so much to tell that the session had to go beyond the scheduled time.

Such a situation made the note-taker's work difficult and the recorded tapes difficult to transcribe. However, getting women and men to talk from their hearts was something that was unusual in China and something that a quantitative survey could never achieve. The human touch of the qualitative approach requires the investigators to place themselves in an equal position with the participants. A key lesson that we learned is that FGD sessions could not be successful unless participants were convinced that they could trust the investigators and that the study would bring some improvement to their lives.

Successful fieldwork requires the support and cooperation of local government, particularly because management of the highly sensitive subject of family planning is devolved to local government leaders in China. Acutely aware of the implications, the field team met first with local program leaders and managers to explain the purpose of the study and detail procedures, including how participants would be selected and their desired characteristics. We emphasized that the study would not assess the performance of the local program, but that the people interviewed would provide information to make general improvements in the China family planning program. Local assistance is not only necessary to gain the cooperation of the local government but also to recruit local field assistants for the FGDs.

A questionnaire survey that complemented the FGDs was carried out in the same project areas. The combined quantitative and qualitative methods provided rich, complementary information and helped us to interpret our findings in a more convincing way than we might have in using either methodology alone. This triangulation of data strongly helped the leaders and managers of the family planning programs to understand the need to hear women's own views of the relationship between family planning and other aspects of their lives.

This research was conducted at a time when China is considering how to shift away from its long-time emphasis on demographic goals. Our study provided a context to understand the need for a client-centered orientation in family planning, and helped pave the way for an innovative quality of care experiment that has been conducted by China's State Family Planning Commission (SFPC) since 1995. This study took the rare step of listening to individuals' voices, a departure for China's family planning program in the mid-1990s. Since our work was implemented, understanding and meeting clients' needs for quality reproductive health care has increasingly become the central theme of the family planning program in China. The voices of women and men from south Jiangsu, north Anhui, and central Yunnan were heard clearly by family planning leaders not only in their own provinces, but also by national leaders in Beijing.

from different intervention strategies" (Rist 2000, 1005). Make use of the power of your conversational partners' words and stories to engage those who influence policy. Select the "face" or aspect of the problem that is most relevant to the interests of your particular audience: A simplified understanding of the problem is crucial in generating support for solutions (Porter and Hicks 1995, 31).

Include an executive summary to accompany a more lengthy report if you want busy policy-makers to learn about your work. An executive summary should state: (1) what was studied; (2) why the study was conducted; and (3) the major findings, conclusions, and recommendations you have generated. Some readers may not have the time or expertise to read through your report, but they will want to know what you found and how it applies to them.

Identify locally credible champions — not necessarily experts, but respected individuals able to convey research-based information — to make the case for change with those who can actually influence reproductive health policies and their implementation. Working to influence policy is a form of behavior change intervention, a field in which both theory and data point to the importance of: (1) participative decision-making; and (2) face-to-face interactions that lead to commitments to change (Stevens and Tornatzky 1980). Never underestimate the importance of personal contact in your policy dissemination efforts.

Oral Presentation of Qualitative Findings

Oral presentation of qualitative findings is very similar to presentation of quantitative study results, with the distinction that treatment of quotes from participants usually replace statistical summaries of the data. As with all dissemination formats, be sensitive to audience needs and expectations (e.g., determine the time your audience has to listen and speak less than the maximum allotted time); know

> *Box 8.5*
> ## Policy Dissemination Tips
>
> - Keep reports brief
> - Provide talking points to policy stakeholders who may either use or disseminate your study results
> - Recognize that research results may have larger political implications, requiring consensus of many stakeholders before action can occur
> - Encourage policy-makers to weigh data from different sources
> - In planning for use of information for policy purposes, consider the availability of resources, the institutional capacity to change practices, and political risk (Rist 2000, 1013-1014)

whether overhead slides or projection images will be better received and what contextual information will be important to provide; and focus on the main question, paying attention to the quality of what you say. When structuring your oral presentation, include the following sections:

Opening. Set the scene by telling a story that will interest your audience.

Introduction. Tell your listeners what your presentation will cover:

- What reproductive or sexual health issue did you study?
- Why did you conduct the study (objectives)? Why was it important?
- What questions did you ask, and how did they evolve as you analyzed initial responses?
- What methods did you use and how close did you get to the participants in the study setting?
- The number of results you will discuss.

Body of the talk. Discuss your results sequentially, and relate them to your theoretical framework. Clarify each point by using examples and presenting selected short quotes from study participants to illustrate major findings. Offer your interpretation of how applicable the findings may be to other settings, and describe the limitations of your work.

Summary. Summarize for the audience the important points in your talk. Articulate any unanswered questions, and identify areas that need further study.

The two most important elements of successful presentations are: (1) to keep overheads, slides, or other visuals short and simple; and (2) to practice giving your talk beforehand. To hold your audience's interest, and to share ownership of the findings, consider inviting a key informant or other stakeholder to co-present the findings. Remember that you are sharing words and experiences of people who entrusted their stories to you. Do not be afraid to try presentation formats that convey the drama and emotion of their lives.

Outcome Indicators for Dissemination

Since you do not know precisely where the research will lead you or to whom the findings will be important, you cannot define outcome indicators for effective dissemination at the outset of your qualitative study. Nevertheless, as you proceed with your study, do your best to identify appropriate indicators for utilization of the results. Defining possible ways to measure the effect of your dissemination will help focus your efforts on activities with greater impact.

To develop indicators, make use of existing theoretical frameworks developed by scientists who study knowledge dissemination and utilization. For example, Havelock, who reviewed 4,000 studies on knowledge dissemination and utilization, framed how individuals and groups use knowledge in terms of: (1) problem-solving; (2) social interaction; and (3) research, development, and diffusion (Havelock 1969). Try to visualize how your study might be used by different groups to address reproductive health or service delivery problems; how the findings might influence relationships among individuals or groups concerned with your topic; and how your study findings might affect future research, public awareness, or community empowerment to improve health. These possible outcomes may become your dissemination indicators. They may include changes in the information resources available to stakeholders or changes in their knowledge base, information-seeking behavior or decision-making processes (Menou 1993; Menou 1999; Thorngate 1995).

Dissemination

Process indicators for dissemination of study findings are data and indicators compiled at the program level. What might the application of your findings mean to program planning, allocation of resources, procedures, or functions (Buckner et al. 1995, 43, 63)? Process indicators for the short-term or intermediate outcomes (or effects) of reproductive health research dissemination may include:

- publication of study findings in-country as well as internationally

- presence of study reports in local, national, and international libraries

- news media coverage of study findings

- number of individuals or groups who need the information reached with summaries of results

- locally initiated translation of study findings into local languages or easier-to-read formats

- increase in the number of ongoing opportunities for and instances of communication between community stakeholders and health researchers or policy-makers

- number of short courses or conferences where study results are disseminated

- funds allocated for additional communication of results

- adoption by sister research agencies of future research priorities suggested by your study

The long-term or ultimate outcomes (or impacts) of qualitative research dissemination are harder to measure, but nevertheless important (Beck and Stelcner 1996a; 1996b). They may include:

- the number, variety, and mutuality of relationships between those interested in the reproductive health issues you studied and those who are in a position to help them out (Cernada 1982, 14, 139; Havelock 1969; The Human Interaction Research Institute 1976)

- persistent enhancement of, and level of, mutual understanding of terminology or language used by different groups (researchers, politicians, community members) to describe reproductive health concepts

- increased accuracy in the information that stakeholders share in dialogue or debate (Communications Initiative 2000)

- persistent enhancement of respect among research stakeholders for each other's perspectives, manifested in greater degree or regularity of consensus on action steps favoring improved reproductive health

- the number, variety, frequency, and persistence of forces that can be mobilized to utilize the knowledge generated (Havelock 1969)

- changes in reproductive health services or policies attributable to your research

- a high level of citations of your report in scientific papers and international bibliographic indexing databases

- increased long-term news media coverage of the topic you studied (as measured through content analyses over time)

- allocation of funds or government support for further research on aspects of the topic you studied

- systematic use of study findings in public health, educational, and training institution curricula

- the percentage of organizations that subsequently offered an evidence-based model of services in line with your research findings

Common sense tells us that if we know where we want to go, we are more likely to arrive at our intended destination. Identifying outcome indicators for dissemination is one way to keep your sights on the potential use of your study findings by people who need them.

Conclusion

The biggest challenge to disseminating qualitative research may lie within ourselves and our conceptions of our roles as researchers. If we do not perceive communication as an explicit research responsibility or are uncomfortable in the role of dissemination, it is unlikely that our work and the insights it generates will make a difference to people's well-being or to the reproductive health programs and policies that serve them.

Even if your orientation, interests, and resources allow you to develop ambitious research dissemination objectives and plans, you will likely face challenges and frustrations as you proceed. A participatory approach to collaboration with stakeholders in the iterative process of dissemination or materials development takes more time than implementing dissemination unilaterally or limiting dissemination to publication of a scientific paper. Community members or health service delivery staff may not be convinced that change is desirable or possible. Recommendations suggested by the findings may be considered too innovative for the political climate of the time. Or research findings may not be focused enough to provide guidelines for action, and you may need to confer again with stakeholders able to create and take responsibility for disseminating action-oriented recommendations.

Research dissemination is both an ethical obligation and practical necessity for qualitative researchers and is most effective when planned and implemented from the outset with significant involvement of research stakeholders. We urge qualitative researchers to challenge existing conceptions of their role in dissemination, to incorporate ideas into dissemination plans as they surface in the research process, and to take active steps to bridge the information gap between the research community, health practitioners, health advocates, and policy-makers.

Neither academic nor medical and health research institutions … regard it as their responsibility to communicate their research findings to local policy-makers, practicing health professionals, or the public.

(Kitua et al. 2000, 821)

Dissemination

APPENDIXES

Appendix 1
Samples of Behavioral Frameworks

Theoretical frameworks from the behavioral sciences can be a valuable source of ideas for developing a research problem and a way of linking one's research to a wider theoretical context. In qualitative research, however, the investigator must take care not to impose structure at the expense of spontaneity and new insight into the problem. Nevertheless, frameworks that have been developed, tested, and refined in numerous studies of a common behavioral phenomenon, such as taking action to reduce health risk, contain useful concepts and relationships that can add clarity to a research problem without constraints on the methodology.

Qualitative researchers should also note a common limitation of most behavioral frameworks, namely their focus on individual behavior. For instance, many women feel at risk of HIV, not due to their own behavior but because of the behavior of their sexual partners. Qualitative designs that use concepts drawn from behavioral models must also encompass the wider social and cultural context — economic constraints, normative influences, and as always, gender and power differences that could explain or contradict the findings of a study limited by a predetermined model.

Below are summaries of four frameworks that have been useful to researchers in sexual and reproductive health.

■ Health Belief Model

One of the most commonly used frameworks in health behavior research, the Health Belief Model, offers useful guidance for understanding sexual risk behaviors (Rosenstock et al. 1994). Basic premises of the model are that individuals differ in: (1) how they perceive the personal benefits or value of avoiding illness or getting well; and (2) their expectations that a specific action can prevent illness. People are more likely to take action to prevent or control an ill-health condition, if:

- they believe it to have potentially serious consequences
- they believe that a course of action available to them would be beneficial in reducing either their susceptibility to or the severity of the condition
- they believe that the anticipated barriers to (or costs of) taking the action outweigh its benefits (Glanz 1997, 44; VanLandringham et al. 1995)

This model can address programmatic or practical questions, such as "Why are women discontinuing the use of intrauterine devices?" or "Why are commercial sex workers not using condoms with their steady partners?" Key concepts are:

Perceived susceptibility. People's perception of their chance of getting a condition such as pregnancy, HIV infection (Brown et al. 1991).

Perceived severity. Opinions of how serious are the medical, social, or financial consequences of a health condition.

Perceived benefits. Perceptions of the efficacy of the recommended action (e.g., abstinence, condom use, contraception) to reduce health risks.

Perceived barriers. Perceptions of the psychological, social, or financial costs of adopting the new health behavior.

Cues or triggers to action. Events that increase the likelihood of action, including symptoms of infection or exposure to family planning messages on the radio.

Self-efficacy. The conviction that one can successfully carry out an action, such as consistent use of dual methods, required to produce the outcomes (e.g., prevention of pregnancy and STI) (Bandura 1977a as cited in Glanz 1997, 47).

Other variables. Especially socio-demographic factors such as educational attainment, as they influence an individual's perceptions and thus indirectly influence health-related behavior.

■ Stages of Change Theory

In this framework, behavior change occurs as a sequence of stages that vary by individual. It can be a useful tool for tailoring health interventions to the needs of target groups — segmented by behavioral stage — and for evaluating programs by measuring behavior change at different stages (Prochaska et al. 1997).

Key concepts are:

Precontemplation. The stage in which an individual is at risk but with no intention to modify behavior (e.g., sexually active adolescents who do not believe they can get pregnant, diabetic women who are uninformed about the dangers of repeated pregnancies, or men with multiple partners who ignore the consequences of their high-risk behavior).

Contemplation. The stage at which an individual recognizes the need for change but is ambivalent.

Preparation for action. Individuals at this stage intend to take action and may have initiated limited behavior change (occasional use of condoms); they may be good candidates for behavior change programs that focus on action steps (consistent use of condoms).

Action. The individual has made specific modifications in behavior or lifestyles sufficient to reduce the risk (correct and consistent use of abstinence or other contraception).

Maintenance. Sustained behavior change for more than six months.

Factors that influence movement through this sequence of changes may also come from other frameworks; for example, perceived severity of risk or sense of self-efficacy as in the Health Belief Model.

■ AIDS Risk Reduction Model

The AIDS Risk Reduction Model (ARRM) provides a framework for explaining behavior change in relation to the sexual transmission of HIV/AIDS (Catania et al. 1990). It incorporates several variables from other behavior change frameworks, including several from the Health Belief Model: self-efficacy and theoretical understanding of interpersonal processes. Like the Stages of Change framework, ARRM hypothesizes a sequence of three stages of change: (1) recognizing and labeling one's behavior as high-risk; (2) making a commitment to reduce high-risk sexual contacts and to increase low-risk activities; and (3) taking action. The last stage is further classified as information-seeking, obtaining remedies, and enacting solutions. Phases may occur concurrently or may be skipped, depending on the individual.

Variables that influence movement through these stages include:

- knowledge of sexual activities associated with AIDS transmission, belief in personal susceptibility, believing that AIDS is undesirable

- costs and benefits of action, self-efficacy, knowledge of the health utility and pleasure of a sexual practice

- social networks and problem-solving help, prior experience with problems and solutions, self-esteem, verbal communication with sexual partner, partner's beliefs and behaviors

In addition to the influences above, ARRM postulates other motivators to change such as public education campaigns, informal support groups, or an image of a person dying from AIDS. In the past ten years, ARRM studies have examined a variety of populations, including people attending HIV-testing clinics, gay and bisexual men, unmarried heterosexuals, and adolescent women attending family planning centers. Results from a published study revealed how difficult it was for women in Zaire to label their high-risk behavior as problematic; only one-third of the study participants felt personally at risk for contracting HIV/AIDS (Bertrand et al. 1992).

Locus of Control

This theoretical construct is derived from social learning theory. It has been used to conceptualize the distinction between the belief that events in one's life are the result of one's own action and the belief that such events are governed by forces independent of oneself (Wallston et al. 1978; Lau 1982). Health locus of control has been measured by a scale composed of items that determine the relative strength of external or internal health beliefs about health and illness. Key concepts are:

External locus of control. Belief that outcomes are under the control of powerful others or are determined by fate, luck, or chance.

Internal locus of control. Belief that outcomes are directly the result of one's behavior.

Locus of control is relevant to research problems that focus on behavior change to reduce the risk of HIV. For example, a fatalistic attitude toward one's risk of acquiring the HIV virus (internal locus of control) is likely to be associated with inconsistent or incorrect use of condoms, in contrast to consistent use of condoms by individuals who believe they offer protection against disease (external locus of control). However, a woman who believes in the efficacy of condoms might also believe that she has no power to control the decision to use them. For her, behavior change is limited by an external locus of control, in this case the perceived influence of "powerful others."

Appendix 2

Examples of Oral Consent Forms

Example 1

Family Health International (FHI)

Oral Informed Consent for Focus Groups (to be read to the group by the Moderator)

Name of Research Study:

Principal Investigator:

Reason for the Research

We would like to talk to you about taking part in discussion group(s) conducted by (*name of organization*) to (*objectives of the research study in easily understood words*).

You are being asked to take part in a group that will have a trained leader. The groups will talk about:

Your Part in the Research Study

About (*# women/men/couples*) will take part in this research (*specify at this site and/or at # of sites*).

If you agree to take part in the research, you will be in ___ groups lasting ___ hours each.

Your participation is voluntary and there is no penalty for refusing to take part. (If you do not take part, it will not affect any health care that you would normally receive.) Also, you may quit being in the groups at any time.

How you were identified

We are asking you to participate because we are talking to people who use the (*name of clinic*).

Possible Risks and Benefits

There is a small chance that what people talk about in the group will make you feel uncomfortable. There is also a small chance that others in the group may tell someone you were taking part or report what you said.

Confidentiality

No one except the group leaders and the other group members will know that you took part in the research. The groups will be tape recorded with voices only. [To protect confidentiality of research participants, state what will be done with the audiotapes after being used for focus groups.] Note-takers will write down opinions and what group thinks during the sessions. We will not record your name or any other personal things about you during the groups. **We ask that participants not reveal outside the group information they may have heard in the group.** Even though we will ask people in the group not to reveal anything to others, we cannot guarantee this. We will protect information about you and your taking part in this research to the best of our ability. If the results of this research are published, your name will not be shown.

Compensation

You will be paid ____(or given gifts worth____) per session for taking part in this research.

Contact for Questions

(Give separate list of contact numbers to subjects when oral consent is used.)

Consent Form to Be Signed by Moderator

1. Read and review the Oral Consent for Focus Groups with each participant in a private setting.
2. Ask the following: "Are you willing to be in a focus group to talk about _____?"
3. Read the Oral Consent for Focus Groups to the group before the first session begins. Whenever possible, this reading before the group should be (voice) tape-recorded.

I have reviewed the Fact Sheet with the research participants, and they have fully agreed to be in this focus group research. I further agree to keep confidential anything that is said in the discussion group.

Please print clearly:

_____   _____
(Moderator's name)   (Signature of Moderator)

_____
(Date)

Example 2
Family Health International (FHI)
Oral Informed Consent for Surveys/Interviews
[Title of Research Study — may be simplified]

This interview is for a research study that is being done by (*name of organization*).

This research will gather information on (*how people in this city think about AIDS and HIV*). We are talking to people who use the (*name of clinic*).

The interview will include questions on (*sexually tramsitted diseases, AIDS, condom use*). It will take most people about _____ minutes/hours to answer the questions.

The names of people who agree to be interviewed (*will not be recorded without their permission*).

Your participation is voluntary and there is no penalty for refusing to take part. (If you do not take part, it will not affect any health care that you would normally receive.) You may refuse to answer any question in the interview or stop the interview at any time.

(Give separate list of contact numbers to subjects when oral consent is used.)

- -

Every aspect of the research outlined above has been fully explained to the volunteer in his/her native language, (*specify*).

_____   _____
(Signature of Person Obtaining Consent)   (Date)

Appendix 3

Example of a Qualitative-Quantitative Research Design

Unintended Pregnancy and School Drop-out among Women Students in an Urban Secondary School

This partial research design shows the progression from an area of research linked to a policy issue to development of research questions and selection of methods. Note that the full design would also include a conceptual framework and plans for data analysis and dissemination.

Area of Research

Unintended pregnancy and consequent discontinuation of studies among female adolescents attending secondary school.

Policy Issue

Immediate punitive suspension of pregnant students for one year from date that pregnancy is discovered by school authorities.

Research Problem

- To explore and compare the experiences of sexually active young adults with respect to: (a) pregnancy prevention; (b) the effect of pregnancy on school achievement; (c) vocational goals; and (d) perceptions of personal control in their lives
- To explore attitudes of school authorities toward female students who become pregnant while still in school

Study Objectives

- To identify patterns of sexual activity, contraceptive use, contraceptive help-seeking, and pregnancy experience in a sample of adolescent women
- To compare academic and vocational aspirations of: (a) sexually inactive women students; (b) sexually active women students who have never been pregnant; (c) women students with histories of pregnancy; and (d) women (former

students) who left school permanently because of pregnancy
- To explore young women's sense of personal control in relation to pregnancy prevention, school achievement, and vocational goals
- To identify the potential for policy change regarding suspension of pregnant students
- To describe the experiences of adolescents who seek contraceptive information and service

Examples of Research Questions

Objective 1: Patterns of sexual activity
- Quantitative: At what ages did women in the study population become sexually active?
- Quantitative: To what extent have sexually active young women used contraception (age, methods, consistency, continuity)?
- Quantitative: What have been the outcomes of pregnancy when it occurs (births, abortions, live children)?
- Quantitative/Qualitative: How and where have young women sought contraceptive methods and at what ages?
- Qualitative: To what extent do young women believe they have been successful in obtaining contraceptive information and methods? If not successful, why?
- Qualitative: What were young women told or advised to do when they sought contraceptive information and methods?

Objective 2: Academic and vocational aspirations
- Qualitative: In what ways do students and former students believe their academic and vocational goals have changed since they began secondary school?
- Qualitative: How do current academic and vocational goals differ among sexually active students who have never been pregnant, students

who have ever been pregnant, and former students who dropped out due to pregnancy?
- Qualitative: How do students perceive the policies and attitudes of school authorities toward student pregnancy?

Objective 3: Personal control
- Qualitative: How do women in the four study categories differ with respect to their beliefs that they can act on their own desires or decisions regarding: (a) having sex; (b) becoming pregnant; (c) pursuing education; and (d) choosing a vocation?
- Qualitative: What influences or circumstances do women in each category perceive as encouraging and discouraging their ability to control their reproductive, academic, and vocational decisions?

Objective 4: Potential for policy change
- Qualitative: What are the opinions of school teachers and administrators concerning the suspension policy?
- Qualitative: In the views of school authorities, how should the school respond to a pregnant student?

Objective 5: Contraceptive information and service
- Qualitative: How do women students describe their experiences in pharmacies and clinics when they have sought help for pregnancy prevention?
- Qualitative: How do students' accounts compare with observed behavior of pharmacists and clinic personnel?

Sources of Information

Quantitative: Phase I
School sample: 800 female students, 15-18 years of age, enrolled in a large urban secondary school; all eligible respondents.

Community sample: 75 women factory workers, 25 years of age or less, who say they discontinued schooling because of pregnancy.

Qualitative: Phase II
Subsamples of phase I respondents, purposively selected to represent:
- sexually inactive women students
- sexually active women students who have never been pregnant
- students who have dropped out of school during a pregnancy and returned
- former students who dropped out of school due to pregnancy and did not return

Key informants, purposively selected:
- four school administrators from a different but demographically similar school
- four school teachers from a different but demographically similar school
- four family planning providers from a reproductive health clinic in the study community
- four pharmacists from the study community

Total: three family planning clinics and three pharmacies.

Methods

Quantitative: Phase I
Structured questionnaire, multiple-choice responses with skip patterns, administered to all phase I respondents in one session (n=800).

Qualitative: Phase II
- Focus group discussions with two groups of participants from each of the phase II subsamples, repeated in a total of three discussions with each group, or 24 discussions
- In-depth interviews with key informants: school administrators, teachers, family planning providers, and pharmacists
- Mystery client observation in family planning clinics and pharmacies serving the study community

Anticipated Ethical Issues

Sensitivity to preference of some students not to participate. Prospective participants need full explanation of the nature and purpose of the research, possible risks (breach in confidentiality), and what will be expected of them as respondents to the phase I survey questionnaire, as well as in phase II if they are selected and agree to participate.

Parental consent if required by an Institutional Review Board. Informed consent of adolescent participants in social (nonclinical) research may be sufficient. If parental consent is required, the researcher must take great care not to suggest that any individual student is or is not sexually active. Emphasis should be on healthy reproductive decisions in relation to educational and vocational achievement. If possible, the request will come from the school as part of an ongoing health education program.

Protection of confidentiality. Survey questionnaires will be administered by researchers, not school personnel. School personnel will not be present during any data collection. Only researchers will have access to data, which will be secured in a locked place. Participants in phase II will sign a pledge to respect the confidentiality of their peers. Focus group moderators will guide discussion toward normative aspects of the research problem by inviting participants to comment on common experiences and feelings of young women. They will not ask for disclosure of personal experience. Selecting key informants from schools other than the study site will minimize possible student anxiety about school officials being in the study.

Deceptive nature of mystery client observation. This technique will be used only if pharmacists and clinic personnel grant permission to conduct occasional anonymous and unannounced observation visits by simulated customers or clients over a six-month period.

Appendix 4

Procedural Guidelines for Managing Focus Group Discussions

Before Leaving for the Site

Review notes
Include notes from focus group discussions conducted earlier for this study, including team debriefings if they were done.

Review study protocol and topic guide

Gather materials
Tape recorder, extra tape recorder, sufficient cassettes, extra batteries, notepads and pens, labels, nametags, topic guides, gifts, snacks or travel reimbursements for participants, other materials.

Test tape recorder

At the Site before Discussion Begins

Set up room
Refreshments should be available before focus group discussion begins. Ensure that participants help themselves or are served. Arrange mats or chairs in a circle. A table may or may not be present, depending on cultural norms of conversation.

Test tape recorder
Label cassette with date and group identification code; load and test.

Greet participants

Collect socio-demographic data informally
Make labels with numbers corresponding to data sheets if using them to identify individual speakers during recording and note-taking.

Starting the Discussion

Introduce yourself and invite participants to introduce themselves
If names are used, use first name only.

Summarize the purpose of the study

Describe the focus group discussion process
No right or wrong answers; all should participate; all should respect the opinions of others; help to keep discussion on track; use of tape recorder; notes will be taken. Advise group that the discussion will last approximately 1-1/2 hours. Invite questions.

Review the statement of informed consent
Make sure everyone understands.

Encourage confidentiality
Ask participants to guard the confidentiality of others in the group.

Conducting the Discussion

Begin with warm-up questions

Be aware of who is talking and who is not
Do not allow one or two individuals to dominate; bring silent participants into the discussion.

Use broad, open-ended questions
Avoid yes or no or short-answer questions in a questionnaire format. Frame the discussion with more general questions and encourage participants to raise issues that are important to them.

Always probe
On some occasions moderators may want to probe for additional information when a participant's initial answer appears incomplete. Probing does not mean suggesting a more interesting answer. Probes that suggest answers are leading probes and must be avoided.

Examples of leading probes not to use:
• Do you mean ... ?
• Are you saying that ... ?
• Is that the only thing you can think of?
• You do not mean that ... ?

Good non-leading probes are usually general inquiries such as:

- How do you mean?
- In what way?
- What other methods/means of/do you know?
- There is no hurry. Take a moment to think about it and tell me all that comes to your mind.

Do not hesitate to use silence (waiting expectantly while a speaker thinks through her idea) and non-verbal prompts (raising your eyebrows, nodding your head, saying "hmmm," etc.). They tell the respondent that you are listening and interested in whatever she has to say.

Note any questions that are not understood well by the group, as well as questions that stimulate good discussion. Revise the topic guide after the session if necessary for future discussion.

Record body language, nonverbal communications
Participant's tone of voice or physical movements may communicate more than she is actually voicing. An idea stated forcefully or even angrily might emphasize the strength of a participant's convictions. A hesitant manner might suggest the participant is not sure about the idea she is stating, or that she anticipates disagreement from others in the group. Rivalries or "one-upmanship" between group members may also be communicated non-verbally. Such dynamics should be noted. Body language and nonverbal communications, just as verbal expression, should also be noted.

Use the guidelines flexibly; return to topics that were not fully discussed or that needed more thought.

End of Discussion
Thank participants

Explain how discussion information will be used

Remunerate discreetly
Distribute travel reimbursement, small gifts, or honorarium if used.

Collect tape recorder, tapes, socio-demographic data sheets if used
Check that all cassettes are appropriately identified with coded information.

After Discussion
Expand notes in outline form
Note-taker and moderator should do this together immediately following the session if possible, or at least on the same day as the focus group discussion. Record in writing any nonverbal data.

Transcribe tapes
May take four to eight hours. The task may be shared or rotated from note-taker to moderator. Develop a system to transcribe tapes as quickly as possible.

Review transcribed notes
Add researcher's comments in parentheses. These could include observations about the group, remarks to probe in later discussions, or methodological problems.

Translate

Sample Budget Categories for Planning Focus Group Discussions

The following budget categories have been developed for focus group proposals. Estimated costs should be based in part on the number of discussions to be conducted, which will depend on the purpose of the study and the range of characteristics of people whose participation will be needed.

❏ Planning (possible extra sessions with representatives of implementing agencies or target groups, including transportation and meeting space)

❏ Recruitment of participants (recruitment questionnaire, transportation)

❏ Payment or gifts for participants (incentives)

❏ Refreshments

❏ Rental for space where discussions are held

❏ Child care

❏ Moderator fee and assistant moderator or note-taker fees; transportation; possible feedback sessions with moderators or assistant moderators after the data collection

❏ Transportation for participants to and from the site

❏ Transcription of tapes (full day of secretarial service for each discussion held)

❏ Translation, if not included in transcription

❏ Data management (including computer software such as *Ethnograph* or *NUD*IST* if used for coding and analysis; computer time; data entry personnel)

❏ Analysis, interpretation, and report preparation

❏ Typing and photocopying report

❏ Supplies and equipment (tape recorders, tapes, paper, overhead, etc.)

❏ Oral presentation of results (may involve meeting space, transportation, per diems, equipment rental, photocopying)

❏ Technical assistance (may involve multiple visits at several stages throughout the research)

Adapted from a resource allocation tool developed by Dr. Michele G. Shedlin, Sociomedical Resource Associates, Westport, CT.

Topic Guides for Focus Group Discussions on Reproductive Health

The following sample topic guides are intended to provide project managers with ideas for series of questions that could be asked of a variety of types of focus group participants. The number of questions used varies widely. All question topic guides should be pretested prior to administration with a small group of participants similar in characteristics to those who will participate in the focus groups discussions.

A. Sample topic guide for research examining the features of social relationships among homosexual and bisexual men at risk for AIDS (O'Brien 1993)

The goals of the long-term program were to identify which features of social ties enhance the psychological health of men in this population as well as the ability to adhere to widely publicized behavioral guidelines for preventing transmission of HIV. Only four questions were used in a "funneling" sequence leading from a general topic to the specific interest — the influence of social relationships on psychological health and on safer sex practices.

1. How is your life different because of the HIV/AIDS epidemic? (This first question is the "ice breaker," which allowed each participant to speak and helped the researchers to learn the language used by participants for talking about their experiences.)

2. When people get involved sexually, why is it that sometimes they have safer sex and sometimes they don't? (This question helped to focus the discussion on safe sex experiences and to allow the conversation to move toward a discussion of social interactions.)

3. What are some things other people have done that you have found supportive in dealing with the HIV/AIDS epidemic?

(The researchers asked this question so that specific interventions, such as expressions of support for safer sex activities, could be identified.)

4. How can we best recruit men for the large-scale questionnaire phase of this study?

B. Sample topic guide for a study to explore opinions on sexual practices (WHO 1990)

1. Have you ever heard of people of the same sex having sex together in your society/community?

2. In general, do people in society accept that? Why or why not?

3. In general, which is more common: men having sex with men or women having sex with women? Why?

4. What do men do with each other when they have sex? (Try to elicit information on oral and anal sex.)

5. What do men and women do when they have sex? (Try to elicit information on oral and anal sex; differences between age groups; urban/rural differences.)

6. How common is it for men to go to prostitutes?

C. Sample topic guide to explore perceptions concerning norms governing sexual decision-making and behavior associated with the risk of HIV transmission to women in Haiti (Ulin, Cayemittes, and Metellus 1993)

The format involves the use of a story to prompt discussion among the participants. This technique allows the participants to discuss the behavior of the story characters rather than their own personal behavior, thus revealing perceptions on social norms for sexual behavior.

Story for discussion:

Moderator: *Joujou is living with a man by the name of René. René is working in a factory, but Joujou is not working. Joujou has four kids at home; the oldest one is seven years old, the youngest one and a half and she is again pregnant. Before Joujou got pregnant with this last child, she wanted to start using family planning, but René did not want her to. René gives money for food in the house, but it is he who decides what to cook. When the children are sick, Joujou must ask René's permission before she takes them to the clinic.*

1. What do you think about the way René and Joujou are living? (Kinds of decisions men and women make together, women's decisions, men's decisions)

2. Who makes the decision when a man and woman "make love?"

3. If a man feels like making love with his woman and the woman does not want to, what can she do? How does the man react? (Women's right to refuse sex, refusal strategies, partners' response)

4. What reasons might there be for a woman to refuse to make love with her man? (Women's rights under specific conditions, bargaining)

Moderator: *There is another part to the story of Joujou and René. Let's continue it and see what happens ...*

Joujou is worried. She has learned that when René goes to town, he often goes to the houses of other women with whom he is having affairs. Joujou does not know what she should do. She does not want to leave René, but she is afraid he will give her AIDS.

5. What do you think this woman should do? (Expectations of behavior for women at risk of HIV)

6. If the woman does what you are saying, how do you think the man will react? (Expectations of male response to protective behavior)

7. Do you think that the woman should talk to the man about the fears she has of contracting AIDS? How can she bring up the subject? How will he react? (Male-female communication on AIDS and AIDS prevention)

8. If the man is having an affair with another woman, can he give the disease to his woman (at home)? How? (Knowledge of HIV transmission)

9. As far as you know, how do people (in general) get AIDS? (Knowledge of HIV transmission)

10. What kind of people get AIDS? Do you fear AIDS? (Transmission, belief in severity, sense of vulnerability, personal fear, appearance of HIV-infected people)

11. What are the consequences of this disease for the family? (Knowledge of the disease, belief in severity)

12. If a woman knows nothing about this disease, how can she get information? What do women want to know? (Formal and nonformal sources of information, desire for information)

13. (Women only) Do women talk to each other about AIDS? When? How do they feel in these discussions? (Nature and circumstances of informal discussion, emotional responses to discussion, level of interest)

Moderator: *The woman in the story (Joujou) is afraid that her man may give her AIDS because she knows that he is having affairs with other women ...*

14. How can she protect herself? How will the man react? (Knowledge of prevention, spontaneous reference to condoms, right of women to protect themselves, initiating behavior change, barriers to prevention)

15a. Does the woman have the right to ask the man to use condoms? How can she ask him? How will he respond?

15b. If the man does not want to use condoms can the woman convince him? How? (Empowerment, communication, male response, barriers)

16. In general, are women willing to use condoms? (Women's attitudes toward condoms, response of women to men who initiate condom use)

17. Where can a person get condoms?

18. Are women able to obtain (buy) condoms on their own? (Condom availability, barriers to obtaining condoms)

19. We have heard that not all women have the right to ask a man to use condoms. What can you tell us about that? (Types of women who have/do not have the right to demand condoms)

20. As far as you know, are young people in their teens in danger of contracting AIDS? Why? (Beliefs about adolescent sexual behavior and AIDS risk)

21. How do you think you might help young people avoid getting AIDS? (Responsibility of adults to counsel adolescents, appropriate advisors, nature of advice)

22. If you knew they were sexually active, would you advise young people to use condoms? (Belief in the appropriateness of condoms for adolescents)

23. Some parents say they would not talk to their children about sex. What do you think about that? (Responsibility of parents for sex education)

24. (Women only) You women know what AIDS is about. Do you believe you have a responsibility to protect yourselves? To protect your unborn babies? Please explain what you mean. (Responsibility for prevention, risk of perinatal transmission)

25. (Women only) How do you think women might help each other to be stronger in their relationships with men? (Mutual support for protection against AIDS, sense of collective responsibility)

26. (Men only) You men know what AIDS is about. Do you feel that you have a responsibility to protect your wives? Other women that you may be seeing? Yourselves? Please explain. (Responsibility for prevention, stable and casual partners)

27. As far as you know, would people benefit from talking about AIDS in small groups like this one? (Networking and support)

(translated and abbreviated)

D. Sample FGD topic guide for female youth exploring knowledge about AIDS, sexual activity, and condom use to guide development of a KABP survey (AIDSCAP/FHI 1993)

The following topic guide was designed for FGDs among female youth to assist in questionnaire development. In-country researchers collaborating with AIDSCAP adapt the guide to local situations, translate it into the language in which the guide will be used, and pretest it prior to use. The main objective is to investigate the dynamics of sexual behavior among young women in order to identify the vocabulary and phrasing used to describe relationships and sexual activity, particularly condom negotiation and use. Using the FGD results, researchers then adapt core questionnaires for collecting data to establish the prevalence within target populations of various aspects of sexual behavior.

Following an introductory statement appropriate for the local context, the following questions could be used to elicit information about sexual beliefs and practices among young women:

Sexual Activity:

1. Where do girls your age meet boys or men?

2. Is there an age difference between most of your female friends and their boyfriends/partners?

3. What kind of relationships are common among your female friends — for example, are many of your friends engaged, have regular boyfriends, have casual boyfriends, etc?

4. Tell me about couples who are _____ (regular, casual partners, etc.) How long do these arrangements usually last? Is it common for girls your age to have sexual relations with their boyfriends? About what age do girls your age have sexual intercourse for the first time? Why does it vary?

5. Before a girl reaches the age where she has sexual intercourse, are there other non-penetrative sexual activities which are commonly practiced among girls and boys/men? Can you describe some of these activities? With whom might a girl practice these activities? (What is their relationship, partner's age?) At what age do girls your age begin these activities?

6. If a girl has a regular boyfriend, about how often might she see him during a week? About how many times might she have sexual intercourse with him during a one week/month period?

7. Where might a couple your age go to have sex?

8. Is it common for girls your age to have sexual relations with more than one man, that is to be with one man one night and another man on a different night?

9. Is it common for your female friends' boyfriends/partners to have sexual relationships with more than one girl/woman?

10. Have sexual practices among people your age changed over time? For example, are the common practices we have discussed today different than what your parents or grandparents might have experienced? How are they different? Which practices are the same?

Condom Use:

1. Do girls your age who are having sex use anything to keep from getting pregnant? If so, what, which methods of birth control? Where do they obtain these methods?

2. Does anyone know what these are? (Show condom in and out of the package) What else are they called?

3. Who uses condoms, in your opinion? What kind of man/boy? What kind of woman/girl? Why?

4. Is it common among your female friends to use condoms? Why? Why not?

5. Among your friends who use condoms, who do you think initiates using a condom?

6. What would girls your age think if a man stated that he was going to use a condom?

7. What would a man/boy think if a girl asked him to use a condom? What would a man/boy think if a girl had a condom with her? Why? Can you explain that further?

8. Would you be insulted if a man said he wanted to use a condom? Do you think your partner would be insulted if you asked him to use a condom?

9. Have you ever used a condom before? Why? Why not?

10. Where could you go today to get a condom? How much do they cost?

11. Do you think using a condom is a good idea? Why? When? Why not?

12. Have you ever asked a partner to use a condom? Do you know if any of your friends have ever asked their partners to use a condom? What happened?

13. Can you imagine any circumstances under which you would ask a man to use a condom? Tell me about that.

14. If you were planning to have sex with a man, are there any circumstances under which you would change your mind and refuse to have sex with him? Under what circumstances?

15. How could you ask a man to use a condom, that is, what could you say?

16. If he refused, how might you respond to try and convince him?

Lodging:

1. With whom are you living now?

2. Who pays for your:

food
clothing
transportation
health care
school fees
incidental expenses/pocket money

Questionnaire review:

One of the objectives of this project is to do a survey of people your age to learn about the kinds of issues we have discussed today. What I would like to do now is to read you some questions from the questionnaire and see if you can suggest ways to improve the wording of the questions. I also want your opinion on whether you think young people will respond honestly to these questions.

1. If someone came to your home and asked you to participate in this survey, would you agree?

2. Please listen to the introduction of the questionnaire. What is this study about? How will the information be used?

3. After listening to this statement, are you confident that this information will not be shared with anyone? If yes, why? Which statements convinced you? If not, why? Which statements made you suspicious?

4. If you were doing the study and you knew that none of the information would ever be released to anyone outside of the staff, what would you say to convince respondents?

Adapted with permission from Hogle et al. 1994.

Sample Interviewer Training Program Agenda

NORPLANT STUDY
QUALITATIVE METHODS WORKSHOP
Dakar, Senegal
June 5-8, 1996
Eight Participants

WEDNESDAY, JUNE 5

Morning

Coffee and introductions
About Norplant
- Introduction to the method: what it is, how it works
- Findings of other studies: common concerns
- Norplant in Senegal
  Handout: Fact sheet on Norplant

Break

Goals and objectives of the Norplant study
Study design
- Record review
- Focus groups discussion
- In-depth interviews
- How data will be analyzed
Discussion of ethical issues
  Handout: Overview of the Norplant Study

Lunch

Techniques
- How to use a topic guide
- Asking questions in interviews and discussions
- Probes: verbal and nonverbal
Focus group discussion demonstration

Break

Observations and discussion: managing interviews and focus groups
  Handout: Steps in Leading a Focus Groups Discussion
  Assignment: Develop a topic guide for an in-depth interview or a focus group on Thursday morning

THURSDAY, JUNE 6

Morning

Role-play: interviews and note-taking
  Handout: Tips for Interviewers

Break

Role-play: focus group discussion and note-taking

Handout: Tips for Focus Group Moderators and Note-takers

Lunch

Preliminary analysis
- Group level
- Individual level
- Coding

Break

Review of study topics guides

Assignment: Review techniques and prepare to conduct an interview

FRIDAY, JUNE 7

Morning

Field practice (by prearrangement at two clinics): Participants will observe and conduct one interview each and write up notes

Afternoon

Presentation of findings from morning interviews

Group discussion and critique
- Additional probing
- Revisions to guide
- Preliminary coding

Assignment: Each team prepares to conduct one focus group

SATURDAY, JUNE 8

Morning

Field practice (by prearrangement at two clinics): Each team will pretest the Continuing Client FGD guide and transcribe tape for two focus groups discussions. Each participant will observe one focus group and moderate or take notes in the other.

Lunch

Afternoon

Presentation of FGD findings

Group discussion and critique
- Additional probing
- Revisions to guide
- Preliminary coding

Summary and evaluation of training

Common Errors in Moderating Focus Groups

Facilitating a focus group discussion on a sensitive topic is never easy, but for moderators who are new to qualitative data collection, hearing all points of view and keeping the discussion on track can be especially challenging. It is not unusual for an interviewer to begin a qualitative project with a strong background in survey work. Many find it difficult at first to replace the structure of a quantitative interview with the flexibility demanded by qualitative research — asking open-ended questions, probing answers, and following the participants' lead while keeping the discussion focused on the research problem.

Common errors that appear in focus group transcripts are:

- Allowing one or two participants to dominate the discussion, or not enabling reticent participants to speak
- Remaining too long on a topic; continuing to repeat questions even after participants have nothing additional to say
- Using the same words to repeat a question instead of probing what has just been said or noticing new ideas and asking participants to elaborate
- Interrupting people who begin to express a different point of view by repeating the original question as if the speaker were not addressing it
- Accepting comments on what people should do without probing what they actually do and why there is a difference
- Not probing the logical conclusions of ideas ("If that, then what?" or simply, "Why?")
- Not probing assumptions to see where they come from ("Why do people say that?")
- Letting a good question drop if it is not answered immediately
- Failure to explore vague or nonspecific terms, or to clarify vernacular expression that may not

be familiar to the researchers
- In certain studies, allowing the group to talk only about married (more stable) relationships and to ignore casual (less stable) unions
- Asking leading questions that might bias the answers; for example, "Don't you think that … ?" or "Would you agree that … ?"

The examples below are taken from the transcripts of focus group discussions conducted in Haiti for the purpose of understanding women's perspectives on sexual decision-making in relation to HIV/AIDS protection. Although they come from focus groups, most of these points apply equally to in-depth interviewing or any interactive technique in which the researcher must probe sensitive information.

Example 1

A group of women in casual relationships with male sexual partners are talking about protecting themselves if they suspect a partner is HIV-infected.

Moderator: *Do you think you have a responsibility to protect yourself from getting AIDS?*

Group (in unison): *No.*

Moderator: *You don't feel you have any responsibility? Why do you think you don't have any responsibility?*

Participant 1: *Because we don't have husbands.*

Moderator: *You don't feel you have a responsibility to protect yourself from AIDS? Is that what you are saying?*

Participant 2: *I personally feel I should be using condoms. I have children and I wouldn't like to have any more.*

Comment
This moderator correctly probed the group's denial of responsibility, but she kept repeating the word when it may not have been clear what "responsibility" meant to participants. Her probe also seems

like a leading question — as if the participants have given an unacceptable answer. She might have asked, "What do we mean by 'responsibility for protection?'" Or she could have restated the question, probing the idea with different words: "Whose responsibility is it to protect the woman from AIDS? Is it up to the man? The woman? Someone else? What do you think that person should do to protect herself or himself?"

The answer "because we don't have husbands" offers another important clue that was missed. The moderator should have probed this response with such questions as, "Why does having a husband or not having a husband make any difference?" "What is the responsibility of a woman with a husband?" "What about a woman without a husband?" "What about the responsibility of the husband, himself — or the man who is not her husband?" The moderator could also have clarified what the term "husband" meant to the participants, since in Haiti multiple relationships, both stable and non-stable, are common.

Participant 2 did not answer the question directly. The moderator could then have explored views on the uses of condoms and gradually brought the discussion back to the use of condoms as protection against sexually transmitted infection.

Example 2
A group of men are talking about the causes of AIDS.

Moderator: *What are some of the ways that people can get AIDS?*

Participant 1: *If a man has sex with several women and the women have sex with several men, they will get AIDS.*

Participant 2: *If you go to the hospital and get an injection and the syringe has AIDS on it …*

Participant 3: *We know there is something called voodoo in our country. The [voodoo] priest prepares all kinds of diseases. He can prepare a powder … he sends it to you … you get a different kind of AIDS.*

Moderator: *What are some other ways you can get AIDS?*

Comment
The moderator did not pursue this reference to a different form of AIDS. He should have asked in what way AIDS from powder is different from sexually transmitted AIDS, whether a person with voodoo AIDS can pass it to another person by sexual contact, whether it can be cured, and so forth. He then could have invited other participants to add to the discussion of this different kind of AIDS.

Example 3
A group of men are discussing a situation in which a man may have acquired the AIDS virus.

Participant: *Superstitious people say that this infected person has supernatural AIDS.*

Group: *(Laughs)*

Moderator: *Do you think he could give his AIDS to other people?*

Comment
Again, the moderator let an important theme drop. The group's laughter suggests a strong reaction to the comment. Is it excitement? embarrassment? fear that the response might be socially unacceptable? The transcript did not say. The moderator might have asked the participants to talk more about what superstitious people and the transmission of supernatural AIDS mean to them and to others in the community. How do the consequences of supernatural AIDS differ from the consequences of other kinds of AIDS?

Example 4

A group of women in married or stable sexual relationships have been discussing women's vulnerability to AIDS.

Moderator: *Can a woman protect herself from AIDS?*

Participant: *We are afraid because now men do not want to stay with one woman; they want to live with them.*

Moderator: *When that happens, is there any way the woman can protect herself?*

Comment

While keeping the discussion on the topic of protection, the moderator missed an opportunity to probe the implication that men are more promiscuous now than they used to be. She could have asked, "Why do men not stay with one woman?" "How has this changed?" "Why has it changed?" She might have been able to develop a new theme, namely that women think men have more partners than they used to, and to identify factors that might contribute to the perceived change.

Example 5

A group of women in married or stable relationships have just agreed that many women do not use condoms.

Moderator: *Why do women not use condoms?*

Participant: *I have other things I use.*

Moderator: *Are there others here who also will not use condoms?*

Comment

The moderator missed the clue that: (a) women may believe there are other ways to prevent HIV transmission; (b) women may be thinking of condoms only as contraception; or (c) women may have other ideas about condoms that were not expressed. She should have asked, "What other

things?" and "In what ways do these protect the woman?" The question she did ask could be perceived as a leading question. The participant did not say she would not use condoms, but the moderator's next questions reflects refusal and the possible implication that such behavior by others in the group would be unacceptable.

Example 6

A group of women in married or stable sexual relationships are talking about women's vulnerability in the AIDS epidemic.

Moderator: *What can a woman do to protect herself from AIDS?*

Participant: *I can't imagine taking precautions myself, because I can't avoid making love. The only thing that could prevent me from making love would be if he would come on too strong; but as long as it isn't rape, there should be love and affection. If AIDS really exists, I will get it anyway from making love.*

Moderator: *Does anyone else have something to say?*

Comment

In this relatively complex comment there were at least two important clues that the moderator did not follow. First, she could have asked how a woman chooses between her duties as a wife or sexual partner and her need to protect herself from AIDS? And does she have any choice in the matter? The discussion might have taken a different turn at this point, expanding on the potential subordination of women in the sexual relationship and its effect on women's well-being.

A second clue was the participant's question as to the existence of AIDS. The moderator might have gently probed whether women in the group doubted its existence, whether other women they knew might suspect that it did not exist, and if so, what alternatives they would offer for the current widespread concern about this disease.

Example 7

A group of men are sharing what they know about HIV/AIDS transmission.

Moderator: *What are some ways people get AIDS?*

Participant: *The person could have AIDS, and I can eat and drink with that person and never contract it — I am not susceptible. Another can just touch the person with AIDS and contract it.*

Moderator: *What do you mean by "not susceptible?"*

Comment

The moderator did the right thing to probe perception of susceptibility, but the participant never answered his question. The moderator should have come back to it, asking why some people seem more susceptible than others, what made the speaker feel safe, whether this difference in susceptibility includes other kinds of sexual transmission, and so forth.

Example 8

A group of women in non-stable sexual relationships are talking about how women get AIDS.

Moderator: *What are some ways that women can get AIDS?*

Participant 1: *If you're trying to survive by living on the streets and you're poor, you have no protection against it [AIDS]; it can happen to you more easily.*

Participant 2: *Women of ill repute [can get AIDS].*

Moderator: *Are those the only women who can catch the disease?*

Comment

The moderator turned the discussion away from a very important theme: the ability of women with multiple partners to protect themselves and their partners. These participants were poor and in casual and other non-stable relationships. They were beginning to talk about the pressure on poor women to exchange sex for money or other support. The moderator should have probed the idea that poor women are more susceptible. She should have asked them to talk more about what it means to be a single woman and what poor and economically dependent women might do to protect themselves from AIDS. Probing responses in greater depth might have provided richer information on sexual decision-making and barriers to protection in this highly vulnerable group.

Critical Appraisal Skills Programme (CASP):
Ten Questions to Help You Make Sense of Qualitative Research

GENERAL COMMENTS

- The first two questions are screening questions and can be answered quickly. If the answer to both is "yes," it is worth proceeding with the remaining questions.
- A number of italicized hints are given. These are designed to remind you why the question is important. It is important to emphasize that all of these prompts need not necessarily be met.
- Several of the questions ask for a response on a scale ranging from "yes" to "no." Where there are sub-questions, try to answer these first and then summarize the sub-questions into one overall response by marking a cross on the scale.
- The 10 questions have been developed by the national CASP collaboration for qualitative methodologies.

SCREENING QUESTIONS	
1. Was there a clear statement of the aims of the research? HINTS: What are/were they trying to find out? Why is it important? What is its relevance?	Yes ——————— No
2. Is a qualitative methodology appropriate? HINT: Does the research seek to understand or illuminate the subjective experiences or views of those being researched?	Yes ——————— No

---

DETAILED QUESTIONS	
3. Sampling strategy	

Is it clear:
  a. From where the sample was selected and why?
  b. Who was selected and why?
  c. How were they selected and why?
  d. Was the sample size justified?
  e. Is it clear why some participants chose not to take part?
HINT: Consider saturation of data.	

Was the sampling strategy appropriate to address the aims?	Yes ——————— No

4. Data collection	

Is it clear:
  a. Where the setting of the data collection was, and why that setting was chosen.
  b. How was the data collected and why?
HINTS: Focus group, structured interview, etc.
  c. How the data were recorded and why?
HINTS: Recorded, made notes, etc.
  d. If the methods were modified during the process and why?	

Were the data collected in a way that addresses the research issue?	Yes No
5. Data analysis	

Is it clear:
  a. How the analysis was done?
  b. How the categories/themes were derived from the data? Is there adequate description?
  c. If steps have been taken to test the credibility of the findings?
  d. Are you confident that all the data were taken into account?
 	
HINTS: Is there adequate discussion of the evidence both for and against the researchers arguments? Have attempts been made to feed results back to respondents, and/or using and comparing different sources of data about the same issue where that is appropriate (triangulation). Was the analysis repeated by more than one researcher to ensure reliability?	

Was the data analysis sufficiently rigorous?	Yes No

6. Research partnership relations	

Is it clear:
  a. If the researchers critically examined their own role, potential bias, and influence?
  b. Where the data were collected and why that setting was chosen?
  c. How the research was explained to the participants?
 	
HINT: Consider confidentiality, ethics, implications, and consequences for research findings for all of the above.	

Has the relationship between researchers and participants been adequately considered?	Yes No

7. Findings	
HINTS: What were the findings — are they explicit, easy to understand?	
Is there a clear statement of the findings?	Yes No

8. Justification of data interpretation	
a. Is there sufficient data presented to support the findings? b. Do the researchers explain how the data presented in the paper were selected from the original sample? HINTS: Criteria for the selection of the quote, some details of the respondent, what is the role of the data — example, illustration, "nice" quote to share, etc.	
Do the researchers indicate links between data presented and their own findings on what the data contain?	Yes No

9. Transferability	

HINTS: Consider:
  a. Whether the context and setting in which the study was performed is described in sufficient detail to determine similarities and differences to your own.
  b. If all the relevant clinically important outcomes were considered.	

Are the findings of this study transferable to a wider population?	Yes No
10. Relevance and usefulness	

a. In terms of addressing the research aim?
  b. In terms of contributing something new to understanding/new insight/different perspective?
  c. In terms of suggesting further research?
  d. In terms of impacting on policy/practice?	

How relevant is the research?
  a. To your patient/problem/scenario.
  b. To you personally.
	Very Not at all

How important are these findings to your practice?	Very Not at all

Reproduced with permission from:
  CASP, Institute of Health Sciences
  Old Road, Headington
  Oxford, OX3 7LF UK
  Tel: 0 1865 226968
  Fax: 0 1865 226959
  E-mail: ann.davis@phru.anglox.nhs.uk

Where to Publish

An increasing number of scientific journals that cover reproductive health issues are accepting articles that report on qualitative studies. The journals and presses listed below represent a selection of publishing venues for qualitative researchers to consider.

JOURNALS

African Journal of Reproductive Health
Editor
Women's Health and Action Research Centre
4 Alofoje Avenue, Off Uwasota Street
P.O. Box 10231, Ugbowo
Benin City, Edo State Nigeria
Telephone: 234 52 602334/600151
Fax: 234 52 60209
E-mail: wharc@warri.ncl.nih.com
Web site: *http://www.wharc.freehosting.net*

AIDS Education and Prevention
Francisco S. Sy, M.D., Dr.P.H., Editor
Publications, Inc.
Centers for Disease Control and Prevention
1600 Clifton Road, N.E., Mailstop E-59
Atlanta, GA 30333 USA

American Anthropologist
American Anthropological Association
1703 New Hampshire Avenue, N.W.
Washington, DC 20009 USA
Telephone: (202) 232-8800

American Ethnologist
Carol Greenhouse, Editor
Department of Anthropology
Student Building 130
Indiana University
Bloomington, IN 47405 USA
Telephone: (812) 855-8473
Web site: *http://www.ameranthassn.org/aes/ae/ae.htm*

American Journal of Public Health
AJPH Submissions
800 I Street, N.W.
Washington, DC 20001-3710 USA
E-mail: ajph.submissions@apha.org

American Journal of Sociology
Andrew Abbott, Editor
5835 S. Kimbark Avenue
Chicago, IL 60637-1684 USA
Telephone: (773) 702-8580
Fax: (773) 702-6207

Cross Cultural Research (formerly *Behavior Science Research*)
Melvin Ember, Editor
Sage Publications, Inc.
2455 Teller Road
Thousand Oaks, CA 91320 USA
Telephone: (805) 499-0721
Fax: (805) 499-0871

Culture, Medicine and Psychiatry
Byron J. Good, Editor-in-Chief, or
Mary-Jo Delvecchio Good, Associate Editor
Department of Social Medicine
Harvard Medical School
641 Huntington Avenue
Boston, MA 02115 USA

Field Methods
Dr. H. Russell Bernard
Department of Anthropology
University of Florida
1112 Turlington Hall
Gainesville, FL 32611 USA
Telephone: (352) 392-3139
Fax: (352) 392-6929
E-mail: ufruss@nersp.nerdc.ufl.edu

Health Education and Behavior
Marc A. Zimmerman, Ph.D., Editor
Department of Health Behavior and Health Education
University of Michigan
School of Public Health
1420 Washington Heights
Ann Arbor, MI 48109-2029 USA
Web site: *http://www.sph.umich.edu/hbhe/heb*

Human Organization
Journal of the Society for Applied Anthropology
Robert V. Kemper, Editor
c/o Department of Anthropology
Southern Methodist University
Dallas, TX 75275 USA
Web site: *http://www.smu.edu/~anthrop/humanorg/html*

International Quarterly of Community Health Education
Dr. George P. Cernada, Editor
Baywood Publishing Co., Inc.
26 Austin Avenue, Box 337
Amityville, NY 11701 USA

Telephone: (516) 691-1270
Fax: (516) 691-1770
E-mail: baywood@baywood.com
Web site: *http://www.baywood.com*

Journal of Contemporary Ethnography
Robert D. Benford, Editor
Southern Illinois University
Mailcode 4524
Carbondale, IL 62901 USA
Telephone: (618) 453-7614
Fax: (618) 453-8926
E-mail: rbenford@siu.edu

Journal of Family Practice
Mark H. Ebell, M.D., M.S.
B101 Clinical Practice Center
Department of Family Practice
Michigan State University
East Lansing, MI 48824-1315 USA
Telephone: (517) 432-5128
Fax: (517) 432-5129
E-mail: jfp@ht.msu.edu
Web site: *http://www.jfponline.com*

Journal of Health and Population in Developing Countries
Editor
Department of Health Policy and Administration
CB#7400
University of North Carolina at Chapel Hill
Chapel Hill, NC 27599-7400 USA
Telephone: (919) 966-1938
Fax: (919) 966-6961
E-mail: HPJournal@unc.edu

Journal of Immigrant Health
Kluwer Academic/Plenum Publishers
Ms. Mariclaire Cloutier, Senior Publishing Editor
233 Spring Street
New York, NY 10013-1578 USA
Telehone: (212) 620-8013
Fax: (212) 463-0742
E-mail: cloutier@plenum.com
Web site: *http://www.wkap.nl/contact_pub.htm/1096-4045+NY0006*

Journal of Interpersonal Violence
Jon R. Conte, Editor
School of Social Work JH-30
University of Washington
4101 15th Avenue, N.E.
Seattle, WA 98195 USA

Journal of Women's Health and Gender-based Medicine
(formerly *Journal of Women's Health*)
Ms. Grey Osterud, Managing Editor
215 Meadows Edge
Acton, MA 01718 USA
Telephone: (978) 266-9588
Fax: (978) 266-0090
E-mail: jwomenhealth@aol.com

Lancet
The Lancet Publishing Group
84 Theobald's Road
London, WC1X 8RR UK
Telephone: 44 020 7611 4100
Fax: 44 020 7611 4101

650 Avenue of the Americas
New York, NY 10011 USA
Telephone: (212) 633 3800
Fax: (212) 633 3850

Medical Anthropology
Stacy Leigh Pigg
Department of Sociology and Anthropology
Simon Fraser University
8888 University Drive
Burnaby, BC V5A1S6 Canada

Medical Anthropology Quarterly
American Anthropological Association
4350 North Fairfax Drive, Suite 640
Arlington, VA 22203 USA

Psychology and Health
Gordon and Breach Publishing
P.O. Box 32160
Newark, NJ 07102 USA
Telephone: (800) 545-8398
Fax: (973) 643-7676
E-mail: info@gbhap.com

Qualitative Health Research
Dr. Janice Morse, Editor
International Institute for Qualitative Methodology
6-10 University Extension Centre
Edmonton, Alberta T6G 2T4 Canada
E-mail: Judy-norris@ualberta.ca

Qualitative Inquiry
Norman K. Denzin, Editor
Department of Sociology
326 Lincoln Hall

University of Illinois
Urbana, IL 61801 USA
Telephone: (217) 333-1950
Fax: (217) 333-5225
E-mail: n-denzin@uiuc.edu

Qualitative Sociology
University of Baltimore
1420 North Charles Street
Baltimore, MD 21201 USA
Telephone: (301) 625-3000
Fax: (301) 539-3714

Reproductive Health Matters
Marge Berer, Editor
444 Highgate Studios
53/79 Highgate Road
London, NW5 1TL UK
Telephone: 44 020 7267 6567
Fax: 44 020 7267 2551
E-mail: editor@rhmjournal.org.uk

Social Science and Medicine
Dr. Sally MacIntyre
MRC Social and Public Health Sciences Unit
4 Lilybank Gardens
Glasgow, G12 8RZ UK
Telephone: 44 0 1865 843900
Fax: 44 0 1865 843905
E-mail: authors@elsevier.co.uk

Sociological Quarterly
Kevin T. Leicht, Editor
Department of Sociology
505 Seashore Hall
University of Iowa
Iowa City, IA 52242-1401 USA
E-mail: tsq@uiowa.edu
Web site: http://www.ucpress.edu/journals/tsq/edsub.htm

Studies in Family Planning
Julie Reich, Managing Editor
Population Council
One Dag Hammarskjold Plaza
New York, NY 10017 USA
Web site: http://www.popcouncil.org/sfp

Symbolic Interaction
Kathy Charmaz, Editor
Department of Sociology
Sonoma State University
Rohnert Park, CA 94928 USA
Telephone: (219) 239-7367

BOOKS AND MONOGRAPHS
Alta Mira Press
Ethnographic Alternatives
Rosalie M. Robertson, Senior Editor
Anthropology, Ethnic Studies
1630 North Main Street, #367
Walnut Creek, CA 94596 USA
Telephone: (925) 938-7243
Fax: (925) 933-9720
E-mail: rrobertson@altamirapress.com

Duke University Press
Ken Wissoker, Editor-in-Chief
905 West Main Street, Suite 18B
Durham, NC 27701 USA
Telephone: (919) 687-3600
Fax: (919) 688-4574
E-mail: kwiss@duke.edu

Indiana University Press
Janet Rabinowitch, Editorial Director
601 North Morton Street
Bloomington, IN 47404 USA
Telephone: (812) 855-5063
Fax: (812) 855-8507
E-mail: jrabinow@indiana.edu

New York University Press
Qualitative Studies in Psychology Series
Eric Zinner, Editor-in-Chief
838 Broadway, 3rd Floor
New York, NY 10003-4812 USA
Telephone: (800) 996-6987
Fax: (212) 995-3833
E-mail: eric.zinner@nyu.edu
Web site: http://www.nyupress.nyu.edu/

Oxford University Press
Executive and Editorial Offices
198 Madison Avenue
New York, NY 10016 USA
Telephone: (212) 726-6000
Web site: http://www.oup-usa.org/

Routledge
11 New Fetter Lane
London, EC4P 4EE UK
Telephone: 44 020 7583 9855
Fax: 44 020 7842 2298
Web site: http://www.routledge.com

29 West 35th Street
New York, NY 10001 USA
Telephone: (212) 216 7800
Fax: (212) 564-7854
Web site: *http://www.routledge-ny.com*

Rutgers University Press
Jill Stuart, Editorial Assistant, Sciences and Social Sciences
100 Joyce Kilmer Avenue
Piscataway, NJ 08854-8099 USA
Telephone: (732) 445-7762
Fax: (732) 445-7039
E-mail: jbstuart@rci.rutgers.edu

Sage Publications, Ltd.
6 Bonhill Street
London, EC2A 4PU UK
Telephone: 44 020 7374 0645
Fax: 44 020 7374 8741
E-mail: info@sagepub.co.uk

2455 Teller Road
Thousand Oaks, CA 91320 USA
Telephone: (805) 499-0721
Fax: (805) 499-0871
E-mail: info@sagepub.com
Web site: *www.sagepub.com*

M-32 Market
Greater Kailash-1
New Delhi, 110024 India
Telephone: 91 11 6419884/6444958
Fax: 91 11 6472426
E-mail: sageind@giasdl01.vsnl.net.in
Web site: *http://indiasage.com/*

Temple University Press
Janet M. Francendese, Editor-In-Chief
1601 North Broad Street, USB 305
Philadelphia, PA 19122-6099 USA
Telephone: (215) 204-8787
Fax: (215) 204-4719
Web site: *http://www.temple.edu*

University of Chicago Press
Editorial Department
1427 East 60th Street
Chicago, IL 60637 USA
Telephone: (773) 702-7700
Fax: (773) 702-9756
Web site: *http://www.press.uchicago.edu*

University of Michigan Press
P.O. Box 1104
839 Greene Street
Ann Arbor, MI 48106-1104 USA
Telephone: (734) 764-4388
Fax: (734) 936-0456
E-mail: umpress-www@umich.edu
Web site: *http://www.press.umich.edu*

University of North Carolina Press
P.O. Box 2288
Chapel Hill, NC 27515-2288 USA
Telephone: (800) 848-6224
Fax: (919) 966-3829
Web site: *http://uncpress.unc.edu*

University of Pennsylvania Press
Peter A. Agree or Walda Metcalf, Social Science Editors
4200 Pine Street
Philadelphia, PA 19104-4011 USA
Telephone: (215) 898-6261
Fax: (215) 898-0404
Web site: *http://www.upenn.edu/pennpress*

Zed Books
7 Cynthia Street
London, N1 9JF UK
Telephone: 44 020 7837 0384
Web site: *http://www.zedbooks.demon.co.uk*

Appendix 11

Sample Research Brief on the Female Condom

Lessons from a Female Condom Community Intervention Trial in Rural Kenya

What impact will a general distribution of the female condom have on sexually transmitted infection (STI) rates in a rural area? To address this question, FHI conducted a community intervention trial and follow-up service delivery assessment in rural Kenya, collaborating with the University of Nairobi, Department of Medical Microbiology, and the Family Planning Association of Kenya. The researchers concluded:

- The availability of the female condom did not reduce STI rates, relative to the reductions achieved by distribution of the male condom alone.
- Female condom users generally liked the device, recognized its dual protection properties and appreciated its advantages over the male condom.
- Provider preconceptions may have limited opportunities for women to use the device.

The community intervention trial was conducted in six matched pairs of tea, coffee and flower plantations, each served by at least one primary health care clinic. Each matched pair comprised an intervention and a control site. In the intervention areas, providers and outreach workers received training in providing male and female condoms, STI risk reduction and treatment, and were supplied with free male and female condoms. The control areas received training, supplies and training only on the male condom. A thorough educational campaign reached residents throughout all sites with activities in control sites covering only the male condom.

The study followed about 1,600 women, testing and treating them at baseline, six months and 12 months for three infections — gonorrhea, chlamydia, and trichomoniasis. At both control and intervention plantations, about 24 percent of the women tested and treated had one or more of the three STIs at the beginning of the study. After 12 months, STI rates had declined to about 18 percent at both the intervention and control sites.[1] These results indicate that adding the female condom to the male condom distribution system did not contribute to any additional reductions in disease prevalence. At the same time, the intensive promotional campaign in the male-condom-only distribution system was not sufficient to have an important impact on disease rates either.

Reported female condom use was not sufficiently frequent to make a substantial difference in the overall number of protected sex acts in the intervention sites. Also, providing female condoms did not result in more overall condoms distributed in intervention sites. At the end of the study, 58 percent of study participants in intervention sites reported that they had not used the female condom at all in the previous six months.[2]

Service delivery impact
To assess why so few women used the female condom, researchers visited 16 of the 23 sites participating in the community trial, including a balance of high- and low-performing intervention and control sites. At each site, surveys were conducted with all available clinicians, outreach workers, recent family planning clients, and community key informants. Also, researchers observed all family planning service delivery encounters in the clinic on the day of the visit.[3]

A gap existed between clinicians' reported condom promotion activities and their observed behaviors. In 42 observed family planning visits, the woman in every case chose a hormonal method, but only once did a provider suggest a condom as a supplemental method for STI protection. Moreover, 91 percent of providers interviewed said they had a major influence on whether clients used condoms. Many clinicians viewed the female condom as a feasible method only for single women and sex workers, not for women in stable unions. This provider opinion regarding appropriate female condom users may have contributed to inadequate interest on the part of clients. Only one of 10 intervention site clinics distributed female condoms all 12 months of the trial as called for by the protocol.

Despite the provider behaviors, outreach workers reported that the female condom was viewed by clients as an acceptable method, credited for being warmer, roomier, and stronger than the male condom. Some women felt safer with the female condom because it was perceived as being less prone than the male condom to break. Further, women appreciated being able to insert the female condom themselves, avoiding the risk of men tampering with the device, as was suspected with the male condom.

At the same time, social norms and personal preferences appeared to limit true acceptability of the female condom and impede its introduction into sexual relationships. Community members expressed concern that the female condom may allow women too much freedom, enabling them to "move around" on their husbands. Some feared that intensified distribution of condoms might lead to increased prostitution.

With limited understanding of female anatomy, some users expressed fears that it could "slip into the stomach," get "lost inside the womb," or get "stuck in the vagina." Others rumored it was laced with HIV or that the lubricant could cause infertility or produce infections. Some men worried that a woman can take semen captured in the female condom to a witch doctor and put a hex on the partner.

When considering the introduction of the female condom in rural areas, program planners need to take into consideration the local culture and address the negative influence that traditional gender roles can have on female condom use.

1. Feldblum PJ, Kuyoh MA, Bwayo JJ, et al. Female condom introduction and sexually transmitted infection prevalence: results of a community intervention trial in Kenya. AIDS 2001 May 25;15(8):1037-1044.
2. Welsh MJ, Feldblum PJ, Kuyoh MA, et al. Condom use during a community intervention trial in Kenya. Int J AIDS STDs 2001 July;12(7):469-474.
3. Toroitich-Ruto C. Assessment of the Intervention: Was It Implemented as Intended? Presented at Conference on Female Condom and STDs: A Community Intervention Trial, May 9, 2000, Nairobi, Kenya.

FHI produced these research briefs as part of an information dissemination effort supported by the Bureau for Africa/Office of Sustainable Development, U.S. Agency for International Development. For more information, please visit FHI's Web site at *http://www.fhi.org*. Copyright Family Health International, 2001.

Appendix 12

Who Is an Author?

In qualitative research, data collection and analysis phases tend to be less temporally distinct than in quantitative research, and team members who collect study data are called on to conduct iterative analysis as they go. Such active participation by all study team members in refining questions, coding data, and generating insights has implications for authorship roles on study papers. Although different journals have different rules for authorship, this one by the International Committee of Medical Journal Editors, is most widely accepted:

All persons designated as authors should qualify for authorship, and all those who qualify should be listed. Each author should have participated sufficiently in the work to take public responsibility for appropriate portions of the content. One or more authors should take responsibility for the integrity of the work as a whole, from inception to published article.

Authorship credit should be based only on: (1) substantial contributions to conception and design, or acquisition of data, or analysis and interpretation of data; (2) drafting the article or revising it critically for important intellectual content; and (3) final approval of the version to be published. Conditions 1, 2, and 3 must all be met. Acquisition of funding, the collection of data, or general supervision of the research group, by themselves, do not justify authorship.

Authors should provide a description of what each contributed, and editors should publish that information. All others who contributed to the work who are not authors should be named in the acknowledgments, and what they did should be described. Increasingly, authorship of multicenter trials is attributed to a group. All members of the group who are named as authors should fully meet the above criteria for authorship. Group members who do not meet these criteria should be listed, with their permission, in the acknowledgments or in an appendix.

The order of authorship on the byline should be a joint decision of the coauthors. Authors should be prepared to explain the order in which authors are listed.

Reprinted from International Committee of Medical Journal Editors 2000.

Sample Brochure to Share Qualitative Study Findings with Participating Communities

This brochure was developed by Susan Settergren and the staff of the POLICY Project to share findings with members of the communities in Zimbabwe where a qualitative study on unsafe abortion and postabortion care was conducted. It is reprinted with permission from the POLICY Project, an international effort funded by the U.S. Agency for International Development and undertaken by The Futures Group International, Research Triangle Institute, and The Centre for Development and Population Activities in 1999. For more information, see: *http://www.policyproject.com/pubs/policymatters/pm-01.pdf.*

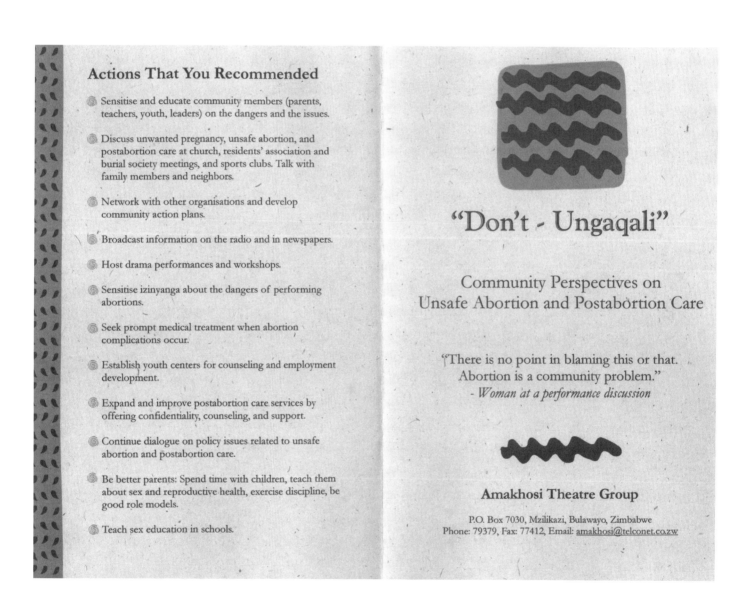

Actions That You Recommended

- Sensitise and educate community members (parents, teachers, youth, leaders) on the dangers and the issues.

- Discuss unwanted pregnancy, unsafe abortion, and postabortion care at church, residents' association and burial society meetings, and sports clubs. Talk with family members and neighbors.

- Network with other organisations and develop community action plans.

- Broadcast information on the radio and in newspapers.

- Host drama performances and workshops.

- Sensitise izinyanga about the dangers of performing abortions.

- Seek prompt medical treatment when abortion complications occur.

- Establish youth centers for counseling and employment development.

- Expand and improve postabortion care services by offering confidentiality, counseling, and support.

- Continue dialogue on policy issues related to unsafe abortion and postabortion care.

- Be better parents: Spend time with children, teach them about sex and reproductive health, exercise discipline, be good role models.

- Teach sex education in schools.

"Don't - Ungaqali"

Community Perspectives on Unsafe Abortion and Postabortion Care

"There is no point in blaming this or that. Abortion is a community problem."
- *Woman at a performance discussion*

Amakhosi Theatre Group

P.O. Box 7030, Mzilikazi, Bulawayo, Zimbabwe
Phone: 79379, Fax: 77412, Email: amakhosi@telconet.co.zw

Performances, Discussions, and Interviews

In November and December 1998, Amakhosi Theatre Group performed the play, *Don't - Ungaqali*, in communities throughout Bulawayo and Hwange. The play tells the story of a teenage couple who engages in sex and the girl becomes pregnant. The girl has an illegal abortion and suffers complications. Her life is saved because she gets medical attention in time, but she can bear no more children.

Over 2,500 people saw the play and nearly 500 of them participated in discussions on unsafe abortion following the performances. We took notes on those discussions and also interviewed 60 community members to learn more about your views on unsafe abortion and postabortion care.

What We Heard From You

■ Unsafe abortion is a well-known problem, although most abortions are done secretly. It's often only when someone dies or gets sick that the problem becomes known.

■ Young girls are at highest risk of unwanted pregnancy and unsafe abortion. However, women of all ages induce abortions.

■ Causes of unwanted pregnancy are many. They include economic hardship that leads to sex for income, poor parenting, ignorance about sex and reproductive health, early physical maturity and experimentation with sex, promiscuity, unprotected sex, peer pressure to have sex, shift from traditional to modern societal values, inaccessibility of contraceptives, women's lack of control of their sexuality, inadequate family accommodation, boys and men cheating girls into having sex by promising marriage, and lack of respect between a man and a woman.

■ Men's denial of responsibility for the pregnancy and fear of family members finding out about the pregnancy are major causes for abortion.

■ Abortions are obtained from a variety of sources, including izinyanga, community elders, and medical doctors. They also are self-induced, sometimes with assistance from friends and other community members. Most abortionists are unskilled, although some are more qualified than others.

■ The law requires health care facilities to report abortion cases to the police. However, the practice of reporting appears to vary among service delivery sites and individuals. Parents and community members also report cases to authorities. Frequently, they file these reports because they want the abortionist to be arrested.

■ Those who experience complications of induced abortion often delay, or do not seek, medical treatment. Fear of being reported to the police by clinic or hospital staff; fear of harsh treatment and exposure by nurses, and fear of reactions from parents, friends, and community members are the primary reasons for avoiding medical attention. People reported that nurses gossip and treat clients, especially youth, harshly. On the other hand, nurses expressed frustration with a client's failure to explain the reason for her condition and her delay in seeking treatment until complications were severe.

Making Study Findings Accessible to Other Researchers

There are four important ways that you can make your study findings more accessible to other researchers nationally, regionally, and internationally:

- Add standardized cataloguing information to the title page or inside cover of your report.
- Submit your report or article to bibliographic indexing databases and information clearing-houses.
- Make your study report or data set available to other researchers through physical and electronic libraries.
- Ask a reproductive health organization or research partner organization to post your report on their Web site.

Below are some general guidelines based on advice from qualitative researchers and librarians. Where you submit your materials may depend on your study topic and region.

Cataloguing Information

1. ISBN. If your institution is registered as a publisher with the International Standard Book Number (ISBN) system, assign an ISBN number and print the number with other title-page or cover information in your document.

2. U.S. Library of Congress. The U.S. Library of Congress (LC) database is used throughout the world by people searching for information on publications. There are two options for getting your book into the LC database. Both require providing information to LC before publication:

(a) Register the book electronically by completing the LC Preassigned Control Number Program form before publication. You will receive an LC Control Number (LCCN) that should be printed in the book, usually on the back of the title page. You are required to send a copy of the book to the Library of Congress when it is published. When the library receives the book, they will catalog it and add it to

their database. The LCCN and the database make it much easier for libraries and dealers to find your book and the catalog information. For more information and electronic registration forms go to: *http://pcn.loc.gov/pcn.*

(b) Register with the LC Cataloging In Publication (CIP) program. Before printing, generally at the final draft stage, you send the complete text of the book in electronic form to the Library of Congress to be cataloged. They will send you the complete bibliographic record of your book, including classification numbers and subject headings. This information should be printed in the book when it is published. Having the catalog record in the book makes it much easier for libraries to process the book and for anyone to select, locate, and order the book. You must send a copy of the book to the Library of Congress once it is published. For more information on the CIP, contact:

Mr. John Celli, Chief
Cataloguing in Publication Division (CIP)
Library of Congress
101 Independence Avenue, S.E.
Washington, DC 20540-4320 USA
E-mail: jcel@loc.gov

For general information or to view the forms and register, go to: *http://cip.loc.gov/cip.*

Bibliographic Indexing Databases and Information Clearinghouses

Consider submitting your report or article to bibliographic indexing databases and information clearinghouses, such as:

1. POPLINE. (POPulation information onLINE) is the world's largest bibliographic database on population, family planning, and related health issues. POPLINE provides citations with abstracts for over 275,000 records representing published and unpublished literature in the field.

POPLINE Digital Services (PDS) provides authoritative, accurate, and up-to-date reproductive health information in electronic formats for developing-country health professionals and policy-makers. Full-text copies of most of the documents cited in POPLINE are available to individuals or institutions in developing countries free of charge, upon request. PDS also provides full-text documents via the Internet. For more information, contact:

POPLINE Digital Services
111 Market Place, Suite 310
Baltimore, MD 21202 USA
Telephone: (410) 659-6300
Fax: (410) 659-6266
E-mail: popline@jhuccp.org

2. SOSIG. Social Science Information Gateway (SOSIG) at *http://www.sosig.ac.uk* is a fully searchable subject-based catalogue of international Internet resources on social science. This service, funded by the Economic and Social Research Council of the United Kingdom, offers access to a catalog of thousands of high-quality social science resources from around the world including:

- Research reports and papers
- Electronic journals and texts
- Statistics and software
- Databases and data
- Learning and teaching resources
- Internet links to university social science departments

If you would like to recommend that SOSIG post your study citation or data sets or publicize information related to your work, you must complete registration information at the SOSIG Internet address at *www.sosig.ac.uk/about_us/contacts.html* or write to:

The Social Science Information Gateway
Institute for Learning and Research Technology
University of Bristol
8-10 Berkeley Square
Bristol, BS8 1HH UK
Telephone: 44 0 117 928 7117
Fax: 44 0 117 928 7112

3. *Development Experience Clearinghouse (DEC).* If your research is done with support from the U.S. Agency for International Development, (USAID) you may submit your study reports or documents for inclusion in the DEC Development Experience System (DEXS). This database was developed to ensure that valuable USAID experience is preserved and gains wider exposure. Once processed into the DEXS system, your documents will be searchable and accessible online over the Internet, and paper copies can be ordered by the public at any time. For instructions on how to submit your material, see *http://www.dec.org/submit/submit.htm* or contact:

Document Acquisitions
USAID Development Experience Clearinghouse
1611 North Kent Street, Suite 200
Arlington, VA 22209-2111 USA
Telephone: (703) 351-4006, ext. 106
E-mail: docorder@dec.cdie.org

4. *Asia-Pacific POPIN.* Asia-Pacific POPIN is a decentralized network involving regional, sub-regional, national, and nongovernmental population information centers in the Economic and Social Commission for Asia and the Pacific (ESCAP) region. To submit studies conducted in Asia or the Pacific to the ESCAP directory of current population research, contact:

Director, Population and Rural and Urban Development Division
ESCAP, United Nations Building
Rajdamnern Avenue
Bangkok, 10200 Thailand
Telephone: 66-2 288-1536
Fax: 66-2 288-1009
E-mail: ertuna.unescap@un.org

For more information, visit the ESCAP Web site at: *http://www.unescap.org/pop/popin/index.htm* or the main POPIN Web site at: *http://www.undp.org/popin.*

5. *U.S. Library of Congress.* The size and variety of its collections make the Library of Congress the largest library in the world. Collections include research materials in more than 450 languages. By sending a copy of your research report to the Library of Congress, you contribute to the preservation of knowledge and public access to your materials — whether available in hard copy or in a full-text electronic version. To submit your report, send a copy to:

Mr. Michael Albin, Chief
Anglo/American Acquisitions Division
(LS/ACQ/ANAD)
Library of Congress
101 Independence Avenue, S.E.
Washington, DC 20540-4170 USA
Telephone: (202) 707-5361
Fax: (202) 707-9440
E-mail: malb@loc.gov

For more information, see: *http://www.loc.gov/rr/ collects.html*.

6. U.S. National Library of Medicine. The U.S. National Library of Medicine provides online access to MEDLINE, PubMed and other specialized databases on HIV/AIDS, bioethics, public health, and health services research at: *http:// www.nlm.nih.gov/hinfo.html*. To request that your publication or document be catalogued and made accessible through the NLM, we suggest contacting:

The National Library of Medicine
Cataloging Section
8600 Rockville Pike
Bethesda, MD 20894 USA
Telephone: (301) 496-5497
Fax: (301) 402-1211
E-mail: custserv@nlm.nih.gov

7. WorldCat. Submit your publication to the WorldCat database, the most consulted database in higher education. WorldCat is managed by the Online Computer Library Center, Inc. (OCLC), a global library cooperative. It holds over 46 million

cataloging records created by libraries around the world, with 400 languages represented. Request that your publisher send your document to a participating library to catalog. Libraries that participate in the OCLC may submit the record to the WorldCat database, and may be willing to undertake the cataloguing work in exchange for a free copy of your material. To locate a member library, visit: *http://www.oclc.org/contacts*. For more information, contact:

OCLC Online Computer Library Center, Inc.
6565 Frantz Road
Dublin, OH 43017-3395 USA
Telephone: (614) 764-6000/(800) 848-5878
(USA/Canada)
Fax: (614) 764-6096
E-mail: oclc@oclc.org

8. BIREME's Scientific Electronic Library Online (SciELO). BIREME is a project of the Centro Latino-Americano e do Caribe de Informação em Ciências da Saúde (Latin American and the Caribbean Center on Health Sciences Information) and the Fundação de Amparo à Pesquisa do Estado de São Paulo (FAPESP) — a governmental foundation in Brazil aimed at supporting scientific research. The BIREME project promotes a common methodology for the preparation, storage, retrieval, and evaluation of electronic publications through the use of information and communication technologies. One of the applications of the methodology is the Scientific Electronic Library Online — SciELO, a virtual library comprising scientific publications produced in Latin America and the Caribbean. For more information on how to submit your study report to SciELO, contact:

FAPESP/BIREME Project for Electronic Scientific Publications
Centro Latino-Americano e do Caribe de Informação em Ciências da Saúde
Rua Botucatu, 862-04023-901

São Paulo SP, Brazil
Telephone: 55 11 576 9863
Fax: 55 11 571 1919/575 8868
E-mail: scielo@bireme.br

Depositing Data Sets

To make your research permanently available to the international community, seek opportunities to deposit your data set at a national or regional university library or faculty of social sciences.

1. Inter-University Consortium for Political and Social Research (ICPSR). The Inter-University Consortium for Political and Social Research (ICPSR), established in 1962, is the main repository for social science research in the United States. ICPSR maintains and provides access to a vast archive of social science data for research and instruction, and offers training in quantitative methods to facilitate effective data use. ICPSR preserves data to ensure that data resources are available to future generations of scholars, migrating the data to new storage media as changes in technology warrant. In addition, ICPSR provides user support to assist researchers in identifying relevant data for analysis and in conducting their research projects.

ICPSR, a unit within the Institute for Social Research at the University of Michigan, encourages researchers to deposit their own computer-readable data in the archive for long-term preservation and for use in secondary analysis by other social science researchers.

For instructions on how to prepare a data set for deposit, visit the ICPSR Web site at *http://www.icpsr.umich.edu/ACCESS/deposit.html*. This Web site explains ICPSR guidelines for depositing data, including how to prepare data for archiving during the research stage. When a data collection arrives at ICPSR, it is prepared for public release and archived in perpetuity, thus benefiting the entire social science research community. For more information, contact:

The Inter-University Consortium for Political and Social Research
P.O. Box 1248
Ann Arbor, MI 48106-1248 USA
Telephone: (734) 998-9900
Fax: (734) 998-9889
E-mail: netmail@icpsr.umich.edu

2. The Social Science Data Archives (SSDA). Located in the Research School of Social Sciences at the Australian National University, the SSDA was established in 1981 to collect and preserve computer-readable data and to make the data available for further analysis. SSDA actively seeks deposit of data sets from research by academic, government, and private organizations in order to preserve them for future use. For information on how to deposit data, see: *http://ssda.anu.edu.au/SSDA/depositing-data.html*.

3. Dublin Core Metadata Initiative. The Dublin Core is a directory of directories. One way to help other researchers find your report or locate your data sets — if these materials are posted on the Internet by you or someone else — is to make sure the final HTML Web pages are annotated with Dublin Core metatags or indexing information. Dublin Core metadata supplement existing methods for searching and indexing Web-based metadata, regardless of whether the corresponding resource is an electronic or physical document. Adding Dublin Core metatags promotes greater access to your information by anyone searching the World Wide Web. Even if your study report will not immediately be posted on the Internet, you can add bibliographic descriptors to your data set or report using the Dublin Core Metadata Element Set. Some people also use Dublin core elements for cataloging.

To download the Dublin Core metadata, see: *http://dublincore.org/documents/2000/07/16/usageguide*. For a copy of this guide in French, see: *http://www.bibl.ulaval.ca/DublinCore/usageguide-200000716fr.htm*.

Web Sites

1. i-biblio. If your organization — or a research partner's organization — has posted your material on a Web site, explore their interest in permitting a major Web hub such as *www.ibiblio.org* to replicate the material in the social or applied sciences sections of its collections. i-biblio, a collaboration of the Center for the Public Domain and The University of North Carolina at Chapel Hill, is home to one of the largest collections of freely available full-text online information used for teaching, research, and public service. For more information, visit: *http://ibiblio.org/collection.html*.

2. AMEDEO. If you own the copyright to your research report, do not plan to submit your data to a peer-review journal, and would like to see your findings made freely available to the public, consider submitting your text electronically to AMEDEO, The Medical Literature Guide. The editors will post your report on the following Web sites, which archive scientific research and ideas: *http://publiclibraryofscience.com* or *http://www. FreeMedicalJournals.com*. For more information, contact AMEDEO's senior editor, Bernd Sebastian Kamps, M.D. at Bernd.Sebastian.Kamps@ AMEDEO.com.

Suggested Readings and Selected Internet Resources

I. General Texts on Qualitative Research Methods

Bernard HR. Research methods in anthropology: qualitative and quantitative approaches. 2nd ed. Walnut Creek, CA: Altamira Press; 1995.

Campbell O, Cleland JG, Collumbien M, et al. Social science methods for research on reproductive health. Geneva: World Health Organization; 1999.

Denzin NK, Lincoln YS, editors. Handbook of qualitative research. Thousand Oaks, CA: Sage; 1994. (Also available in a 3-volume paperback series.)

Hudelson PM. Qualitative research for health programmes. Geneva: World Health Organization; 1996.

Patton MQ. Qualitative evaluation and research methods. 2nd ed. Newbury Park, CA: Sage; 1990.

Rossman GB, Rallis FR. Learning in the field: an introduction to qualitative research. Thousand Oaks, CA: Sage; 1998.

Schensul JJ, LeCompte MD, editors. Ethnographer's toolkit. Vols. 1-9. Walnut Creek, CA: Altamira Press; 1999.

Yoddumnern-Attig B, Allen-Attig G, Boonchalaksi W, et al., editors. Qualitative methods for population and health research. Institute for Population and Social Research, Mahidol University, Thailand; 1993.

II. Theoretical Basis of Qualitative Research

Kelle U. Theory-building in qualitative research and computer programs for the management of textual data. Sociological Research Online 1997;2(2). Available from: *http://www.socresonline.org.uk/socresonline/2/2/1.html*

Patton MQ. Variety in qualitative inquiry: theoretical orientations. Chapter 3. In: Patton MQ. Qualitative evaluation and research methods. 2nd ed. Newbury Park, CA: Sage; 1990.

Strauss A, Corbin J. Basics of qualitative research: grounded theory procedures and techniques. Newbury Park, CA: Sage; 1990.

Trotter RT II. Anthropological midrange theories in mental health research: selected theory, methods and systematic approaches to at-risk populations. Ethos 1997;25(2):259-274.

III. Participant Observation

Bernard HR. Participation observation. Chapter 9. In: Bernard HR. Research methods in anthropology: qualitative and quantitative approaches. 2nd ed. Walnut Creek, CA: Altamira, 1995.

DeWalt KM. Participant observation: a guide for fieldworkers. Walnut Creek, CA: Altamira Press; 2001.

Schensul SL, Schensul JJ, LeCompte MD. Exploratory or open-ended observation. Chapter 5. In: Schensul SL, Schensul JJ, LeCompte MD. Essential ethnographic methods: observations, interviews, and questionnaires. In: Schensul JJ, LeCompte MD, editors. Ethnographer's toolkit. Vol. 2. Walnut Creek, CA: Altamira Press; 1999.

Spradley JP. Participant observation. New York: Holt, Rhinehart, and Winston; 1980.

IV. In-depth Interviewing

Rubin HJ, Rubin IS. Qualitative interviewing: the art of hearing data. Thousand Oaks, CA: Sage; 1995.

Patton MQ. Qualitative interviewing. Chapter 7. In: Patton MQ. Qualitative evaluation and research methods. 2nd ed. Newbury Park, CA: Sage; 1990.

V. Focus Group Research

Debus M. Handbook for excellence in focus group research. Washington: Academy for Educational Development; 1986.

Morgan DL, Krueger RA, editors. The Focus Group Kit. Thousand Oaks, CA: Sage; 1998.

VI. Social Network Analysis

Scott J. Social network analysis: a handbook. Newbury Park, CA: Sage; 1991.

Trotter RT II. Friends, relatives, and relevant others: conducting ethnographic network studies. Chapter 1. In: Schensul JJ, LeCompte MD, Trotter RT II, et al. Mapping social networks, spatial data, and hidden populations. In: Schensul JJ, LeCompte MD, editors. Ethnographer's toolkit. Vol. 4. Walnut Creek, CA: Altamira Press; 1999.

VII. Data Management and Analysis

Huberman AM, Miles MB. Data management and analysis methods. In: Denzin NK, Lincoln YS, editors. Handbook of qualitative research. Part IV, Methods of collecting and analyzing empirical materials. Thousand Oaks, CA: Sage; 1994.

Kreuger, RA. Analyzing and reporting focus group results. In: Morgan DL, Krueger RA, editors. The Focus Group Kit. Vol. 6. Thousand Oaks, CA: Sage; 1998.

Miles MB, Huberman AM. Qualitative data analysis: an expanded sourcebook. 2nd ed. Thousand Oaks, CA: Sage; 1994.

Patton, MQ. Enhancing the quality and credibility of qualitative analysis. Health Serv Res 1999; 34(5):1189-1208.

Silverman D. The quality of qualitative health research: the open-ended interview and its alternatives. Soc Sci Health 1998;4(2):104-117.

VIII. Combining Qualitative and Quantitative Methods

Caracelli V, Greene J. Data analysis strategies for mixed-method evaluation designs. Policy Anal 1993;15(2):195-207.

Morgan DL. Practical strategies for combining qualitative and quantitative methods. Qualitative Health Res 1998 May;8(3):362-376.

Pedersen D. Qualitative and quantitative: two styles of viewing the world or two categories of reality? In: Scrimshaw NS, Gleason GR, editors. Rapid assessment procedures: qualitative methodologies for planning and evaluation of health-related programmes. Boston: International Nutrition Foundation for Developing Countries; 1992.

Sandelowski M. Combining qualitative and quantitative sampling, data collection, and analysis techniques in mixed method studies. Res Nurs Health 2000 Jun;23(3):246-255.

Tashakkori A, Teddlie C. Mixed methodology: combining qualitative and quantitative approaches. Thousand Oaks, CA: Sage; 1998.

IX. Ethical Issues

Alty A, Rodham K. The ouch! factor: problems in conducting sensitive research. Qualitative Health Res 1998;8(2):275-282.

Association of Social Anthropologists of the Commonwealth. Ethical guidelines for good research practice. Available from: *http://www. asa.anthropology.ac.uk/ethics2.html*. 1999.

Ringheim K. Ethical issues in social science research with special reference to sexual behavior research. Soc Sci Med 1995;40:1691-1697.

Rivera R, Borasky D, Rice R, et al. Research Ethics Training Curriculum. Research Triangle Park, NC: Family Health International; 2001.

Seal DW, Bloom FR, Somlai AM. Dilemmas in conducting qualitative sex research in applied field settings. Health Educ Behav 2000 Feb;27(1):10-23.

World Health Organization. Putting women's safety first: ethical and safety recommendations for research on domestic violence against women. Geneva: World Health Organization; 1999.

X. Writing Qualitative Reports

Wolcott HF. Writing up qualitative research: qualitative research methods. No. 20. Newbury Park, CA: Sage; 1990.

Richardson L. Writing strategies: reaching diverse audiences. Newbury Park, CA: Sage; 1990.

XI. Special Issues and Applications

Chambers R. Shortcut methods of gathering information for rural development projects. In: Cernea M, editor. Putting people first: sociological variables in rural development. New York: Oxford University Press; 1985.

Green LW, George MA, Daniel M, et al. Study of participatory action in health promotion: review and recommendations for the development of participatory research in health promotion in Canada. Vancouver: Institute of Health Promotion Research, University of British Columbia and the B.C. Consortium for Health Promotion Research; 1995.

Knodel J. A case for nonanthropological qualitative methods for demographers. Popul Dev Rev 1997 Dec;23(4):847-853.

Petchesky RP, Judd K, editors. Negotiating reproductive rights: women's perspectives across countries and cultures. London: Zed Books; 1998.

Scrimshaw S, Hurtado E. Rapid assessment procedures for nutrition and primary health care. Tokyo: UN University; 1987.

XII. E-mail Lists

QUALRS-L: Qualitative research for the human sciences
To subscribe, send the following message to listserv@listserv.uga.edu:
subscribe QUALRS-L<your name>

Qual-software: Qualitative analysis computer programs
To subscribe send the follow message to jiscmail@jiscmail.ac.uk:
join qual-software<your name>

PSYCH-NARRATIVE: Discussion of narrative in everyday life
To subscribe, send the following message to majordomo@massey.ac.nz:
subscribe psych-narrative<your name>

XIII. Web Sites

Council for the Development of Social Science Research in Africa (CODESRIA)
http://www.sas.upenn.edu/African_Studies/codesria.html

QualPage: Resources for Qualitative Research
http://www.ualberta.ca/~jrnorris/qual.html

National Centre for Social Research, Qualitative Research Unit
http://www.scpr.ac.uk/units/gru/index.htm

The Center for Social and Behavioral Sciences Research, University of California at Riverside
http://www.chass.ucr.edu/csbsr/qualitative.html

Qualitative Research Resources
http://don.ratcliff.net/qual

XIV. Online Journals

The Qualitative Report
http://www.nova.edu/sss/QR

Forum: Qualitative Social Research
http://www.qualitative-research.net/fqs/fqs-eng.htm

References

Adioetomo SM, Eggleston E. Helping husband, maintaining harmony: family planning, women's work and women's household autonomy in Indonesia. J Popul 1998;4(2, special edition):7-32.

Adrien A, Cayemittes M. Le Sida en Haïti: connaissances, attitudes, croyances, et comportements de la population. Bureau du Coordination du Programme National de Lutte contre le SIDA. Port-au-Prince: Institut Haïtien de l'Enfance; 1991.

Alty A, Rodham K. The ouch! factor: problems in conducting sensitive research. Qualitative Health Res 1998;8(2):275-282.

Association of Social Anthropologists of the Commonwealth. Ethical guidelines for good research practice. Available from: *http://www.asa.anthropology.ac.uk/ethics2.html*. 1999.

Babbie E. The practice of social research. 8th ed. Belmont, CA: Wadsworth; 1998.

Babbie E. The practice of social research. 5th ed. Belmont, CA: Wadsworth; 1989.

Bandura A. Social foundations of thought and action: a social cognitive theory. Englewood Cliffs, NJ: Prentice Hall; 1986.

Bandura A. Perceived self-efficacy in the exercise of control over AIDS infection. In: Mayes VM, Albee GW, Schneider SF, editors. Primary prevention of AIDS: psychological approaches. London: Sage; 1989. p. 128-141.

Barnett B, Eggleston E, Jackson J, et al. Case study of the Women's Center of Jamaica Foundation Program for Adolescent Mothers (WP96-03). Research Triangle Park, NC: Family Health International; 1996.

Basch CE. Focus group interview: an underutilized research technique for improving theory and practice in health education [review]. Health Educ Q 1987 Win;14(4):411-448.

Beck T, Stelcner M. Guide to gender-sensitive indicators. Quebec: Canadian International Development Agency; 1996a.

Beck T, Stelcner M. The why and how of gender-sensitive indicators: a project level handbook. Quebec: Canadian International Development Agency; 1996b.

Bender DE, Baker R, Dusch E, et al. Integrated use of qualitative and quantitative methods to elicit women's differential knowledge of breastfeeding and lactational amenorrhea in Periurban Peru. J Health Popul Developing Countries 1990;1(1):68-84.

Bender DE, Castro D. Explaining the birthweight paradox: Latina immigrants' perceptions of resilience and risk. J Immigrant Health 2000 Jul;2(3):155-173.

Bender DE, Harbour C. Tell me what you mean by "Si": perceptions of quality of prenatal care among immigrant Latina women. Qualitative Health Res 2001 Nov;11(6):780-794.

Bentley M, Fullem A, Srirak N, et al. Acceptability of novel, microbicide BufferGel during a phase I safety trial in Thailand, Zimbabwe, and Malawi. Presentation at the Microbicides 2000 conference, Washington, DC, March 13-16, 2000. Abstract in: AIDS 2001 Feb;15(suppl 1):S30.

Bernard HR. Research methods in anthropology: qualitative and quantitative approaches. 2nd ed. Walnut Creek, CA: Altamira; 1995.

Bertrand J, Brown L, Kinzonzi M, et al. AIDS knowledge in three sites in Bas-Zaire. AIDS Educ Prev 1992;4:251-266.

Blumer H. Symbolic interactionism: perspective and method. Englewood Cliffs, NJ: Prentice-Hall; 1969.

Bogdewic SP. Participant observation. In: Crabtree BF; Miller WL, editors. Doing qualitative research. Vol. 3, Research methods for primary care. Newbury Park, CA: Sage; 1992.

Bond KC, Valente TW, Kendall C. Social network influences on reproductive health behaviors in Urban Northern Thailand. Soc Sci Med 1999 Dec; 49(12):1599-1614.

Brown LK, DiClemente RJ, Reynold LA. HIV prevention for adolescents: utility of the health belief model. AIDS Educ Prev 1991;3(1):50-59.

Bruce J. Fundamental elements of the quality of care. Stud Fam Plann 1990;21(2):61-91.

Bryman A, Burgess RG. Qualitative research. 4 Vols. London: Sage; 1999.

Buckner BC, Tsui, AO, Hermalin AI, et al. A guide to methods of family planning program evaluation: 1965-1990: with selected bibliography. Chapel Hill, NC: The Evaluation Project; 1995.

Burgess RG. In the field: an introduction to field research. London: Allen and Unwin; 1984.

Burrell G, Morgan G. Sociological paradigms and organizational analysis. London: Heinemann; 1979.

Buston K. NUD*IST in action: its use and its usefulness in a study of chronic illness in young people. In: Bryman A, Burgess RG, editors.

Qualitative research. Vol. III, Analysis and interpretation of qualitative date. London: Sage; 1999. p. 183-202.

Cabaraban M. Personal communication with Elizabeth T. Robinson: August 2001.

Cabaraban M, Morales B. Social and economic consequences of family planning use in the Southern Philippines. Research Triangle Park, NC: Family Health International; 1998.

Cáceres CF. La (Re)Configuracion del Universo Sexual. Lima, Peru: REDESS Jóvenes; 1999.

Campbell O, Cleland JG, Collumbien M, et al. Social science methods for research on reproductive health. Geneva: World Health Organization; 1999.

Carey JW. Linking qualitative and quantitative methods: integrating cultutal factors into public health. Qualitative Health Res 1993 Aug;3(3):298-318.

Caro DA. What you count is not what I am: notions of gender in quantitative analysis. Unpublished. GENESYS Project, U.S. Agency for International Development; 1995.

Castle S, Konaté MK, Ulin PR, et al. A qualitative study of clandestine use in urban Mali. Stud Fam Plann 1999;30(3):231-248.

Catania JA, Kegeles SM, Coates TJ. Towards an understanding of risk behavior: an AIDS risk reduction model (ARRM). Health Educ Q 1990;17(1):53-72.

Centers for Disease Control and Prevention. AnSWER analysis software for word-based records. Available from: *http://www.cdc.gov/hiv/software/answr*. Aug 6, 2001.

Centre d'Études et de Recherche sur la Population pour le Développement (CERPOD). Lorsque l'entourage hésite…: résultats d'une étude réalisée dans le district de Bamako. Bamako, Mali: CERPOD; 1999.

Cernada GP. Knowledge into action: a guide to research utilization. Vol. 1, Community health education monographs. Farmingdale, NY: Baywood Publishing Company; 1982.

Cicourel AV. Cognitive sociology. Language and meaning in social interaction. London: Penguin Education; 1973.

Cobas JA, Balcazar H, Benin MB, et al. Acculturation and low-birthweight infants among Latino women: a reanalysis of the HHANES data with structural equation models. Am J Publ Health 1996;86(3):394-396.

Coffey A, Holbrook B, Atkinson P. Qualitative data analysis: technologies and representations. In: Bryman A, Burgess RG, editors. Qualitative research. Vol. III, Analysis and interpretation of qualitative data. London: Sage; 1999. p. 165-181.

Communications Initiative Partners Meeting. Transcript of meeting at the Rockefeller Foundation: May 15-17, 2000; New York. Tapes 9-10.

Cornwall A, Jewkes R. What is participatory research? Soc Sci Med 1995;41(12):1667-1676.

Crabtree BF, Miller WL, editors. Doing qualitative research. Vol. 3, Research methods for primary care. Newbury Park, CA: Sage; 1992.

Dagron AG. Making waves: stories of participatory communication for social change. New York: The Rockefeller Foundation; 2001.

Debus M. Handbook for excellence in focus group research. Washington: Academy for Educational Development; 1986.

Denison J. Behavior change: a summary of four major theories. Arlington, VA: Family Health International; 1996.

Denzin NK. The practices and politics of interpretation. In: Denzin NK, Lincoln YS, editors. Handbook of qualitative research. 2nd ed. Part V, The art and practices of interpretation, evaluation, and representation. Thousand Oaks, CA: Sage; 2000. p. 897-922.

Denzin NK, Lincoln YS, editors. Handbook of qualitative research. Thousand Oaks, CA: Sage; 1994.

Devers, KJ. How will we know "good" qualitative research when we see it? Beginning the dialogue in health services research. Health Serv Res 1999;34(5):1153-1188.

Díaz M, Simmons R. When is research participatory? Reflections on a reproductive health project in Brazil. J Women's Health 1999;8(2):175-184.

Dickin K, Griffiths M, Piwoz E. Designing by dialogue: a program planner's guide to consultative research for improving young child feeding. Washington: Academy for Educational Development, Health and Human Resources Analysis (HHRAA) Project; 1997.

Fetterman DM. A walk through the wilderness: learning to find your way. In: Shaffir WB, Stebbins RA, editors. Experiencing fieldwork: an inside view of qualitative research. Newbury Park, CA: Sage; 1992.

Fishbein M, et al. Factors influencing behavior and behavior change; final report — theorist's workshop. Washington: American Cancer Society; 1991. In: Glanz K, Lewis FM, Rimer BK, editors. Health behavior and health education: theory, practice and research. 2nd edition. San Francisco: Jossey-Bass; 1997.

Flick U. An introduction to qualitative research. Thousand Oaks, CA: Sage; 1998.

Gans H. The participant observer as a human being: observations on the personal aspects of fieldwork. In: HS Becker, B Greer, D Reisman, et al., editors. Institutions and the person. Chicago: Aldine; 1968.

Gergen MM, Gergen KJ, editors. Qualitative inquiry: tensions and transformations. In: Denzin NK, Lincoln YS, editors. Handbook of qualitative research. Part VI, The future of qualitative research. Thousand Oaks, CA: Sage; 2000. p. 1025-1046.

Gilchrist VJ. Key informant interviews. In: Crabtree BF, Miller WL, editors. Doing qualitative research. Vol. 3, Research methods for primary care. Newbury Park: Sage; 1992.

Glantz NM, Halperin DC, Hunt LM. Studying domestic violence in Chiapas, Mexico. Qualitative Health Res 1998 May;8(3):377-392.

Glanz K, Lewis FM, Rimer BK, editors. Health behavior and health education: theory, practice and research. 2nd edition. San Francisco: Jossey-Bass; 1997.

Glaser B, Strauss A. The discovery of grounded theory. Chicago: Aldine; 1967.

Golden-Biddle K, Locke L. Appealing work: an investigation of how ethnographic texts convince. In: Bryman A, Burgess RG, editors. Qualitative Research. Vol. III, Analysis and interpretation of qualitative data. London: Sage; 1999. p. 369-396.

Goldstein E, Wrubel J, Faigles B, et al. Sources of information for HIV prevention program managers: a national survey. AIDS Educ Prev 1998;10(1):63-74.

Greenhalgh S. Methods and meanings: reflections on disciplinary difference. Popul Dev Rev 1997;23(4):819-824.

Grimes DA. Communicating research. In: O'Brien PM, Pipkin FB, editors. Introduction to research methodology for specialists and trainees. London: FCOG Press; 1999. p. 210-217.

Guba EG, Lincoln YS. Competing paradigms in qualitative research. In: Denzin NK, Lincoln YS, editors. Handbook of qualitative research. Part II, Major paradigms and perspectives. Thousand Oaks, CA: Sage; 1994. p. 105-117.

Harris E, Tanner M. Health technology transfer. Br Med J 2000 Sep 30; 321(7264):818.

Havelock RG. Planning for innovation through dissemination and utilization of knowledge. Ann Arbor, MI: Center for Research on Utilization of Scientific Knowledge, Institute for Social Research; 1969.

Heise L, McGrory CE, Wood SY. Practical and ethical dilemmas in the clinical testing of microbicides. New York: International Women's Health Coalition; 1998.

 Helitzer-Allen D, Makhambera M, Wangel AM. Obtaining sensitive information: the need for more than focus groups. Reprod Health Matters 1994 May;3:75-82.

Hess DJ. Teaching ethnographic writing: a review essay. Anthropol Educ Q 1989;20;163-176.

Hogle J, Stalker M, Hassig S, et al. Conducting effective focus group discussions. Arlington, VA: Family Health International; 1994.

Holstein JA, Gubrium JF. Active interviewing. In: Bryman A, Burgess RG. Qualitative research. Vol. II, Methods of qualitative research. London: Sage; 1999. p. 105-121.

Huberman AM, Miles MB. Data management and analysis methods. In: Denzin NK, Lincoln YS, editors. Handbook of qualitative research. Part IV, Methods of collecting and analyzing empirical materials. Thousand Oaks, CA: Sage; 1994. p. 428-444.

Hudelson PM. Qualitative research for health programmes. Geneva: World Health Organization; 1996.

Hull T. Personal communication with Priscilla R. Ulin: Jun 2001.

Human Interaction Research Institute. Putting knowledge to use: a distillation of the literature regarding knowledge transfer and change. Los Angeles: Human Interaction Research Institute; 1976.

International Committee of Medical Journal Editors. Uniform requirements for manuscripts submitted to biomedical journals. Available from: *http://www.icmje.org.* 2000.

Janesick VJ. The choreography of QR design: minuets, improvisations and crystallization. In: Denzin NK, Lincoln YS, editors. Handbook of qualitative research. Part III, Strategies of inquiry. Thousand Oaks, CA: Sage; 2000. p. 379-399.

Janowitz B, Holtman M, Hubacher D, et al. Can the Bangladeshi family planning program meet rising needs without raising costs? Int Fam Plann Perspect 1997 Sep;23(3):116-121.

Janowitz B, Jamil K, Chowdhury J, et al. Productivity and costs for family planning service delivery in Bangladesh: the NGO program. Research Triangle Park, NC: Family Health International; 1996.

Kaler A. "It's some kind of women's empowerment": the ambiguity of the female condom as a marker of female empowerment. Soc Sci Med 2001; 52(5):783-796.

Kelle U. Theory-building in qualitative research and computer programs for the management of textual data. Sociological Research Online 1997;2(2). Available from: *http://www.socresonline.org.uk/socresonline/2/2/1.htm*l.

Kelly JA, Somlai AM, DiFranceisco, WJ, et al. Bridging the gap between the science and service of HIV prevention: transferring effective research-based HIV prevention interventions to community AIDS service providers. Am J Public Health 2000 Jul;90(7):1082-1088.

Kidder LH. Qualitative research and quasi-experimental frameworks. In: Brewer MB, Collins BE, editors. Scientific inquiry and the social sciences. San Francisco: Jossey-Bass; 1981.

Kimani L. Personal communication with Priscilla R. Ulin: Nov 1990.

King G, Keohane RO, Verba S. Designing social inquiry. Princeton, NJ: Princeton University Press; 1994. p. 26-27.

Kirk J, Miller ML. Reliability and validity in qualitative research. Newbury Park, CA: Sage; 1986.

Kitua AY, Mashalla YJS, Shija JK. Coordinating health research to promote action: the Tanzanian experience. Br Med J 2000 Sep 30;321(7264):821-823.

Knodel J. A case for nonanthropological qualitative methods for demographers. Popul Dev Rev 1997 Dec;23(4):847-853.

Knodel J. Conducting comparative focus group research: cautionary comments from a coordinator. Health Transition Rev 1994;4(1):99-104.

Koo HP, Woodsong C. Conceptual model for study of the dynamics and meaning of unintended pregnancy. Unpublished. Research Triangle Institute; 1997.

Kreuger, RA. Analyzing and reporting focus group results. In: Morgan DL, Krueger RA, editors. The Focus Group Kit. Vol. 6. Thousand Oaks, CA: Sage; 1998.

Lau RR. Origins of health locus of control beliefs. J Personality Soc Psych 1982;42(2):322-334.

Lewis M. Personal communication with Elizabeth E. Tolley: Aug 2000.

Lincoln YS, Guba EG. Naturalistic inquiry. Beverly Hills, CA: Sage; 1985.

Lofland JH. Styles of reporting qualitative field research. Am Sociologist 1974 Aug;9(3):101-111.

Mason J. Qualitative researching. London: Sage; 1996.

Menou MJ. Impact of the Internet: some conceptual and methodological issues, or how to hit a moving target behind a smoke screen. In: Nicholas D, Rowlands I, editors. The Internet: its impact and evaluation. London: ASLIB; 1999.

Menou MJ. Measuring the impact of information on development. Ottawa: International Development Research Centre; 1993.

Merton RK, Fiske M, Kendall PL. The focused interview: a manual of problems and procedures. 2nd ed. New York: The Free Press; 1956.

Miles MB, Huberman AM. Qualitative data analysis: an expanded sourcebook. 2nd ed. Thousand Oaks: Sage; 1994.

Miller WL, Crabtree BF. Clinical research. In: Denzin NK, Lincoln YS, editors. Handbook of qualitative research. Part III, Strategies of inquiry. Thousand Oaks, CA: Sage; 2000. p. 607-631.

Morgan DL. Focus groups as qualitative research. Newbury Park, CA: Sage; 1988.

Morgan DL. Practical strategies for combining qualitative and quantitative methods. Qualitative Health Res 1998 May;8(3):362-376.

Morris LL, Fitz-Gibbon CT, Freeman ME. How to communicate evaluation findings. Newbury Park, CA: Sage; 1987.

National Bioethics Advisory Committee. Ethical and policy issues in international research. Bethesda, MD: National Bioethics Advisory Committee; 2001.

Obermeyer CM. Qualitative methods: a key to better understanding of demographic behavior? Popul Dev Rev 1997;23(4):813-818.

Olesen VL. Feminisms and qualitative research at and into the millennium. In: Denzin NK, Lincoln YS, editors. Handbook of qualitative research. Thousand Oaks, CA: Sage; 2000.

Pan American Health Organization. Workshop on gender, health, and development: facilitator's guide. Washington: Regional Program on Women, Health, and Development, Pan American Health Organization; 1997.

discussion of mixed methodologies

☆ Patton MQ. Qualitative evaluation and research methods. 2nd ed. Newbury Park, CA: Sage; 1990.

Patton, MQ. Enhancing the quality and credibility of qualitative analysis. Health Serv Res 1999;34(5):1189-1208.

Paulson S, Gisbert ME, Quiton M. Case studies of two women's health projects in Bolivia. Research Triangle Park, NC: Family Health International; 1996.

Pedersen D. Qualitative and quantitative: two styles of viewing the world or two categories of reality? In: Scrimshaw NS, Gleason GR, editors. Rapid assessment procedures: qualitative methodologies for planning and evaluation of health-related programmes. Boston: International Nutrition Foundation for Developing Countries; 1992.

Petchesky RP, Judd K, editors. Negotiating reproductive rights: women's perspectives across countries and cultures. London: Zed Books; 1998.

Pino R, Schensul J, Romero M. The roles of cousins in the social networks of drug-using youth in Hartford. Presentation at the American Anthropological Association Annual Meeting; Chicago, Illinois, 1999.

Piotrow PT, Kincaid DL, Rimon JG, et al. Health communication: lessons from family planning and reproductive health. Westport, CT: Praeger; 1997.

Population Council. Communication strategy: the Africa operations research and technical assistance project II. Unpublished. Population Council; 1994.

Porter RW, Hicks I. Knowledge utilization and the process of policy formation: toward a framework for Africa. Washington: Academy for Educational Development; 1995.

Porter RW, Prysor-Jones S. Making a difference to policies and programs: a guide for researchers. Washington: Academy for Educational Development; 1997.

Potter J, Wetherell M. Discourse and social psychology: beyond attitudes and behaviour. London: Sage; 1987.

Prochaska JO, DiClemente CC, Norcross JC. In search of how people change: applications to addictive behaviors. Am Psychologist 1992;47(9): 1102-1114.

Prochaska JO, Redding Ca, Evers KE. The transtheoretical model and stages of change. In: Glanz K, Lewis FM, Rimer BK, editors. Health behavior and health education: theory, practice and research. San Francisco: Jossey-Bass; 1997. p. 60-84.

Richardson L. Writing strategies: reaching diverse audiences. Newbury Park, CA: Sage; 1990.

Rist RC. Influencing the policy process with qualitative research. In: Denzin NK, Lincoln YS, editors. Handbook of qualitative research. 2nd ed. Thousand Oaks, CA: Sage; 2000.

Rogers EM, Storey JD. Communication campaigns. In: Berger CR, Chafee SH. Handbook of communication science. Beverly Hills, CA: Sage; 1987. p. 817-846.

Ronai CR. Multiple reflections of child sex abuse: an argument for a layered account. J Contemp Ethnography 1995 Jan;23(4);395-426.

Rosenstock I, Strecher V, Becker M. The health belief model and HIV risk behavior change. In: Clemente RJ, Peterson JL, editors. Preventing AIDS: theories and methods of behavioral interventions. New York: Plenum Press; 1994. p. 5-24.

Rossman GB, Rallis FR. Learning in the field: an introduction to qualitative research. Thousand Oaks, CA: Sage; 1998.

Rothman J. Using research in organizations. Beverly Hills, CA: Sage; 1980.

Rubin HJ, Rubin IS. Qualitative interviewing: the art of hearing data. Thousand Oaks, CA: Sage; 1995.

Rutter M. Resilience: some conceptual considerations. J Adol Health 1993;14(8):626-631.

Ryan GW, Bernard HR. Data management and analysis methods. In: Denzin NK, Lincoln YS, editors. Handbook of qualitative research. 2nd ed. Part V, The art and practices of interpretation, evaluation, and representation. Thousand Oaks, CA: Sage; 2000. p. 769-802.

Schensul JJ, LeCompte MD, Hess GA Jr., et al. Using ethnographic data: interventions, public programming and public policy. Vol. 7. In: Schensul JJ, LeCompte MD, editors. Ethnographer's toolkit. Walnut Creek, CA: Altamira Press; 1999.

Schensul SL, Schensul JJ, LeCompte MD. Essential ethnographic methods: observations, interviews, and questionnaires. Vol 2. In: Schensul JJ, LeCompte MD, editors. Ethnographer's toolkit. Walnut Creek, CA: Altamira Press; 1999.

Schuler SR, McIntosh EN, Goldstein MC, et al. Barriers to effective family planning in Nepal. Stud Fam Plann 1985 Sep/Oct;16(5):260-270.

Scribner R, Dwyer JH. Acculturation and low birthweight among Latinos in the Hispanic HANES. Am J Publ Health 1989;79(9):1263-1267.

Seidel R. Notes from the field in communication for child survival. Washington: Academy for Educational Development; 1993.

Selltiz C, Wrightsman LS, Cook SW. Research methods in social relations. New York: Holt, Rinehart and Winston; 1976.

Shah MK. Listening to young voices: facilitating participatory appraisals of reproductive health with adolescents. Washington: FOCUS on Young Adults; 1999.

Sharma RR. An introduction to advocacy: training guide. Washington: Academy for Educational Development; 1996.

Smith JB. Personal communication with Elizabeth T. Robinson: Aug 2001.

Smith PH, Earp JAL, DeVellis R. Measuring battering: development of the Women's Experience with Battering (WEB) scale. Women's Health: Research on Gender, Behavior, and Policy 1995;1(4):273-288.

Smith PH, Tessaro J, Earp JAL. Women's experiences with battering: a conceptualization from quantitative research. Women's Health Issues 1995 Win;5(4):173-195.

Smith WA. Mass communication for health: a behavioral perspective. Presentation at the National Academy of Sciences Expert Meeting on Reproductive Health, np, January 25, 1995.

Spradley JP. The ethnographic interview. New York: Holt, Rinehart and Winston; 1979.

Steckler A, McLeroy KR, Goodman RM, et al. Toward integrating qualitative and quantitative methods: an introduction. Health Educ Q 1992 Spr;19(1):1-8.

Stevens WF, Tornatzky LG. The dissemination of evaluation: an experiment. Eval Rev 1980 Jun;4(3):339-354.

Strauss A. Qualitative analysis for social scientists. New York: Cambridge University Press; 1987.

Strauss A, Corbin J. Basics of qualitative research: grounded theory procedures and techniques. Newbury Park, CA: Sage; 1990.

Tashakkori A, Teddlie C. Mixed methodology: combining qualitative and quantitative approaches. Thousand Oaks, CA: Sage; 1998.

Tesch R. Qualitative research: analysis types and software tools. New York: Falmer; 1990.

Thomas WI, Thomas DS. The child in America. New York: Knopf; 1929.

Thorngate W. Measuring the effect of information on development. In: McConnell P, editor. Making a Difference: measuring the impact of information on development. Ottawa: International Research Centre; 1995.

Timyan J. Guidelines for gathering qualitative data for HAPA PVO grants project evaluation. Baltimore, MD: Johns Hopkins University, Institute for International Programs, School of Hygiene and Public Health; 1991.

Tolley E, Dev A, Hyjazi Y, et al. Context of abortion among adolescents in Guinea and Côte d'Ivoire. Research Triangle Park, NC: Family Health International; 1998.

Tolman DL, Szalacha LA. Dimensions of desire: bridging qualitative and quantitative methods in a study of adolescent sexuality. Psych Women Q 1999 Mar;23(1):7-39.

Tourigny SC. Some new dying trick: African American youths "choosing" HIV/AIDS. Qualitative Health Res 1998 Mar;8(2):149-167.

Trotter RT II. Anthropological midrange theories in mental health research: selected theory, methods and systematic approaches to at-risk populations. Ethos 1997;25(2):259-274.

Trow M. Comment on participant observation and interviewing: a comparison. Human Org 1957;16:33-35.

 Ulin, PR, Cayemittes M, Metellus E. Haitian women's role in sexual decision-making: the gap between AIDS knowledge and behavior change. Research Triangle Park, NC: Family Health International; 1995.

UNAIDS (Joint United Nations Programme on HIV/AIDS). Ethical considerations in HIV preventive vaccine research. Geneva: Joint United Nations Programme on HIV/AIDS; 2000a.

UNAIDS (Joint United Nations Programme on HIV/AIDS). Report on the global HIV/AIDS epidemic. Geneva: World Health Organization; 2000b.

United Nations. Programme of Action for the International Conference on Population and Development. New York: United Nations; 1994.

United Nations. Platform for Action of the Fourth World Conference on Women. New York: United Nations; 1995.

VanLandringham MJ, Suprasert S, Grandjean N, et al. Two risky views of sexual practices among northern Thai males: the health belief model and the theory of reasoned action. J Health Soc Behavior 1995;36(2);195-212.

Varga, CA. The condom conundrum: barriers to condom use among commercial sex workers in Durban, South Africa. Afr J Reprod Health 1997 Mar;1(1):74-88.

Wallston KA, Wallston BS, DeVellis R. Development of the multidimensional health locus of control (MHLC) scales. Health Educ Monographs 1978;692):160-170.

Wang CC. Photovoice: a participatory action strategy applied to women's health. J Women's Health 1999 Mar; 8(2):185-192.

Wang CC, Burris M. Photovoice: concept, methodology, and use for participatory needs assessment. Health Educ Behavior 1997; 24(3):369-387.

Webb EJ, Campbell DT, Schwartz RD, et al. Unobtrusive measures: nonreactive research in the social sciences. Chicago: Rand McNally; 1966.

Werner EE. Risk, resilience and recovery: perspectives from the Kauai Longitudinal Study. Dev Psychopathology 1993;5:303-315.

Williams WC. The Doctor Stories. Coles R, compiler. New York: New Directions Books; 1984.

Williamson N. Protecting study participants in social science research versus biomedical research. Unpublished. Research Triangle Park, NC: Family Health International, 1995.

Winch PJ, Wagman JA, Malouin RA, et al. Qualitative research for improved health programs: guide to manuals for qualitative and participatory research on child health, nutrition, and reproductive health. Washington: Academy for Educational Development; 2000.

Wolcott HF. Writing up qualitative research: qualitative research methods, No. 20. Newbury Park, CA: Sage; 1990.

Wolff B, Knodel J, Sittitrai W. Focus groups and surveys as complementary methods: examples from a study of the consequences of family size in Thailand. Research report no. 91-213. Ann Arbor, MI: Population Studies Center, University of Michigan; 1991.

Woodsong C. Personal communication with Elizabeth T. Robinson: Feb 2001.

World Health Organization. Preparing a research project proposal: guidelines and forms. 3rd edition. Geneva: World Health Organization; 2000.

World Health Organization. Revised 1990 estimates of maternal mortality: a new approach by WHO and UNICEF. Geneva: World Health Organization; 1996.

Xie Z, Gu B, Hardee K. Family planning and women's lives in three provinces of the People's Republic of China. Final report. Research Triangle Park, NC: China Population Information and Research Center, Family Health International, and The Futures Group; 2000.

Yin RK. Case study research: design and methods. Thousand Oaks, CA: Sage; 1994.

Yoddumnern-Attig B, Allen-Attig G, Boonchalaksi W, et al., editors. Qualitative methods for population and health research. Institute for Population and Social Research, Mahidol University, Thailand; 1993.

Authors and Contributors

Sri Moertiningsih Adioetomo, Ph.D., is Director of the Demographic Institute, Faculty of Economics, University of Indonesia. She received her doctorate in demography from Australian National University, Canberra, in 1994. She has conducted research and analysis in demography, population, and related issues, was principal investigator of a study in Indonesia on women's work and women's household autonomy for FHI's Women's Studies Project, and has published numerous articles on family planning and fertility. From 1993 to 1994 she served as chief editor of the English version of the *Indonesian Journal of Population.*

Patricia Bailey, Ph.D., has been a researcher with FHI for 18 years, focusing largely on programmatic evaluation in the areas of maternal health, adolescents, and HIV prevention. She is experienced in both quantitative and qualitative research methods and has provided technical assistance to colleagues in the field on study design, sampling, questionnaire development, and data management systems and analysis, using both complex statistical techniques and text analysis. Since 1996, she has focused on safe motherhood efforts, working in Mozambique, Nicaragua, and Peru on Columbia University's Averting Maternal Deaths and Disability Program, and in Guatemala and Honduras with Mothercare and the Maternal and Neonatal Project. As a senior researcher with FHI's Women's Studies Project, she collaborated on a manual for reproductive health providers in Bolivia to incorporate a gender perspective into services and conducted a study of adolescents in Brazil to determine the impact of abortion or motherhood on educational status, self-esteem, and family relationships.

David Bell, M.A., Ed.D., is an educator and psychologist who, for the past 10 years, has worked in community development projects throughout Southern Africa. His particular interest focuses on the power relationships and dynamics inherent in community development in developing country settings.

Deborah E. Bender, Ph.D., M.P.H., is a professor in the School of Public Health at the University of North Carolina at Chapel Hill. Her research interests focus on reproductive health issues for Latina women in the Americas. She has worked extensively in the Andean region and with immigrant Latina populations in North Carolina. Her methodological strength lies in the integration of quantitative and qualitative methods of data collection. Through this linkage, her findings have enriched the validity of women's explanations and strengthened the generalizability of findings related to specific reproductive issues.

Marge Berer, M.A., has been the editor of the journal *Reproductive Health Matters* for nine years. Since 1996, she has served as chairwoman of the World Health Organization's Gender Advisory Panel, Department of Reproductive Health and Research. She is also the editor of *Safe Motherhood: Critical Issues, Women and HIV/AIDS: An International Resource Book,* and the author of numerous articles on making abortion safe and legal. For the past 25 years, she has been a feminist and international advocate for women's reproductive rights.

Sarah Castle, Ph.D., is a lecturer in the Centre for Population Studies at the London School of Hygiene and Tropical Medicine. She has conducted research for more than 13 years in Mali, where she first started doing field-work on infant feeding and illness management. More recently, her research interests have focused on reproductive health. She is currently involved in setting up and evaluating a peer education program to improve sexual health among the young people of the Mopti region in Mali.

Dina C. Castro, M.P.H., Ph.D., is a researcher at the Frank Porter Graham Child Development Center at the University of North Carolina at Chapel Hill. She has worked for 20 years in public health and education research and has conducted interventions to improve the quality of life of low-income families in her native Peru and in the United States. Her current work focuses on issues affecting Latino children and access to and utilization of health and education services by families.

Edmond Bagdé Dingamhoudou, a journalist and social worker with the Population Council in Senegal, formerly served at the Centre d'Etudes et de Recherche sur la Population pour le Développement (CERPOD) in Bamako, Mali, where he was responsible for communicating and disseminating findings from the institute's regional research.

Baochang Gu, Ph.D., is Senior Associate at the China Population Information and Research Center (CPIRC), Beijing. He is a member of the Population Advisory Committee of State Family Planning Commission of China, and adjunct professor at Peking University. Dr. Gu served as principal investigator of a study in China on the effect of family planning on women's lives for FHI's Women's Studies Project. The main topics of his work are population dynamics and fertility trends, family planning and reproductive health, sex ratio at birth and women's status, quality of care and informed choice, and urbanization and migration. He has served as deputy chair and associate professor of the Department of Sociology, Peking University, Beijing; United Nations Population Fund advisor on population and development to the Democratic People's Republic of Korea; and Senior Program Associate, the Population Council, New York. He received his Ph.D. in sociology and demography from the University of Texas at Austin.

Theresa Hatzell, Ph.D., is a Senior Research Associate in FHI's Health Services Research group. Dr. Hatzell's recent research supports programming and policy formulation regarding male and female condom promotion as an STI/HIV prevention strategy. Dr. Hatzell has worked in Niger, Senegal, Zaire, Philippines, Sri Lanka, South Africa, Kenya, Tanzania, and Madagascar. She earned her doctorate from the Department of Health Policy and Administration at the University of North Carolina (UNC) at Chapel Hill. She holds a master's degree in public health, specializing in maternal and child health, also from UNC.

Barbara Janowitz, Ph.D., is director of Health Services Research at FHI, where she has worked since 1977. In recent years she has concentrated her research on cost analysis and cost effectiveness analysis. Her published work in economics includes a paper exploring the impact of introducing contraceptive implants into the Thailand family planning program, on the costs and outputs of community-based distribution programs in Tanzania, and on the costs of family planning services in Bangladesh. Her work in both Bangladesh and Tanzania included analyses of the costs of programs that provided family planning services to women in their homes. She has worked on studies to determine the costs of adding reproductive health services to family planning clinics in Zimbabwe; of improving quality of care in Egypt and Uganda; of providing reproductive health services to youths in Kenya; of involving men in the maternity care of their partners, and of preventing vertical transmission of HIV. Dr. Janowitz served on the faculty of Kent State University for several years and received her doctorate in political economy from Johns Hopkins University.

Shireen J. Jejeebhoy, Ph.D., works at the UNDP/UNFPA/WHO/World Bank Special Programme of Research, Development and Research Training in Human Reproduction, Department of Reproductive Health and Research, World Health Organization, Geneva. She is involved in and provides technical support to investigators conducting science research on sexual and reproductive health in developing countries, with a focus on issues relating to adolescent sexual and reproductive health. Prior to joining the World Health Organization, she worked in India as an independent researcher in the field of reproductive health. She has focused on social science research in reproductive health issues, female autonomy, and gender issues. She has published extensively in areas relating to women's education and reproductive behavior, women's autonomy in India, and adolescent sexual and reproductive health. She holds a Ph.D. in demography from the University of Pennsylvania.

Naveeda Khawaja, M.Sc., M.P.H., is the coordinator of the Technical Alliance for Social Change, Pakistan, a technical resource unit that focuses on building nongovernmental and private-sector capacity to use community-based information, education, and communications strategies to improve reproductive health and early child care. She has held leadership positions on projects and for organizations such as UNICEF, the British Council, MotherCare/John Snow, Inc., and the U.S. Agency for International Development (USAID). She held a USAID Jefferson Fellowship, and has served as a consultant to the Asia Foundation, the World Bank, and the World Food Program. She is a graduate of Punjab University and Emory University's Rollins School of Public Health, where she specialized in international health and behavioral sciences.

Kate MacQueen, M.P.H., Ph.D., is a senior scientist with FHI, where her work focuses on qualitative approaches, ethics, and community-based research. Prior to arriving at FHI she was a researcher and senior scientist with the U.S. Centers for Disease and Control and Prevention (CDC), where she worked on a variety of topics, including preparations for domestic and international HIV-vaccine efficacy trials, public health ethics, and community-based participatory research models. She is one of the developers of

AnSWR, a CDC-based qualitative data management and analysis software program, and is a strong proponent of research that integrates qualitative and quantitative approaches. She has a Ph.D. in demographic anthropology from Binghamton University/State University of New York and an M.P.H. from the Rollins School of Public Health at Emory University.

Erin T. McNeill, Ph.D., is a human scientist who has been working in the field of international reproductive health and rights with the combined power of social and biological science for the last 13 years. After completing her Ph.D. in Edinburgh, Scotland, on steroidal contraception, bleeding and women's well-being, in which she used qualitative, quantitative, and clinical research techniques, she joined the U.S. Agency for International Development (USAID). There, she was the technical advisor for two large USAID-supported contraceptive technology development projects. For more than four years she also played a central role in the gender and development work of USAID's Office of Population and fostered a growing interest in human rights. Since 1997, she has been FHI's representative in Edinburgh, Scotland, and has continued to work on a variety of global research and technical assistance activities, including qualitative research. She delivers an annual Masters in Science lecture series at the University of Edinburgh on "Reproductive Health in the Real World."

Susana L. Rance is a researcher and activist living in La Paz, Bolivia. She teaches courses on gender, health, and qualitative research methods. She coordinates a network of working groups on unwanted pregnancy and abortion in three Bolivian cities. Her publications include books on the family planning debate in Bolivia, and on humane treatment in medical education. She is a doctoral candidate with the Department of Sociology, Trinity College, Dublin, with a thesis on medical discourse concerning abortion.

Elizabeth T. Robinson, M.S., is Associate Director for Information Programs at FHI. She manages FHI publications, information dissemination activities, technical assistance in communications, and the FHI Web site. Since joining FHI in 1985, she has served in various capacities, including as managing editor for FHI's scientific periodicals *Network*, *Network en français*, and *Network en español*; editor of numerous reports, books, and articles; member of FHI's Gender Advisory Committee; and manager of FHI's international health journalism training and scientific paper writing programs. She worked on FHI's Women's Studies Project, codeveloping a process evaluation to determine the inclusion of women's advocates in the research process, and has served on interagency working groups on female genital cutting, emergency contraception, and gender. Ms. Robinson has held consultancies with the World Health Organization, the American Social Health Association, and the International Monetary Fund. Prior to coming to FHI, she worked as a journalist in metropolitan New York, Washington, DC, North Africa, and francophone West Africa, experience that provided rich comparisons with qualitative approaches used to study reproductive health. Ms. Robinson received an M.S. in journalism from the Columbia University Graduate School of Journalism in New York and held a fellowship in the Columbia University School of International and Public Affairs Fellows Program. She speaks French, German, and Spanish.

Suzanne Smith Saulniers, Ph.D., is a rural sociologist and specialist in gender and development planning. She has worked as a development project and program designer for more than 25 years in Pakistan, Asia, and Africa. She has worked directly in reproductive health projects and program design, implementation and evaluation in Haiti, Kenya, and the Democratic Republic of Congo (formerly Zaire). At the time of the study described on page 117, she served as Assistant Representative of the Asia Foundation's office in Pakistan. Dr. Smith Saulniers holds a Ph.D. from the University of Wisconsin in sociology. She taught social research methodology for seven years at Huston-Tillotson College in Texas. She is currently a community development consultant for United Nations Office of Project Services (UNOPS) in Punjab Province, Pakistan.

Iqbal Shah, M.A., M.Sc., Ph.D., is a social scientist working with the Department of Reproductive Health and Research at the World Health Organization (WHO) in Geneva. He has worked at WHO since 1985, and is primarily responsible for the implementation of activities on social science and operations research in reproductive health. His recent publications include articles on dynamics of contraceptive use, infant mortality, abortion, condom use, and indicators for reproductive health. His academic training is in sociology, public health, and demography. Prior to joining WHO, Dr. Shah worked for the World Fertility Survey (WFS), International Statistical Institute.

Michele G. Shedlin, Ph.D., President of Sociomedical Resource Associates, Inc., is a medical anthropologist with U.S. and international experience in qualitative health research. She consults for community-based organizations, policy institutions, governmental agencies, and the private sector in program design, evaluation, teaching, and training in qualitative research methodology. Her experience in Latin America and with Latino populations in the United States and her work in maternal and child health, substance abuse, and HIV/AIDS have resulted in numerous reports and publications.

Nancy Stark, R.N., Ph.D., is a medical anthropologist with experience in international health, particularly maternal and child health and reproductive and family planning decision-making. Dr. Stark is currently a Research Associate and Cancer Control Fellow at Wake Forest University School of Medicine. Her research interests include breast and other reproductive cancers, symptom management, quality of life, and complimentary and alternative medicines. Recent publications by Dr. Stark include articles on reproductive health and family planning.

Elizabeth E. Tolley, M.A., is a senior research associate at FHI and a full-time doctoral student at the School of Public Health, University of North Carolina at Chapel Hill. She was first introduced to the use of qualitative methods for research in health in 1991 while living in Mumbai, India, where she became involved in a project funded by the Ford Foundation and administered by Johns Hopkins University School of Public Health to train Indian researchers in the use of qualitative methods. The project enabled her to learn side-by-side with her Indian counterparts from an internationally recognized team of experts including Dr. Margaret Bentley, Dr. Perti Pelto, Dr. Joel Gittelsohn and Dr. Moni Nag. Since joining FHI in 1995, she has used qualitative research methods to examine a range of topics, including access to early removal of Norplant, the context of adolescent abortion in West Africa, and women's experiences with menstrual changes related to contraceptive use. She is especially interested in exploring ways to make qualitative analysis more systematic and rigorous and ways to make qualitative and quantitative approaches more compatible. Ms. Tolley received her M.A. in Social Change and Development from Johns Hopkins University Nitze School of Advanced International Studies. She is fluent in French and proficient in German, Arabic, and Hindi.

Priscilla R. Ulin, M.N., Ph.D., is a senior research scientist at FHI. She first discovered the power of qualitative methods while conducting survey research in Botswana in 1970. Since then, she has combined qualitative and quantitative techniques in research, teaching, and technical assistance in sexual, reproductive, and maternal and child health in the United States and developing countries. A medical sociologist, her focus is primarily on social change and health decision-making, especially in relation to the influence of gender in reproductive health decisions and protection against HIV/AIDS and other sexually transmitted infections. Dr. Ulin worked in Haiti under the auspices of FHI's AIDSTECH project, where she used qualitative methods to explore women's sense of vulnerability in the AIDS epidemic. She was the deputy director of FHI's Women's Studies Project, a multinational program of social and behavioral science research, both qualitative and quantitative, on the consequences of family planning for women's lives. In this capacity, she also directed research in sub-Saharan Africa on women's strategies to adopt modern family planning in the face of community opposition; on the impact of family planning on women's participation in economic development; and on the influence of family on contraceptive decisions. Dr. Ulin received a master's degree in nursing from Yale University and a Ph.D. in sociology from the University of Massachussetts at Amherst.

Cynthia Woodsong, Ph.D., a medical anthropologist, is a senior scientist at FHI, where her work focuses on qualitative methodology, vaginal microbicides and reproductive health, including STIs/HIV. Prior to coming to FHI, she served as the deputy director for the Population and Health program at Research Triangle Institute's Center for International Development. There, she was responsible for the design, training, monitoring, and conduct of qualitative research in the areas of reproductive health and HIV/AIDS, as well as integrated qualitative/quantitative studies.

Index

toward participants, 4, 35, 61–63, 91, 115, 168, 214
    training in, 122, 248
    See also Confidentiality; Informed consent
Ethnograph (software), 90, 142
Exit interviews, 52, 189

Fact sheets, distribution of, 187, 198, 237–238, 240–241
Family planning, 1
    in China, 200–201
    male role in, 118
    spousal communication in, 89
    support groups for, 90
    See also Condom use; Contraception
Female condom, 2–3, 140–142, 237–238
Feminist theory
    in qualitative analysis, 69
    in qualitative research, 14, 18, 23–24, 25, 26, 28–29, 33
    in research question design, 45
    of subordination, 24
    use of photo narratives, 102
Field
    analysis in, 67, 137
    ethics in, 73, 133
    interventions in, 19, 78, 79, 237
    logistics in, 8, 113–114, 123
Field notes, 82, 127, 131
    in confirmability of data, 166
    payment for, 217
    researchers' perspectives in, 136
    reviewing of, 133
    See also Data management; Documentation; Note-taking; Participant observation
Field staff
    assistants to, 116
    data analysis by, 124, 137
    data collection protocols, 32
    introduction to community, 76, 114
    local participation in, 59, 116, 118, 123, 127
    professional, 119
    in research proposals, 40
    supervision of, 82, 119, 126, 127
    training of, 8, 40, 63, 113, 116, 122
    See also Interviewers
Fieldwork
    cooperation of local governments in, 201
    introductory phase of, 76–77, 114
    logistics of, 113–114
    reporting on, 177
    scheduling of, 123, 131
Findings. *See* Analysis; Data interpretation; Results
Flexibility
    in data collection, 50, 52, 86, 121, 122
    definition of, 27
    in design, 3, 11–12, 90
    in qualitative data analysis, 19, 137
    in qualitative research, v, 3, 27, 90, 111
    in research questions, 65

in timelines, 132
    See also Iterative approach
Focus groups, 38, 69, 92–94
    on AIDS, 95–97, 218, 225–228
    anonymity in, 94, 98, 99
    audiotapes of, 98, 127
    background information in, 94, 98, 99
    on birth-weight paradox, 103
    body language in, 96, 216
    budgets for, 217
    coding of participants in, 94, 98, 99
    composition of, 3, 39, 93–94, 98
    conclusion of, 100
    conduct of, 98
    confidentiality in, 93, 94, 99
    on contraception, 93, 192
    controversial topics in, 93
    conversational partnerships in, 98
    cultural norms in, 102
    data collection from, 41, 46, 94, 95, 96
    data from, 39–40
    debriefing after, 100
    emotional level of, 95–97, 130
    empowerment in, 102
    ground rules for, 96, 99
    homogeneity in, 39, 60, 93
    inappropriate use of, 38–39
    versus interviews, 46, 48, 92
    listening in, 3
    local field team's role in, 115
    management of, 215–216
    marginalization of members, 95
    note-taking in, 98, 99, 201, 216
    number of, 39, 94
    partnership in, 111
    photo narratives in, 102
    planning for, 217
    in population research, 92
    prenatal care in, 103–105
    probes in, 215–16, 225–226, 228
    projective techniques for, 110
    purpose of, 96
    quality of, 38–40
    readings on, 247–248
    results of, 39
    risk behavior in, 95
    sensitive topics in, 95
    sexual decision-making in, 102, 218
    site of, 215
    size of, 93, 94
    socio-demographic data on, 215
    spontaneity in, 101
    storytelling in, 102
    tape recorders in, 98, 99, 127, 215, 216
    topic guides for, 98, 99, 218–222
    topics for, 92–93
    transcripts of, 98, 216
    trust in, 201
    See also Moderators; Participants
Formative research, 117, 128
Frameworks. *See* Conceptual frameworks;

Theoretical frameworks
Freelisting, 8, 101

Gatekeepers, 76
Gender, 4
    bias, 72
    definition of, 23n
    difference, 26, 197
    effect on social behavior, 23–24
    equity, 7, 23
    and HIV risk, 81
    identity, 7, 179
    influence on reproductive issues, 4, 23, 92
    in interviews, 86
    needs assessments, 118
    and social change, 129
    and violence, 6, 49, 89, 195
Generalizability, 32, 161, 166
Generalization, *versus* insight, 57
Grounded theory, 19–20, 137
    See also Theory

Health behavior
    cultural models of, 27
    effect of research on, 185
    observation of, 11
    theoretical frameworks in, 207–208
Health belief model (theoretical framework), 207–208
Health care
    access during pregnancy, 103
    focus groups on, 92
    women's decisions in, 26
Health care workers
    as interviewers, 120
    reports for, 171
Health crises, global, 5
    responses to, 6
Health policy, interactive activities in, 199
HIV
    behavioral change and, 208
    data analysis of, 140–142
    dissemination of research on, 190
    focus group discussions on, 95–97, 218–222, 225–228
    men's ideas of, 187, 228
    participant observation studies on, 81
    reporting on, 180
    risk behavior in, 30, 77, 92, 207, 208
    transmission to women, 11, 36, 218
Human rights
    awareness of issues in, 5, 197
    in reproductive health, 7
Hypotheses
    development of, 37, 82, 131, 158
    preliminary, 41
    reporting on, 171
    verification of, 149, 151, 158
    See also Conceptual frameworks; Theory

i-biblio (web site), 246

cultural, 27, 160
See also Conceptual frameworks
Models, theoretical, 13
AIDS risk reduction, 208–209
complexity of, 149, 151
ecological, 18n
environment in, 41
health belief, 207–208
individual factors in, 41
locus of control, 209
in practice, 27, 30
See also Theory
Moderators (focus groups), 99–100
characteristics of, 119
errors by, 225–228
experience of, 65
fees for, 217
guidelines for, 215–216
male, 98
and note-takers, 98
as observers, 70
training of, 40, 122
Multivariate analysis, 18
for focus group discussions, 39
Mystery client technique, 80, 214

Needs assessments, 194
gender-appropriate, 118
Networks. *See* Social networks
Norms
community, 38
ethical, 167–168
focus group discussions on, 54
sexual, 57
social, 60
surveys of, 38
See also Cultural norms
Norplant, 164–165, 182, 223–224
Note-taking, 71, 82
in focus group discussions, 98, 99, 201, 216
payment for, 217
See also Field notes
NUD*IST (software), 147–148

Objectivity, in quantitative research, 16, 21, 30, 32
See also Bias
Observers
effect on participants, 80
as outsiders, 70–71, 76
self-awareness of, 82
in social networks, 77
See also Participant observation
Operations research, 60
Oral histories, 178
Oral presentations, 202–203, 217
Outliers, 54

PALS Program (Zambia), 108
Paradigms
definition of, 12
theoretical, 18, 28

See also Theoretical frameworks; Theory
Participant observation, 70–71, 72–81
contradictions in, 20
cultural perspective in, 19
gender of data collector, 77
insider's perspective on, 71
interactive techniques in, 69, 76
in introduction of studies, 76
key informants in, 80–81
mystery client technique in, 80
nonreactive techniques for, 69, 70–71, 73–74
note-taking in, 71
outsider's perspective on, 70–71
partnership in, 111
in qualitative research, 23
readings in, 247
sites for, 71, 77
in social network research, 106–107
as source of data, 138–139
training for, 122
See also Field notes
Participants
argumentative, 123
assumptions of, 136
at-risk, 123
coding of, 62, 94, 98, 99
collaboration with researchers, 69
communication with researchers, 187
debriefing of, 100
dissemination to, 170, 199, 240–241
emotional distress of, 95–97
ethical responsibility toward, 35, 61–63, 91, 115, 168
family influences on, 114–115
numbers of, 173
partnership with researchers, 4, 7, 83, 87, 111, 231
points of view of, 36
as problem-solvers, 107
quotations from, 168, 181–184
recruitment of, 59, 217
reimbursement to, 100, 217
review of results by, 189
risks to, 61, 62
selection of, 57, 70, 81, 174
Participatory research, 24–25, 107–109
action research, 6, 16–17, 107–108
probes in, 109
Partnership
conversational, 83, 87, 91, 92, 98
in participant observation, 111
with potential adversaries, 114
of researchers with participants, 4, 7, 83, 87, 111, 204–205, 231
See also Community; Stakeholders
Patterns, identification of, x, 144
Photographs, 27
in birth-weight studies, 103–105
photo narratives, 8, 46, 102
reporting on, 169, 170
Pile sorts, 8, 101

Policy-makers, 60
communication with, 184, 185
dissemination of information to, 170, 187, 188, 190, 199, 202
involvement in research, 115
in participatory action research, 108
as stakeholders, 202
in study design, 37
See also Advocacy
POPLINE (POPulation information onLINE), 242–243
Positivism, 14, 18, 21–22, 28–29, 31
Power relationships, 17, 52, 197
effect on data interpretation, 165
in reproductive health, 23–24, 115
See also Feminist theory
Pregnancy
and abortion, 20, 37, 136–137, 162
adolescent, 45, 179
decision-making in, 162
intendedness, 41–42, 212–214
reporting on, 177, 179
safe, 4
of school drop-outs, 212–214
See also Contraception; Family planning
Prenatal care, 103–105
Press releases, 193
Pre-testing, 117, 126, 127, 128, 165, 198
Priority-Sequence Models, 52–53, 54
Probes, 84, 85, 86
in focus group discussions, 215–216, 225, 228
in participatory research, 109, 110
Problem-solving, in research, 203
Program managers, 60
as key informants, 93
in study design, 37
Projective techniques, 110
Public health, role in reproductive health, 2
Public health messages, 11
interpretation of, 26
Purposiveness
in conversation, 83
in sampling, 54, 58, 59, 61

QSR Nvivo (software), 153
Quality
assurance of, 83, 124, 144, 164–166
criteria for, 31–33
See also Credibility
Questions. *See* Research questions, qualitative
Quotes
explanatory notes with, 183
length of, 184
purpose of, 167
in reports, 167, 170, 176, 181–184
representative, 182
selection of, 182
translation of, 175, 182–183
verbatim, 182–183, 184
See also Language; Transcripts

Credits

Design: Erica King
Production/copyediting: Karen Dickerson
Indexing: Roberta Engleman
Printer: PBM Graphics, Inc.
Photographs:
    Chapter 1 — Trygve Bølstad/Panos Pictures
    Chapter 2 — Richard Lord
    Chapter 3 — Richard Lord
    Chapter 4 — Richard Lord
    Chapter 5 — Richard Lord
    Chapter 6 — Philip Wolmuth/Panos Pictures
    Chapter 7 — Julio Etchart
    Chapter 8 — Heldur Netocny/Panos Pictures
    Appendixes — Sean Sprague/SpraguePhoto.com